Mental Health of Children and Adolescents with Intellectual and Developmental Disabilities

A FRAMEWORK FOR PROFESSIONAL PRACTICE

Dedication

In memory of Garry Dezilva, a much valued colleague and author, who passed away during the creation of this book. Garry embodied the collaborative approach to meeting the mental health needs of young people with intellectual and developmental disabilities and their families. His attitude and career exemplified his great concern for them.

Mental Health of Children and Adolescents with Intellectual and Developmental Disabilities

A FRAMEWORK FOR PROFESSIONAL PRACTICE

Edited by
David Dossetor, Donna White,
and Lesley Whatson

IP Communications
Melbourne 2011

IP Communications, Pty. Ltd.,
Level 1,
123 Camberwell Road,
East Hawthorn, Victoria, 3123,
Australia.

Phone: +61 3 9811 6818.
Fax: +61 3 9813 3979.
E-mail: ipcomm@bigpond.com
www.ipcommunications.com.au

First published 2011.

ISBN: 978-0-9808649-2-2

National Library of Australia Cataloguing-in-publication data

Title: Mental health of children and adolescents with intellectual and developmental disabilities: a framework for professional practice/edited by David Dossetor, Donna White and Lesley Whatson

Edition: 1st ed.

ISBN: 9780980864922 (pbk.)

Notes: Includes bibliographical references and index.

Subjects: Developmentally disabled children—Mental health.
Children with mental disabilities—Mental health.
Teenagers with mental disabilities—Mental health.
Youth with mental disabilities—Mental health.

Other Authors/Contributors: Dossetor, David.
White, Donna, 1968–
Whatson, Lesley.

Dewey Number: 616.890875

Edited by Gillespie & Cochrane, Pty. Ltd., Melbourne
Text design by Club Tractor Production Services, Melbourne
Typeset by Desktop Concepts Pty. Ltd., Melbourne
Cover design by Phillips & Father Printing, Melbourne
Indexed by Gillespie & Cochrane, Pty Ltd., Melbourne
Printed by BPA Print Group, Pty. Ltd., Melbourne

Foreword

This impressive book illustrates all that is special and interesting about the field of intellectual and developmental disabilities, most specifically about the mental health needs of children and adolescents with such disabilities. The book is interdisciplinary in its authorship; it acknowledges the need for many different perspectives within the bio-developmental-psycho-social framework; it is inclusive in recognising the knowledge and wisdom of those who have cared for a son or daughter with a disability; it is a resource for those interested in the science that underpins our present understanding; it provides guidance on services and interventions. In combining these various perspectives it undoubtedly provides a comprehensive 'framework for professional practice'.

What then are the key themes and messages that can be drawn from these diverse perspectives presented in the different chapters? The first must be that of development and the need to understand developmental processes. To meet the mental health needs of children and adolescents with intellectual and developmental disabilities there must be an appreciation of the complex and shifting interplay between the child with a likely atypically developing brain and the experiences and influences of the social, emotional, and physical environments that surround the child as he or she grows. Second, there has to be an acknowledgment that the prevention, assessment, and treatment of mental health and behavioural problems that affect children and adolescents with disabilities requires an appreciation of the scientifically sound conceptual models that exist, including an understanding of the perspectives of applied behavioural analysis, the relevance of neurodevelopmental syndromes and their associated behavioural phenotypes, and the occurrence of physical and psychiatric co-morbidities. A further aspect, well illustrated in this book, is that of the wider 'system' that is the family. Not only should parents' and siblings' needs be considered, but also it is necessary to step back and examine how families, in the context of the emotional and physical demands that are part of their lives, may have particular difficulties, perhaps at key points of transition, and need help to address such issues and to move on. When seeing a child or adolescent with a disability, there is a need to obtain information from previous records, and to undertake a detailed history, direct assessments, observations, and informed investigations – all part of good clinical practice. This information, focussed around the individual, must then be ordered and integrated in the context of existing theoretical knowledge through the process of formulation. The complexity of the situation for many children with a disability is such that to fully understand his or her mental health needs requires a rigorous, comprehensive, and systematic analysis.

The third theme is that of partnerships. The central partnership is that between the child with a disability and his or her parents. However, it goes beyond that and includes siblings and the wider family and friends, and those in various statutory and other services, such as other parents in syndrome support organisations, the paediatrician or child psychiatrist who may identify the cause of the developmental delay and identify co-morbid disorders, the speech and language therapist who helps the parents and others to develop an effective communication environment, the physiotherapist and occupational therapist who help the child to maximise his or her skills, the psychologist and specialist nurses or therapists who provide an understanding of challenging behaviour, and the professionals from other disciplines who might dip in and out of that child's life. Different chapters in the book communicate the powerful sense that this is a life journey that is not easily made when health and other services are too easily focussed around discrete episodes of care, out-patient appointments, and single discipline practices of working. The book challenges us to think about how support can be truly comprehensive and designed in a manner that ensures it is flexible, community oriented and interdisciplinary.

The above three themes – understanding development processes; the need for interdisciplinary practice and theoretically sound interventions; the importance of partnerships between the person with a disability, his or her family, and the myriad of others who may become involved perhaps over a life time – are, for me, central to the provision of support to children, adolescents, and adults with disabilities.

Finally, how should this book be read? I would encourage readers to be daring and to read beyond those chapters that directly relate to their interests and expertise. Individual and family therapists should be aware of changes in the developing brain; practitioners in different disciplines in medicine must fully appreciate what can be done to improve a person's communication environment or to maximise their skills; all concerned must be nuanced in their thinking with respect to delayed and atypical patterns of development that characterise people with intellectual and developmental disabilities. We have finally moved beyond the sterility of the medical versus the social model debate to appreciate that at different times and in different ways various perspectives can contribute. The editors and the contributors are to be congratulated.

Professor Tony Holland
Cambridge Intellectual and Developmental Disabilities Research Group
Academic Department of Psychiatry
University of Cambridge
United Kingdom

Contents

Contributors

Hadia Baassiri is a senior cultural clinical consultant in the Department of Psychological Medicine at The Children's Hospital at Westmead and the Centre for Transcultural Mental Health. She has a background in counselling and couple therapy.

Kate Brearley is a psychologist and senior behaviour support specialist with Metropolitan North Region of Ageing, Disability and Home Care, Department of Human Services, NSW. She was formerly senior clinical consultant with the Statewide Behaviour Intervention Service.

Judy Brewer is a mother of a teenager with autism spectrum disorder, founder of Autism Aspergers Advocacy Australia, and co-patron of Autism NSW.

Mary Ellen Burke is a clinical psychologist in private practice who provides clinical support to individuals, systems, and agencies to address the needs of people with complex and challenging behaviours. She is a professional member of the NSW Guardianship Tribunal.

Teena Caithness is a senior speech pathologist with a special interest in augmentative and alternative communication. She was formerly a senior clinical consultant with the Statewide Behaviour Intervention Service, Ageing, Disability and Home Care, Department of Human Services, NSW.

Louisa Carroll is a clinical psychologist with the Developmental Psychiatry Team, Department of Psychological Medicine, The Children's Hospital at Westmead.

Jodie Caruana is a health program manager and coordinator of the School-Link Initiative at The Children's Hospital at Westmead.

Chris Chapparo is a senior lecturer in the Discipline of Occupational Therapy, Faculty of Health Sciences, University of Sydney. She has expertise in the areas of sensory integration, and assessment and intervention for children with learning and developmental disorders.

Bruce Chenoweth is a senior staff specialist in psychiatry in the Diagnostic and Assessment Service at St George Hospital in Sydney, consultant to disability group homes and residential centres, and has a private practice.

Jane Chivers is a social worker and the manager of education and training with Family Planning NSW.

Debra Corfield is a psychologist and senior clinical consultant with the Statewide Behaviour Intervention Service, Ageing, Disability and Home Care, Department of Human Services, NSW.

The late Garry Dezilva was a psychologist and Manager, Behaviour Support Unit, in the Office of the Senior Practitioner, Ageing, Disability and Home Care, Department of Human Services, NSW. Previously, he was manager at Allambi Youth Services in Newcastle, NSW.

David Dossetor is a child psychiatrist with a special interest in intellectual disability and autism. He is Area Director of mental health at The Children's Hospital at Westmead, and clinical associate professor at the University of Sydney.

Stewart Einfeld is a child psychiatrist, and Chair of Mental Health, Faculty of Health Sciences, University of Sydney. He is also a senior scientist at the Brain and Mind Research Institute.

Louise Ellis is a post doctoral research fellow at the University of Sydney and a psychologist. Her research interests include learning difficulties and disabilities, mental health, self-concept, and peer support.

Yasmin Eris is a mother of a young girl with Smith-Magenis syndrome.

Barbara Fleming is a school counsellor with the South Western Sydney Region of NSW Department of Education. She has a background as a teacher and university lecturer.

Helen Goltzoff is a speech pathologist with Ageing, Disability and Home Care, Department of Human Services, NSW. She was seconded as a Project Officer with the School-Link Initiative at The Children's Hospital at Westmead in 2009.

Victoria Grahame is a clinical psychologist in a specialist clinical service for children and adolescents with complex neurodevelopmental disorders in

Newcastle, UK. She formerly worked with the Department of Psychological Medicine at The Children's Hospital at Westmead.

Wendy Grice is a clinical psychologist and senior clinical consultant with the Statewide Behaviour Intervention Service, Ageing, Disability and Home Care, Department of Human Services, NSW.

Anders Hansson is a psychologist and senior clinical consultant with the Statewide Behaviour Intervention Service, Ageing, Disability and Home Care, Department of Human Services, NSW.

Cheryl Jones is a registered nurse and a senior case manager with Metropolitan North Region of Ageing, Disability and Home Care, Department of Human Services, NSW.

Joseph Macdessi is a general paediatrician with a special interest in developmental medicine and psychiatry. He works with the Department of Psychological Medicine at The Children's Hospital at Westmead.

Meredith Martin is a special educator and a consultant in private practice. She supports people with complex needs, including those with challenging behaviour and mental health issues.

Emma Moore is a senior psychologist with Metropolitan South Region of Ageing, Disability and Home Care, Department of Human Services, NSW. She was formerly senior clinical consultant with the Statewide Behaviour Intervention Service.

Lucinda Mora is an occupational therapist and senior clinical consultant with the Statewide Behaviour Intervention Service, Ageing, Disability and Home Care, Department of Human Services, NSW.

Karen Ollerenshaw is a mother of a young man with Smith-Magenis syndrome.

Brett Owens is a psychologist and senior clinical consultant with the Statewide Behaviour Intervention Service, Ageing, Disability and Home Care, Department of Human Services, NSW.

Cal Paterson is a clinical psychologist in private practice who provides consultation to organisations, and counselling and psychological therapy to individuals, couples, and families. He previously worked with the Statewide Behaviour Intervention Service.

Belinda Ratcliffe is a clinical psychologist with the Emotion Based Social Skills Project at The Children's Hospital at Westmead.

Paul Rhodes is a senior lecturer at the Clinical Psychology Unit, Psychology Department, the University of Sydney, honorary senior clinical psychologist with the Department of Psychological Medicine at The Children's Hospital, Westmead, and coordinating editor of the *Australian and New Zealand Journal of Family Therapy*.

Hebah Saleh is a psychologist and project officer with the School-Link Initiative at The Children's Hospital at Westmead. She was previously a Refugee Support Worker and School Counsellor.

Natalie Silove is a senior staff specialist, developmental paediatrician, head of Child Development Services at The Children's Hospital at Westmead, and senior clinical lecturer at the University of Sydney.

Jacqueline Small is a senior staff specialist, developmental paediatrician, and team leader of the Disability Specialist Unit at The Children's Hospital at Westmead, and clinical lecturer at the University of Sydney.

Kate Tye is a mother of a young man with Smith-Magenis syndrome.

Lesley Whatson is a special educator and coordinator of the Children's Team with the Statewide Behaviour Intervention Service, Ageing, Disability and Home Care, Department of Human Services, NSW.

Donna White is a senior speech pathologist, the manager of the Training Curriculum Project, and senior clinical consultant with the Statewide Behaviour Intervention Service, Ageing, Disability and Home Care, Department of Human Services NSW.

Anthony Zehetner is a general paediatrician with an interest in psychopharmacology, and neurodevelopmental and behavioural disorders. He is also a consultant pharmacist, and a clinical lecturer for the Universities of Newcastle and Sydney.

Acknowledgments

This book came about from the collaborative and combined concerns of a large number of individuals, whom I would like to acknowledge. A two-year grant (2007–09) to develop an educational curriculum in child and adolescent mental health and disability was obtained from the Third National Mental Health Plan, but was enabled through the initiative and advocacy of Sandra Heriot, director of MH-Kids. A third year's funding (2009–10) was provided by Ageing, Disability and Home Care (ADHC), Department of Human Services NSW, through the support of Ethel McAlpine, deputy director general, and Don Ferguson and David Coyne, directors of the Office of the Senior Practitioner. The Office of the Senior Practitioner also provided additional support, through accommodating the project with the Statewide Behaviour Intervention Service (SBIS), supported by Frances Roberts, manager. Within The Children's Hospital at Westmead (CHW) the project partnership was supported by Jean Starling, head of department of Psychological Medicine, Bruce Lord, co-chair of Ambulatory and Emergency Program, and Tony Penna, chief executive officer.

Donna White, senior speech pathologist and project manager, was acclaimed by all for her superlative skills in coordinating and driving the project. The richness of the project arises from the close partnership between the Statewide Behaviour Intervention Service (ADHC) and the Developmental Psychiatry Team of the Department of Psychological Medicine (CHW). Lesley Whatson, coordinator of the Children's Team at SBIS, provided the leadership and relationship skills that facilitated everyone taking pride in contributing to the book.

I am grateful for my friends and colleagues who share the special interest in disability who contributed to the project. I would like to thank all the authors and presenters who helped develop and test out the ideas contained in the book. It is a special pleasure to have contributions from a number of parents, who are extraordinary in their contributions of leadership, initiative, and advocacy for children and adolescents with a disability. An extended group of respected colleagues enabled us to have every chapter peer reviewed. The commitment and energy of many team colleagues was extraordinary. Fundamentally, it is a book by clinicians for clinicians, and it appears that this book is one of the first of its kind. Richard Dawkins suggested that

'Charles Darwin had the greatest idea ever to occur to a human mind' (2009, p. 1). This book argues that the evolution of developmental sequence is primary to understanding the mental health problems of children and adolescents with a disability.

David Dossetor

Introduction

Donna White

Background

Children and adolescents with intellectual disability have impaired cognitive functioning and delayed developmental milestones that may have been caused by a variety of genetic, social, environmental, or unidentified factors (IASSID, 2001). The impact of an intellectual disability on young people can be observed in their developmental outcomes and functional capacity in a range of health, physical, cognitive, communicative, emotional, and social domains. Additionally, children and adolescents with intellectual disability have a high risk of developing comorbid emotional, behavioural, and psychiatric problems (Einfeld & Tonge, 1996a; Emerson, 2003a) that may further reduce their functional abilities (Allington-Smith, 2006). It has been reported that between 30 and 50 per cent of children and adolescents with intellectual disability have mental health problems (Cormack et al., 2000; Einfeld & Tonge, 1996b; Einfeld et al., 2006; Hastings & Mount, 2001). This increases to 73 per cent if children and adolescents with autism spectrum disorder (ASD) and intellectual disability are included in prevalence figures (Brereton et al., 2006).

Dosen (2005b) described psychiatric disorders as 'the consequence of harmful intrinsic and extrinsic stimuli, which in turn cause maladaptive behaviour' (p. 10). It is the vulnerability of young people with intellectual disability to these 'harmful stimuli' that make them at a higher risk of emotional and behavioural disturbances, and psychiatric disorders. Wallander and colleagues (2006) suggested that risk factors for psychopathology fit within the domains of developmental, biological, family, and social-ecological risks.

- *Developmental (intrinsic) risk factors*

  Researchers have found that the risk of children and adolescents having mental health problems decreases with the severity of intellectual disability; that is, those with mild to moderate intellectual disabilities have a higher risk (Einfeld & Tonge, 1996b; Cormack et al., 2000; Koskentausta et al., 2007). Brereton and colleagues (2006) studied children with autism and intellectual disability, and found that those with moderate to severe intellectual disability displayed more self-absorbed behaviours and problems with social relating than those with borderline or normal intelligence. They also found that verbal children had more communication difficulties and problems with antisocial behaviours, whereas nonverbal children had more problems with self-absorbed and social-relating behaviours. Koskentausta and colleagues (2007) also found that difficulties with language comprehension in children with intellectual disability were associated with internalising behaviours and social problems. Additionally, Dekker and colleagues (2002) found that children and adolescents with borderline to mild intellectual disability had more social, attention, withdrawal, and thought problems than children without intellectual disability.

- *Biological (intrinsic) risk factors*
  Children and adolescents with intellectual disability are also vulnerable to biological factors that may increase the risk of psychopathology (Wallander et al., 2006). A review of the literature indicated that individuals with intellectual disability have greater physical and health needs as a result of seizure disorders (Allington-Smith, 2006; Dykens, 2000; Kwok & Cheung, 2007), sensory impairments (Dykens, 2000; Carvill, 2001), sleep disorders (Allington-Smith, 2006), specific aetiologies, and behavioural phenotypes (Dykens, 2000). Gender and age were seen to be predictive of behavioural and emotional problems in children with severe intellectual disability (Brereton et al., 2006; Emerson, 2003a; Hastings & Mount, 2001); however, this was not supported in the study by Koskentausta and colleagues (2007).
- *Family and social-ecological (extrinsic) risk factors*
  There are many external factors that increase the risk of young people with intellectual disability developing emotional, behavioural, and mental health disturbances. Hatton and Emerson (2004) found that the 'most common adverse life events experienced by children with intellectual disabilities were parental separation (39%), serious illness requiring hospitalization (34%), death of a pet (27%) and parental financial crisis (20%)' (p. 111). Other factors that may increase the risk of disturbance include: social deprivation; involvement with the criminal justice system; grief and bereavement; parental mental health; and stress associated with family structure and functioning (such as being a single parent or a parent with intellectual disability) (Allington-Smith, 2006; Dodd et al., 2005; White et al., 2007; Dykens, 2000; Emerson, 2003a; Emerson et al., 2005; Hatton & Emerson, 2004; Herring et al., 2006; Koskentausta et al., 2007). However, it is the cumulative effect of a number of adverse and stressful life events that heightens the risk of disturbances (Hatton & Emerson, 2004; Hulbert-Williams & Hastings, 2008).

As a result of developmental, biological, psychological, social, and cultural difficulties associated with the identified risks for psychopathology, children and adolescents with a disability and their families require support from a range of services. These may include generic (such as community health centres, and general medical centres) or specialised clinical services (such as disability services, and child and adolescent mental health services), non-clinical services (such as social support, personal care, education, and advocacy), and carer services (such as respite programs, counselling, parenting programs, and support groups) (Steitz, 2008). However, these services may not meet the complexities of this population's emotional, behavioural, and mental health care needs (Jess et al., 2008; Scior & Grierson, 2004). It has been posited that professionals within these services lack expertise and confidence that is compounded by inadequate training in disability and mental health disorders (Bates et al., 2004; Burge et al., 2002; Costello et al., 2007; Jess et al. 2008; Mohr et al., 2002; Phillips et al., 2004; Tsiantis et al., 2004; Whitehurst, 2008). Poor interagency collaboration across services also undermines the effectiveness of service delivery to this population (Scior & Grierson, 2004; Worrall-Davies et al., 2004).

Although the literature base is limited, it has been found that training programs can have a positive impact on professionals' awareness of the mental health needs of individuals with a disability: knowledge of psychopathology, assessment and intervention; confidence in working with individuals; and attitudes to services (Costello et al., 2007; Gibbs & Priest, 1999; Mohr et al., 2002; Tsiantis et al., 2004). Furthermore, preliminary evidence (despite limitations in research methodologies) suggests that the transfer of knowledge from training programs into clinical practice can be achieved (Mohr et al., 2002; Whitehurst, 2008). However, there is a lack of clarity in the extent to which the benefits of training can effect actual behaviour change (Costello et al., 2007) in professionals' clinical practices and collaboration across disciplines and agencies that is essential to meeting the complex care needs of this population. Researchers and policy makers have highlighted that interprofessional education (IPE) can enhance collaboration and clinical outcomes (Bates et al., 2004; Noyes-Grosser, 2007; Reeves et al., 2007).

Training curriculum project: an interprofessional education program (IPE)

This book is the culmination of the outcomes from the *Training Curriculum Project (TCP)*, which was instigated to develop a comprehensive IPE program to assist in workforce development and service provision. The TCP was a three-year (2007–10) joint venture between the Department of Psychological Medicine at The Children's Hospital at Westmead (CHW) and the Statewide Behaviour Intervention Service (SBIS, Office of the Senior Practitioner,

Ageing, Disability and Home Care, Department of Human Services, NSW). The focus of the IPE program was the development of a holistic framework that considered the biological, developmental, family, educational, social, and cultural contexts of children and adolescents with a disability. This also provided an evidence-based perspective about the specific interventions that effect change and improve the quality of life of young people with a disability, and their families.

The IPE program was developed using a multiphased approach to formulate and validate a framework of core interventions. A two-day training seminar was also developed, implemented, and evaluated. The training seminar aimed to build staff capacity in order to promote the social, behavioural, and emotional well-being and mental health of young people with a disability. Evaluation of the seminar found that the knowledge base, confidence levels and attitude to collaboration of professionals from multiple disciplines significantly increased following the training. Knowledge transference and practical application of learning to the workplace occurred when professionals were supported by their clinical supervisors and management, and given opportunities to share information and discuss ideas with peers and multidisciplinary team members (White et al., 2009).

The framework of core interventions

The framework was based on a literature review, analyses of clinical and training data, expert opinion on 'what works', a review of existing resources and curricula, and a clinical forum that prioritised interventions and integrated them into five clinical domains. This was then validated through surveying professionals and obtaining a consensus view of the importance of the clinical domains and need to include them in the framework. An important element of the framework was to promote an understanding about developmental processes and sequences to assist professionals and families to understand and influence emotional and behavioural problems in the context of delayed development. Part of this process has been the development of a common language across clinical domains and professional disciplines in order to examine the diverse causes of behaviour and the many perspectives that can be taken when understanding the significance of behaviour. The clinical domains of the framework correspond to the five sections in the book, as outlined below.

Part 1: Foundations

This section explores the underlying issues related to understanding the multifaceted needs of children and adolescents with a disability in order to provide appropriate interventions. It has been identified that there are difficulties in interpreting the scientific literature for this population because of variations in the definitions, terminology, and diagnosis of mental health and psychiatric disorders (Allington-Smith, 2006; Bradley et al., 2004; Dekker et al., 2002; Hemmings, 2007). There have been further difficulties with using traditional classification systems for diagnosis, so researchers and clinicians have used assessment instruments that rely on carer–parent–teacher reports of observable and concrete behaviours. Unfortunately, these assessment techniques have further led to discrepancies in definitions of mental health disorders and diagnostic criteria, when observations of *challenging behaviour* have been equated to or included as a measure of a psychiatric disorder (Allen & Davies, 2007; Hemmings, 2007).

Myrbakk & von Tetzchner (2008) stated that, 'Behaviour problems may be (unconventional) symptoms of psychiatric disorders or reflect a difficult life situation caused by psychiatric disorders, or that a difficult life situation may contribute to both psychiatric disorders and behaviour problems in individuals with intellectual disability' (p. 316). This view reflects the complexity associated with comorbid intellectual disability and psychopathology, and the need for an interdisciplinary approach to meet the needs of young people (Allington-Smith, 2006; Davis et al., 2008; Huang et al., 2007). Thus, in order for professionals to promote a quality of life for young people they need to develop a common language or common ground (Saeed, 2008), identify needs through comprehensive assessments, and formulate family- and person-centred care plans within integrated and specialised services (Davis et al., 2008).

Part 2: Focus on carers and families

How a diagnosis of disability has an impact on family functioning will depend on the resilience of parents, carers, and siblings, and their ability to adjust, accept, and adapt to caring for the young person with a disability. This can be influenced by the family's culture, attachment patterns (Dodd et al., 2005), and the ability of the family to make adaptations, both emotionally and practically, in the care of the child. The burden of caring for the child may be increased by additional support needs, such as chronic health concerns, physical disabilities, and behavioural disturbances.

A child with intellectual disability and emotional or behavioural disturbances presents significant challenges to his or her family (Davis et al., 2008), and has been found to have an impact on mothers' stress and parent mental health problems (Herring et al., 2006). Therefore, families require emotional support, such as being listened to (Douma et al., 2006), practical strategies provided through parent-mediated early intervention (Diggle & McConanchie, 2002), parent training programs (Quinn et al., 2007; Hudson, et al., 2003), and access to respite services (Douma et al., 2006). These strategies should help parents and carers and families maintain their mental health and well-being and prevent family breakdown.

Parts 3 and 4: Interventions to promote skill development and to promote mental health

These sections focus on strategies that promote skill development to address the developmental, emotional, and behavioural needs of young people with intellectual and developmental disabilities. Professionals from multiple disciplines can provide early intervention and prevention programs that assist in reducing risks at times of change and transition in a young person's life, as well as interventions to assist in the management of challenging behaviours and mental health issues. Interventions to promote a young person's mental health and well-being apply biological, social, psychological, and developmental approaches (Allen & Davies, 2007).

Reviewed literature and clinical data in these sections focused on early interventions for cognitive impairments and ASD, promotion of skills in sensory modulation, language development, and use of augmentative and alternative communication (AAC), and emotional regulation and understanding (Davis et al., 2008; Dosen, 2005a; White et al., 2007). Specific interventions for managing diagnosed mental illness included counselling and cognitive behavioural therapy (Di Marco & Iacono, 2007; Hassiotis & Hall, 2008), multimodal models (Davis et al., 2008), and psychotropic medication (Allington-Smith, 2006; Davis et al., 2008; Deb & Unwin, 2007; Huang et al., 2007; Kwok & Cheung, 2007; McCarthy, 2007).

Part 5: Integration of service systems

This section acknowledges the importance of young people's wider social context, including their home, school, and other residential settings (Davis et al., 2008), and the need for coordination and interagency collaboration. The contribution and expertise of different professionals and agencies are essential to ensuring that children and adolescents with intellectual and developmental disabilities develop skills to achieve quality of life, and positive mental health and well-being. This section also identifies the significance of a service structure that enables children, adolescents, and their families to access the generic, specialist, and integrated services that they need in a timely and coordinated way (Dagnan, 2007).

Conclusion

The outcome of the Training Curriculum Project (2007–10) was an IPE program that included a holistic core framework of clinical interventions and an evaluated two-day training seminar. The training seminar was found to have a significant impact on the knowledge, skills, and attitudes of the professionals who attended. Evidence from the seminar evaluation indicated that learning outcomes were translated to the workplace with a positive effect on the provision of services to young people with intellectual and developmental disabilities and emotional and behavioural difficulties. The development of the IPE program also assisted in establishing a network of professionals with expertise in meeting the developmental, behavioural, and emotional needs of these young people. The training seminar, in particular, has become the basis of enhanced partnerships, and has provided a learning environment that has fostered interagency collaboration in new and existing projects, and in clinical work.

This book aims to be a practical guide for professionals to assist in making sense of complicated situations. Extensive review of international literature, available information, and resources provided the foundation of the book's content. Unfortunately, not all clinical interventions identified as influential to the behavioural, emotional, and social development of young people with a disability could be included in the book, such as interventions for physical development (such as mobility, coordination, balance, and control), self-injurious behaviour, and complementary and alternative medicine.

Local experiences and practices are reflected in the chapters, as authors were breaking new ground in focusing on a framework of core intervention skills and approaches for working with children and adolescents with a disability and mental health problems. This book is one of the first in its genre, and will be used locally to supplement learning in the IPE training seminars. The book will also enable dissemination of the framework of core interventions to a national and international audience of professionals from multiple disciplines in the hope that ultimately young people with intellectual and developmental disabilities and their families will benefit from improved mental health outcomes.

Acknowledgments

The author would like to thank David Dossetor and Lesley Whatson for being partners on this journey of discovery, and for being inspirational and supportive in all aspects of the project. Acknowledgment and thanks also to Jessica Farah, Research Assistant, who supported the implementation of the education program, and completed analyses of the training evaluation data.

Part 1

Foundations

1

Aiming for a quality of life: What makes for a 'good enough' life?

David Dossetor

What makes a quality of life?

What does a *quality of life* mean? Quality of life is a subjective and personal perception that means different things to different people. A 'good enough' quality of life is what everyone can and should aspire to. Nonetheless there are consistent objective qualities as to what contributes to that sense for most people of satisfaction with one's life as a whole. The research shows that quality of life satisfaction entails having an adequate standard of living and feeling safe (Cummins, 2005). Generally a 'good enough quality of life' means having reasonable health. It also means being connected to other significant people and having valued relationships. It entails being connected to a community and contributing a worthwhile role, a sense of purpose and productivity, and having a hope for the future. For many, a hope for the future involves having children for whom there are also hopes. This has been summarised as 'being, belonging and becoming' by Renwick and colleagues (1996): *being* related to the basic attributes concerning the individual; *belonging* centred on the fit between individuals and their environments; and *becoming* related to individuals' attempts to attain goals and fulfil hopes.

The empirical research shows the evaluation of quality of life is similar and fairly good for most of the population, generally scored at 75 per cent plus or minus 20 per cent (Cummins, 2005). One extraordinary element is that most people find a 'good enough' quality of life in the face of considerable adversity. For example, most people with chronic ill health adapt to finding an adequate quality of life. Being particularly intelligent or being a slow learner is not a predictor of quality of life, nor is being rich or poor. However, it has been suggested that psychiatric disorders are important 'disorders of quality of life'.

Health services have to justify their interventions by demonstrating that they contribute to health-related quality of life in the context of an affliction. Indeed, the internationally accepted concept of health is not just an absence of disease but a sense of health and well-being in physical, psychological, social, and spiritual or cultural dimensions (WHO, 1948). So what does a quality of life for a child or adolescent with intellectual disability or other developmental disorder mean? There is limited research in this area, but what exists suggests that it has similar domains (Cummins, 2005). Even for the young person with autism (with a central disability of difficulty understanding other people's thoughts and feelings, and difficulty communicating), quality of life still involves the quality (not so much the number) of social relationships. This can occur even if a lack of social skills limits this to a sense of belonging, of friendship, or friendliness, or shared activity (Burgess & Gutstein, 2007). Even for the alienated, hostile, neglected young person living in a refuge, family relationships, despite their problems, are still the more important than other factors (NSW Commission for Children and Young People, 2002). For someone with an intellectual disability, developmental achievement, such as walking or developing functional communication, is as valuable in one context as achieving first place in an exam is to another person in another context.

A prerequisite for a quality of life is recognition of the individual's choice. For someone with a disability, this may include enabling the capacity to express a choice and supporting it, while appreciating values and culture (Brown & Brown, 2005). For children with or without a disability, quality of life also depends heavily on the health and happiness of the family system. The Beach Centre Disability Family Quality of Life Scale (Hoffman et al., 2006; Smith-Bird & Turnbull, 2005) found five important contributing domains of family quality of life: family interaction (such as enjoying spending time together); parenting (such as helping family members with schoolwork and activities); emotional well-being (such as having the support needed to relieve distress); physical and material well-being (the feeling of safety at home, at work, at school, and within the neighbourhood); and disability-related support (the family member with special needs has support to make friends).

A study conducted by the author (Dossetor, 1991), involving indepth interviews of 92 families with teenagers who had severe intellectually disabilities, demonstrated that these families form an extraordinary group of people. The families were able to make the best of circumstances of considerable adversity, but they also valued the relationships with their teenagers with intellectual disabilities and celebrated their achievements, just as they would those of siblings with average development. Nonetheless, there are different or special challenges for a young person with an intellectual disability and their families. Some exceptional families can see these challenges as advantages, but for most they also involve hardship, persistence, and problem-solving.

Having a child with an intellectual disability is an atypical experience for the family involved, with some very significant challenges for the child and his or her family, yet all should aspire to having a 'good enough' quality of life. It is in this context that many families and professionals prefer to emphasise *diffability* rather than *disability* (Jordan, 2001), as what some may experience as a disability, others may see as a gift. It is therefore important to identify and examine what are the specific challenges for the family and child with intellectual disability, and in turn attempt to define what community-based clinicians can do to enable this process, and what skills may be important.

How can clinicians contribute to others' quality of life?

What can a group of experienced clinicians contribute to improving the quality of life of young people with intellectual disability and their families? Clinicians can provide testimony of the ways others have resolved similar challenges. They can interpret what the scientific literature has to say, and take the challenge of making science relevant and meaningful for families. They can also take on the challenging task of demystifying jargon used by different professional disciplines.

Clinicians can use language that is accessible to individuals and families who receive intervention services. They can be holistic in considering the biological, developmental, educational, family, social, and cultural context of a child, and be specific about the evidence that supports interventions that bring about change. Clinicians can also provide information about what families can do themselves to help their child with intellectual disability achieve an adequate quality of life. Through training, knowledge and skills can be shared with community clinicians, so that they are made aware of the professional skills that are required to facilitate this process. Through acquiring experience, clinicians often become experts in what can go wrong for individuals and families, but this knowledge should be used to promote skills to improve situations that are likely to go wrong, and even prevent them from occurring. Increasingly there is literature about how these children and families can get it right, which gives insight into the adaptive, proactive, and preventative components of achieving a quality of life.

What are the main challenges?

One essential ingredient for success in growing up is having expectations that are challenging but achievable. In the same way, for a young person with

Table 1.1 The traps and challenges for a family caring for a child with intellectual disability (ID) through the family lifecycle

Common traps	*Main challenges*
1 Failure of adjustment to a different child • Attunement and developmental understanding and special parenting skills 2 Failure to share the care of a different child • Adapting to the burden of care 3 Problems of psychiatric disorder • Seeking special multidisciplinary help 4 Failure to look after the carer's well-being and family relationships	1 Getting to know the child 2 Sharing the burden of care 3 Managing the system • Accessing specialist disability services • Caring for the carer and family 4 Understanding delayed and uneven development

Source: adapted from Nankervis et al., 2009

an intellectual disability it is important to take on board the elements of what contributes to a quality of life and how this can be applied. A prerequisite for happiness is also accepting what you cannot change.

As mental health clinicians, our aim is not to 'cure' intellectual disability. Although science sporadically discovers miracle cures, it has been frequently demonstrated that a search for the holy grail of a cure has harmful effects on the quality of life of the child and the family. Alternative treatments are not without major costs, risks, side-effects, or time commitments, and yet many families don't subject them to scientific scrutiny. This book tries to take into account some of the main challenges of difference and vulnerability that make achieving a 'good enough' quality of life a special challenge or an individual road for a young person with an intellectual disability and their family. Table 1.1 lists both the traps and the challenges for a family caring with a child with intellectual disability. Although the challenges arise progressively as the child with intellectual disability grows older, for those families that are under threat, several or all traps apply (Nankervis et al., 2009).

Getting to know a special child

Do children grow up too quick or too slow? This perception is very dependent on expectation and the end of the telescope you are looking through. The physical bodies of people with intellectual disability grow old at the same rate (more quickly in some situations, such as the risk of premature Alzheimer's dementia in Down syndrome), but cognitive development is slowed. Indeed some families talk about the advantages of having to spend more of life outside of the fast lane. Central to their quality of life is the high value they place on caring for each other and what this teaches about life and its values (Dossetor, 2001; Stainton & Besser, 1998). Perhaps the first big challenge for members of the family is for them to get to know the child and the differences between their child and the 'average' child. Quality of life is not related to the destination, but about appreciating the journey and marking its milestones and achievements.

For many families, an understanding of early development is an important building block for understanding and accepting how this stage can be slowed, extended, and made uneven as part of their child's disability. Most of what individuals know about being a parent comes from having been parented. Accordingly, individuals are attuned to parenting someone like themselves, and according to whether childhood was happy or not, parents will do the same or the opposite. What is also known is that for most individuals, their parenting response is conditioned to be modified by the genetic nature and temperament of their child (Reiss & Neiderhiser, 2000). However, for a parent of a child that is not developing in a typical manner, or whose relationship with his or her parent is disrupted by complex medical or developmental needs, these intuitive processes are not sufficient. In these situations, parenting becomes a process of modifying expectations to understand this child's needs and his or her developmental journey. This is where it may take more time, thought, and individuality to work out what is involved in parenting in order to understand the child. It may also require breaking down skill development into smaller steps and allowing for mastery of skills to develop in smaller stages.

For the child with an intellectual disability to be accepted and loved not just by his or her parents, but by grandparents, extended family, friends, and neighbours, these family members must also learn to understand the individuality of the child. There are natural and normative stigmatising processes that work against this happening. When dealing with the new and different, understanding and positive challenges are needed for positive support (Sensky, 1985). Accordingly, parents and others who understand the child (including community clinicians) have to find a model that explains what may be atypical, and how to adapt or manage this. Adapting to and understanding the differences enables recognition of the consistent and familiar features of childhood. This process of sharing concern for a child is necessary to open the door to a community of especially caring people. Human nature so often provides surprises when you look for caring qualities. In this way all parents need to be advocates for their child.

The burden of caring

Most children with intellectual disability are generally happy, like typically developing children, or *neurotypicals* (as the community of people with autism spectrum disorder like to call 'average' people). All babes and infants are highly dependent on their parents, needing help with feeding, dressing, and toileting. However, what are probably more important are the attentional and interactive needs of infants to engage with adults who can understand and respond to their preverbal communication. There is no doubt that caring for an infant is hard work, and it is possibly the social role that is least financially valued in our community. For a child with intellectual disability, this phase does not last merely two to four years, but may last five to 75 years. It is this burden of long-term caring that most distinguishes families with a child with intellectual disability.

The process of sharing care for the child with an intellectual disability with family and friends is crucial to having them involved in the child's life. Emotional support and understanding may be valuable, but survival as a parent in the long term depends on having friends or relatives who will provide a practical helping hand (Dossetor et al., 1993). Even having one friend or relative who provides an occasional hour of care makes a critical difference. A baby consumes about seven hours a day of individual parental care time and attention, and for the parent of a child who has a disability, this demand continues for the long term. For children with disabilities who are hyperactive or have poor sleep patterns, this can be a gross underestimate of parental care time. Typically developing children can visit friends, have sleepovers and birthday parties, and visit other homes while parents are shopping or going to the doctor. Having the same resource for a child with an intellectual disability involves the parents placing a special trust on the substitute carer, and a special capacity for care by the carer for the child with the disability.

What clinicians see often is the parental sense of undue responsibility, and a defensive belief that no one else would, could, or should provide substitute or supplementary care for their child. This is probably the single most important determinant to predict parental (usually mother's) coping and survival. It has been found that even having one or two people who can provide even occasional additional special child-minding support can make all the difference (Dossetor et al., 1993). For parents, families, and their social networks to work out the support needed, they need to learn about the needs and future potential for a quality of life for the child with the disability and resolve the practical challenges for the burden of care.

One of the practical challenges associated with the burden of care is meeting the specific needs of the child with intellectual disability concurrently with those of the rest of the family. Balancing these needs can be complex and challenging, and can generate significant levels of stress within a family. Family research indicates that well-being is generally maintained by creating healthy routines that are manageable and sustainable, yet meaningful and able to accommodate the needs of all family members (Gallimore et al., 1993). For example, if sharing the evening meal together is an important routine for a family, scheduling dinner for a time that enables older siblings and parents to arrive home and settle back into the household will be important. The time everyone sits down to eat will need to remain flexible to account for evenings where one parent is delayed by traffic or a meeting, or a sibling is late home from sport. In this way a valued routine remains sustainable for everyone.

Family routines provide stability and predictability, but should also be dynamic, flexible, and responsive to new demands. Such routines should enable members of a family to:

- balance the demands of everyday life, both inside and outside the home
- engage others in the lives of their children
- allow parents and siblings to spend adequate time together in various combinations
- allow time for individual members to pursue their own interests (Schneider et al., 2006).

It is not surprising, therefore, that respite care is seen as a crucial cornerstone of enabling a quality of life for a family with a child with an intellectual disability. Over the last 25 years, since the change in community opinion and government policies about putting children with disabilities into long-term institutions, there has been a very gradual process in making respite care more child and family orientated. Such respite services have included the provision of in-home family-based respite, and funding to develop the skills of families and friends to provide respite. This model is currently being trialled through the Family Solutions project of Uniting Care Burnside, Northern Metropolitan Sydney. However, 'respite' or alternative care and affectional relationships within their own networks, is what families would like to have, if only some of the extra cost involved could be supported by 'the system'.

Managing 'the system' and how to survive it

Systemic thinking is an important part of mental health and survival: the study or contemplation of the way in which everyone is part of a greater whole. As a social species, people may see themselves as individuals, but they are often defined by who they belong to. Furthermore, although people have an influence on groups or organisations they belong to, these groups and organisations also influence their members. In the context of having a child with an intellectual disability, the system can be divided into two parts:

- special challenges of parents maintaining well-being and balance in themselves, and for other members of the family, the extended family, friends, colleagues, and community organisations
- the challenge of gaining access to adequate specialist disability, educational and health services provided by the community, and the government, for the special needs of a child with a disability.

Winnicott (1996) noted that an infant cannot be considered without a parent, because of his or her intimate interdependency on that relationship. In the examination of the difference of disability, society has neglected the greater importance of the relationship of the child with a disability with his or her immediate carers. Accepting and integrating children and adolescents with intellectual disability into our community requires clinicians to put special value on the young person's parents or carers and immediate family. Yet the special challenges of accessing necessary services, in a cost-limiting system (such as managing the rotating front door of trainee clinicians in the government system), requires considerable skills of discrimination and assertiveness. The skills of advocacy are necessary for every parent, but they also need to take on superlative dimensions of patience, skill, persistence, and toughness when providing for the special needs of a child with intellectual disability. The necessity of these life challenges frequently brings out special or even heroic qualities in the parents that clinicians meet.

Understanding delayed and uneven development

This section aims to set the scene for some of the principles behind the shared knowledge base of a team of multidisciplinary clinicians working in disability and mental health.

Development

What distinguishes a child from an adult? Development. What distinguishes child psychiatric disorder from adult psychiatric disorder? Developmental psychopathology. This contrasts with our view of adults, who are seen to have substantially matured and are no longer rapidly developing; indeed, they are seen as autonomous with an egalitarian right of responsibility. Similarly, psychiatric disorders in adults are generally seen as disease equivalents that need treatment so that the adults can resume a previous state of wellbeing, and social and emotional competence. Although adolescents can suffer psychiatric disorders such as schizophrenia, bipolar disorder, depression, and post-traumatic stress disorder, children and adolescents also have an additional range of emotional disorders and behavioural disorders. It is these childhood-specific disorders that are substantially related to development and developmental competence. These childhood disorders of emotions and behaviours are caused by:

- the vulnerability of development and developing temperament, in the context of learning skill competence
- the physical and emotional environment of the family and other relationships (Hudziak, 2008).

Developmental versus psychiatric disorders

Take the example of disruptive behaviour problems, where persistent naughty behaviour is largely a learned behaviour in response to inconsistent management, and where emotional displays get what you want. There are some temperamental and genetic risks factors, but environmental factors, including emotional deprivation or abuse, are important contributors. With the exception of *attention deficit hyperactivity disorder (ADHD)*, these behaviours and angry feelings and thoughts are treatable by an energetic change of the environment, to improve warmth, rewards, supervision, and consistency of contingencies for behaviours.

ADHD (problems of attention, restlessness, impulsiveness with or without hyperactivity) is substantially a genetic and constitutional component of disruptive disorders, but it also occurs on its own, when it can contribute to learning problems. All children have to learn to concentrate, sit still, and think things through. So what are the developmental processes necessary to be able to concentrate, sit still, and think things through? These are complex processes, of which there is little understanding at a scientific level, yet clinicians have lots of experience of what helps children develop skills and mature. ADHD has significance because of its predictive validity; that is, if a person does poorly in the areas of developmental competence, there is a high chance that these features will lead to other problems in academic achievement, emotional and behavioural regulation, and establishing good-quality new affectionate relationships (Reid et al., 2002).

The validity of mental disorders in intellectual disability can be tested. For example, a review of ADHD in mild intellectual disability showed that, although the syndrome features are common (in one-third of the population or even more where there are additional developmental problems), in many ways they act as predictors of other problems, and therefore can be seen as a disorder (Antshel et al., 2006). Conversely, developing a capacity for attention, concentration, sitting still, and thinking things through is a problem that every developing infant has, because these are all challenges of normal development.

We therefore face an ambiguity in trying to determine when a disruptive behaviour in a child with intellectual disability is part of normal variation of behaviour, or a 'challenging behaviour', or a psychiatric disorder? High activity and attention-seeking behaviours in a child with intellectual disability may reflect:

- part of a normal developmental phase, even if chronologically delayed, particularly in the context of abnormal or vulnerable brain structure and function ('it's normal for him')
- the challenges of developing motor coordination, or exploring the external world ('he learns from activity')

- awareness of a difficulty, such as fear or confusion about the language used, or the noise of other features of the environment ('he feels stressed and doesn't understand what is going on')
- frustration at someone else not understanding how they are feeling or what they want ('he is trying to let us know what he thinks or feels')
- abnormal activity levels, fidgetiness, and distractibility, with marked impaired concentration, despite other areas of normal development; that is, specific developmental ADHD or
- a disordered pattern of behaviour with awareness of intent to do harm to others, in the context of a persisting rationale of low worth of self or others ('he has a conduct-disordered pattern of behaviour that is likely to persist; he learned it from his social environment').

Different mental health clinicians might describe any or none of these scenarios as a psychiatric disorder. They all reflect problems of behavioural interaction in the context of developmental impairment, although, the last scenario may emphasise the adaptation to an inconsistent learning environment, rather than the capacity to learn modulation of socially meaningful behaviour. All scenarios require developmentally supportive interventions with different approaches, and all may be better considered as developmental disorders.

Conduct disorder, which is resistant to change and tends to persist, may be more likely to be viewed as a psychiatric disorder. Although it is treatable with environmental changes, these environments of family and community interactions are often difficult to influence. These descriptions also suggest that having calmness, stillness, alertness, and concentration require achievement of key development milestones in motor development, proprioception, and modulation of arousal, receptive and expressive communication skills, and sufficient intellect or mental energy. Closely linked to these is a theory of mind, a sense of one's own thoughts and feelings in relation to one's sense of others. An absence of any one of these is likely to lead to a lack of attention and concentration, which are the key long-term predictors of educational failure.

Accordingly, if development is delayed in various areas, then delay in developing these skills becomes normal for the population of intellectually disabled and not a disorder. Indeed, some disorders, such as language and coordination problems, sequencing and memory problems, ADHD, and autism spectrum disorders, are generally described as developmental problems. This means that it may be as helpful or even more helpful to think about these as developmental challenges or delays rather than as disorders. Such a model also requires a range of caring and educational approaches, and not strictly a psychiatric designation.

'Ontogeny recapitulates phylogeny'

'Ontogeny recapitulates phylogeny' is a well-known quote attributed to Haeckel (1866). It means that developmental sequences that occur in evolution occur in embryology and human development. It implies that developmental processes are central to understanding biology. Heinz Werner described the universal principle of development as 'where there is life there is development in a systematic sequence' (Hodapp & Barack, 2006, p. 237). The second principle is the orthogenic principle: 'development progresses from relative globality and lack of differentiation to increasing differentiation, articulation and hierarchic integration; both individual and context differentiate, leading to a development-transactional approach' (Hodapp & Barack, 2006, p. 237). Real development is complex, and involves relations constantly changing within or transacting with its environment.

One of the truths of human development is that skills in a developmental domain are seen to occur in sequence. The remarkable observation is that, regardless of the genetic or neuroanatomical cause for delayed acquisition of skills (such as motor development or language), progress follows the same sequence of gaining skill competence. For example, head control precedes sitting skills, followed by standing and walking; or preverbal noises precede single words, followed by short word sequences. It is suspected that these sequences are governed by rules of developing mathematical complexity at a level of nerve connectedness, rather than one particular neurone or brain region doing one particular task.

In the same way as the evolution of the eye has been shown to have a functional sequence which can be reproduced by a mathematical computer program, clinicians may need to look for natural sequences of developmental achievement in other areas of human development (Dossetor, 2004). For example, although autism has long been conceptualised as a discrete disease process, the research community has now accepted that it involves differences of a dimension of developmental competence (Constantino & Todd, 2000; Constantino et al., 2000). Dossetor (2004) used the evolution and development of the eye as a helpful analogy to understand the stages of social and emotional development, and used these stages to conceptualise autism as a delay in developmental competence of socioemotional understanding and theory of mind. In this vein, Tanguay and colleagues (1998) found from a factor analysis of the gold standard measure, the Autistic Diagnostic Interview–Revised, that the severity of autism spectrum disorders is related to a developmental sequence. The sequence of these factors is:

- *the presence of affective reciprocity:* the preverbal interactive skills of a child in the first year of life

- *joint attention:* the capacity to perceive whether another person is looking at the same object—a key achievement of a child in the second year of life
- *a theory of mind:* a capacity to appreciate that another person has thoughts and feelings distinct from one's own—a skill that starts in the third year of life.

Such a developmental framework accepts that there are complexities that cannot be seen individually, but allows that promoting development is the key to reducing disorder and promoting health. In the last decade, much of psychology has shifted from focusing on 'challenging the deviant' to 'promoting skills in areas of competence deficits' that help young people better manage the challenges of social, emotional, and cognitive integration (Emerson, 2001). It is also interesting that some of the skills of promoting development that have been developed in the field of psychology of intellectual disability have found a central role in mainstream psychology and psychiatry (such as chaining of skills, differential reinforcement of other behaviours, and contingency conditioning). Such a framework also means that these conditions, although historically recognised as psychiatric, are better understood as delays in developmental sequence. This means that anyone who knows about how children grow up, such as parents, can understand and predict their needs.

Conclusion

Quality of life and ill-health are different, but it is clear that those who have a low quality of life also have marked increased rates of ill-health and psychiatric disorder (McConkey, 2009). Accordingly, clinicians should pay attention to enhancing quality of life, as this will also affect risk, outcome, and relapse of ill-health. The aim of the framework outlined in this book is to describe a range of clinical skills, knowledge, and resources, and make them more accessible to the core workforce of community clinicians who encounter children and adolescents with intellectual and developmental disabilities and emotional and behavioural regulation problems.

This all needs to be understood in the context of families, community, and culture, with an aim of enabling coping competence and a sense of purpose, belonging, and future for these children and their families, and to build a quality of life for this special group of people. Medical diagnoses often help define specific interventions. Emotional, behavioural, and psychiatric disorders have a major influence on, and are influenced by, elements of quality of life. Cohort studies of families with a child with Down syndrome reported that 80 per cent have a good enough quality of life

(Byrne et al., 1988). In the face of apparent interminable disadvantage and disturbance, it is important to remember that all children with intellectual and developmental disabilities and their families can achieve a quality of life, and as clinicians our aim should be to help them understand and aspire to a 'good enough quality of life'.

2

A common language for understanding disability, development, emotions, and behaviour

Teena Caithness and Emma Moore

Introduction

A common language is the exchange of communication delivered without professional jargon, reliance on acronyms, or the assumption that the communication partner shares the same skill set and knowledge base to interpret the information given. Therefore, common language is the use of words, including terminology, that is user-friendly and understood by all communication partners. When considering the individual with an intellectual disability and emotional–behavioural disorder as part of a system (such as a family or service system), the issues to address become multifaceted, with intervention often requiring a range of professional services. Working collaboratively and holistically requires a common understanding between agencies, clinicians, and professionals for any intervention to be successful.

Clinicians within multidisciplinary teams are required to work within a communal framework often made up of professionals from different disciplines and/or backgrounds. There is an expectation that professionals have an understanding or awareness of disciplines other than their own. This can lend itself to greater awareness, but also confusion and misinterpretation of roles, responsibilities, and the presenting problem. Difficulties in communication between professionals occur when supporting children in need (Salmon & Rapport, 2005). These authors found that communication breakdown can occur 'when professionals use the same words as each other, but apportion them with different meanings, in the belief that agreement has been reached in conversation, when in fact those conversing are at odds with one another' (Salmon & Rapport, 2005, p. 430).

An interagency approach requires collaboration and effective exchange of information within clearly defined rules and processes. For example, the National Health Service (NHS) in Scotland required a common usage of the word *integration* for its health services, and attempted to derive a National Framework for Service Change (as cited in Scottish Executive, 2005). The concept of integration was a cornerstone of Scottish health policy and practice. Bell and colleagues (2008) reviewed both the Scottish NHS policy and practices several years later, and found that professionals habitually used the term integration in different ways. More specifically, for practitioners and managers engaged with service development and quality improvement, the rhetoric of integration failed to connect with practice. Bell and colleagues (2008) suggested that there was a need to develop a top-down approach to the change in service delivery, through policy and legislation, as well as a bottom-up approach from the service providers. This attempt to formulate a common usage of *integration* highlighted the complexities involved, and acknowledged that language is dynamic and changeable over time in use and meaning (Bell et al., 2008). This holds true for language use in governments and agencies, as well as among professionals, clients, and their families.

The significance of language

Hebert and colleagues (2009) suggested that the ability to communicate effectively across groups is a result of the willingness to treat individuals from other communities with respect and understanding. Additionally, Nicholson and colleagues (2000) found in their research on working relationships in multidisciplinary settings that *working collaboratively* was described as working together as equals, and valuing and utilising the perspectives and expertise of others. Working in a multidisciplinary framework can also be considered as the coming together of differences. Sheehan (1996) described the differences as being a 'clash of cultures' (p. 76), characterised by differences in values, language, problem-solving strategies, and other elements of professional behaviour. According to Nicholson and colleagues (2000), different disciplines contribute separate and often competing philosophies, diagnoses of need and pathology, and models of the way the world works.

Specific terminology is necessary for different professions, and professional bodies spend a great deal of time ensuring that meaning is readily understood among members of the group. When the terminology is used outside the specific group for which it is intended, knowledge or understanding is assumed. Clinically, it is known that this is not always the case. Language defines the clinicians' observations, assessments, and diagnoses. Working in a multidisciplinary framework invites different skills, experiences, and ultimately different perspectives to describe the same presenting problem. It is important to use language that conveys meaning to others outside professional bodies or organisations so that information is credible for working together in a holistic manner.

A model for working together: establishing a common language

To assist the collaborative process between professionals who work together, it is important to establish a shared terminology that is universal for those involved. To do so is to take up a great challenge, particularly as individual disciplines and professional bodies have their own models of practice, terminology, and rhetoric, which have taken years of learning, research, and experience to achieve. However, before information can be confidently transferred beyond the boundary of any one discipline, it is necessary that within a discipline a common language is derived and adopted wholeheartedly by its members. This may sound self-evident; however, Marks (2005) argued that without a common language, confusion is likely. For example, Marks (2005) promoted the adoption of a common language within psychotherapy. He believed that the absence of a common language led different therapists to use different terms to describe the same procedure, and/or the same term to describe different procedures. Additionally, he insisted that using the same terms for common therapy procedures would enable psychotherapists to better communicate what they do.

Despite recognising the value of better communication and the importance of individual disciplines speaking the same language, there is no assurance that understanding is possible for someone outside the discipline who does not have appropriate training to interpret the meaning and the language accurately. Therefore, professionals who work with children and young persons with disabilities and emotional disturbances need to be able to gather and assess information and knowledge that transcends the boundaries of their disciplines. The real challenge then lies in seeking a common language for both the disability and mental health sectors, but more importantly, a language that families of clients find meaningful, interpretative, and informative in their dealings with all professionals.

A common language for working with children, young people, and their families

Professionals working with children and young people with intellectual disabilities use different and multiple conceptual models or 'lenses' to ascribe meaning to emotional and behavioural difficulties that are seen as challenging. A comment such as 'this child has bizarre language' can be interpreted in many valid ways, depending upon the professional's knowledge, attitude, and skills (Beukelman & Mirenda, 2005). Understanding a child's emotional and behavioural disturbances along with his or her developmental disability reflects understanding and experience in both the mental health and disability fields, and requires familiarity with language used in both sectors. Furthermore, depending upon clinicians' professional training, where they work, and even where they live, not to mention their own cultural and social values, there are subtle influences in the language that is adopted and used when working with clients. Language is used to define and label, as well as interpret and represent the child or young person's presenting issue or problem. In practice, this may involve summarising the presenting problems in the language that the child or family has used, as well as describing it in professional terminology.

When considering abnormal child development, there is an assumption or understanding of what this is, how it is measured, an idea of what the child will be like, and how he or she will present. The child is often given a diagnosis by a qualified professional, who develops a hypothesis and formulates an intervention for the presenting problem. However, not all professionals or family members will observe the same thing or even use the same language to describe what they see. At times, even the child or young person and the clinician can experience difficulties in sharing the same view. This is demonstrated in the case study below.

Case study 2.1

The young child could be seen struggling to find words to answer the question posed by the clinician, who was pointing at the middle-sized circle. On the table in front of the child were three circles, a larger circle, a medium circle, and a smaller circle. The clinician waited, with an expectant look on her face, knowing that a child with intellectual disability may need additional time to process the verbal command. It had taken many weeks to get to this point. This young child was reluctant to attempt new activities, had repeatedly moved away from exciting and enticing novel items, and was now showing signs of increased anxiety. The previous reports had stated that this child was not able to sit still at a table, and therefore could not be formally assessed. With gentle coaxing and much encouragement, the young child and clinician had begun the process of assessment tasks. After what seemed to be a long time, the child triumphantly yelled, 'Its Maurice!' and started to laugh.

This scenario could have been interpreted in various ways. Fortunately, the clinician was experienced in working with children in early intervention and was familiar with the not-so-regular characters from *Playschool*, the Australian Broadcasting Corporation's (ABC) television program and book (see Playschool, 2006). On *Playschool*, Maurice was the middle-sized bear, not 'Little Ted' and not 'Big Ted. Although the child understood the concept of *middle*, the child's answer was incorrect, and could not be scored, as the target answer of 'medium', 'middle-sized', or 'middle' for the assessment item was not achieved. Instead, a note of explanation was added to the score-sheet. The child had used a different viewpoint, or generalisation of knowledge, that he had gained in another context, to apply to this situation. The clinician was familiar with the language used by the child, and did not misinterpret the child's response as irrelevant.

Conceptualising a common language: examining language variation over time

Shared knowledge of the use of language can change over time. Tracking the way words are used allows us to map changes in the way people think and see the world. Acknowledging these changes also provides an understanding of how individuals with mental health issues or intellectual disability have been perceived and supported over time. Riding and colleagues (2005) suggested, 'The way in which we perceive the needs and relative value of vulnerable people has an important influence on the way in which we legislate and provide for them' (p. 7). According to Riding and colleagues (2005), the decision to exclude people with an intellectual disability from the *Mental Health Act* 1983 reflected changing social perceptions and an increased awareness of those with special needs, in particular the needs of people with intellectual disability.

Terminology changes within a profession as time elapses, so that what was once common usage may now be seen as inappropriate. As further information is gathered and more accurate terminology is sought, particular philosophies or frameworks are newly applied, legislation or governmental policies adopt specific terms (or acronyms), state, national, or international groups form, and a consensus on terminology is gained. An example of this is the desire for evidence-based research to inform clinical practice and the creation of web-based databases devoted to 'best practice' interventions and treatment efficacy, such as SpeechBITE and PsycBITE.

Ever-increasing reliance on information technology for exchange of communication and documentation has instilled an expectation that professionals across disciplines share a mutual definition or understanding of the information delivered. By examining the current use of language, many different terms (such as *interdisciplinary, multidisciplinary, transdisciplinary,* or *interprofessional*) are used in the literature without an (unanimous) understanding of their meaning (Nicholson et al., 2000). Furthermore, Graham and colleagues (2006) did a Google search of known terms, such as *knowledge translation, knowledge transfer, knowledge exchange, research utilisation, implementation, dissemination,* and *diffusion,* to describe the application of knowledge to practice. After reviewing the first dozen pages for each term, the researchers had difficulty in finding consistent and meaningful definitions for each of the terms. They also acknowledged that these terms were often interchangeable, sometimes used as a noun to reflect the entire process of gaining knowledge, or as a verb to reflect specific strategies. This example demonstrated that language that is thought to be common is in fact not so. Language that is open to interpretation and processes that are not streamlined makes effective clinical practice difficult. The use of discipline-specific assessments ensures sharing of meaning of a child's or young person's presenting issues, but limits the application and deliverance of information to knowledgeable recipients. Although these assessments may assist to provide clinical insight within a discipline, they fall short of achieving a common language across disciplines.

Deriving a common language for clinical practice

When considering this issue on a global level, there are several universal tools that can be used to derive a clinical framework. The text revision of the fourth edition of the Diagnostic and Statistical Manual of Mental Disorders (DSM-IV-TR) (APA, 2000) lists all known mental disorders, and assumes a common understanding of interpretation and diagnosis, as does the tenth revision of the International Statistical Classification of Diseases and Related Health Problems (ICD-10) (WHO, 2007). A point of difference is that the ICD-10 works in tandem with the International Classification of Functioning, Disability and Health (ICF) (WHO, 2002). The ICD-10 and the ICF are classification tools that assist to provide a common language for professionals working across disciplines and professional bodies. The ICD-10 is 'used to classify disease at the level of the health condition in the ICF model' (Imms, 2006, p. 65), and aims to provide a common interdisciplinary language for communication and understanding of health, health-related outcomes, and health determinants. Simeonsson and colleagues (2003) reported that, because of the disproportionate prevalence of disability in developing countries, with children constituting the largest percentage of those with functional and developmental limitations, there was a need for universal measures that are brief and effective for use in surveillance and screening.

The ICF, at its core, addresses this broad need for a common language and classification of functioning and disability (Simeonsson et al., 2003). Also, Jette (2006) stated that, 'If widely adopted, the ICF framework could provide the rehabilitation field with a common, international language with the potential to facilitate communication and scholarly discourse across disciplines and national boundaries, to stimulate interdisciplinary research, to improve clinical care, and ultimately to better inform health policy and management' (p. 726). Although the ICF may assist in providing a universal language across health and disability services, the classification system is still complex, and questions remain about its practicability (Allet et al., 2008). It would appear that, from reviewing clinical practices and professional disciplines, there are varying degrees in which the ICF and the ICD-10 are used to shape the clinical direction of service delivery. Therefore, it may be necessary to utilise alternate approaches to establishing a common language, approaches that could include clinical frameworks that are not discipline specific, but focus on the client, and identifying and addressing their needs.

Clinical frameworks that assist with establishing a common language

It is important for clinicians to examine a child's or young person's presenting disability and emotional–behavioural issues from a holistic point of view. Brofenbrenner (1979) developed *ecological systems theory* in order to look holistically at a child's development within the context of his or her environment. Brofenbrenner's theory defined complex layers of the child's environment, each of which had an effect on his or her development. Brofenbrenner (1979) argued that the interaction between factors in the child's maturing biology, his or her immediate family and community environment, and the societal landscape directed development. He also argued that changes or conflict in any one layer would ripple through other layers, and may have an adverse impact on the child's developmental trajectory. Therefore, in determining the impact of having a disability on the child's development, the child and his or her immediate environment need to be examined, followed by an exploration of the child's interaction with the larger environment.

The bio-psycho-social model is used within the mental health and disability fields, and provides a framework for considering the child's emotional, behavioural, and developmental well-being. Stokes and colleagues (2006) noted that the ICF used the bio-psycho-social model to help conceptualise and measure health and health-related issues. Therefore, by linking the ICF to child mental health and disability services using the bio-psycho-social model, clinicians can establish a common language for considering predisposing, precipitating, perpetuating, and protective factors in understanding the complexity of a child's or young person's presenting problems (Havighurst & Downey, 2009).

Dossetor and colleagues (2005) took this idea a step further to explore the influence of the psychiatry of intellectual disability on child psychiatry, and conversely, the influence of child psychiatry on the understanding of the mental health needs of those with intellectual disability. Dossetor and colleagues (2005) argued that child psychiatry needed to expand its understanding of the bio-psycho-social approach in the management of young people with intellectual disability. Furthermore, they proposed that a more dynamic and broader conceptual framework of developmental neuropsychiatry was one that encompassed a bio-developmental-psycho-social-cultural model. This enhanced model could then assist in establishing a common understanding of the mental health needs of all children, including implications for assessment, diagnosis, and treatment.

Conclusion: Achieving A Common Language

Establishing a common language in child mental health and disability fields is important and continues to evolve. The challenge has been to achieve a definition and a common understanding of its impact on clinical practice. There is strong agreement that a common language is needed across disciplines and agencies, yet there are varied models and frameworks as to how this can be established. This chapter has highlighted that the need for a common language is evident at all levels of government, within and across agencies, disciplines, and fields, and for families and clients. An awareness of clinical tools and clinical frameworks is also necessary so that communication and collaboration is meaningful for all clinicians across both the child mental health and disability sectors. A common language is central to meeting the complex developmental, emotional, and behavioural needs of children and young people with a disability (see figure 2.1).

Laming (as cited in Salmon & Rapport, 2005) suggested that a common language must be established 'for use across all agencies to help those agencies to identify who they are most concerned about, why they are concerned, who is best placed to respond to those concerns and what outcome is being sought from any planned response' (p. 373). However, there are differences in how a common language is derived. Professionals, agencies, and governments may use the universal clinical tools such as the DSM-IV-TR (APA, 2000), ICD-10 (WHO, 2007), or ICF (WHO, 2002) to inform clinical practice. Or, they may use the clinical frameworks such as ecological systems theory (Brofenbrenner, 1979), or the bio-developmental-psycho-social-cultural model (Dossetor et al., 2005). At the end of the day there is no easy answer as to how to derive a common language. However, it is evident that there is a need for professionals to collaborate, exchange information, have a willingness to work across disciplines, form partnerships, and share knowledge.

Nicholson and colleagues (2000) argued that, for professionals to achieve a common language, it is necessary to have a multidisciplinary, collaborative

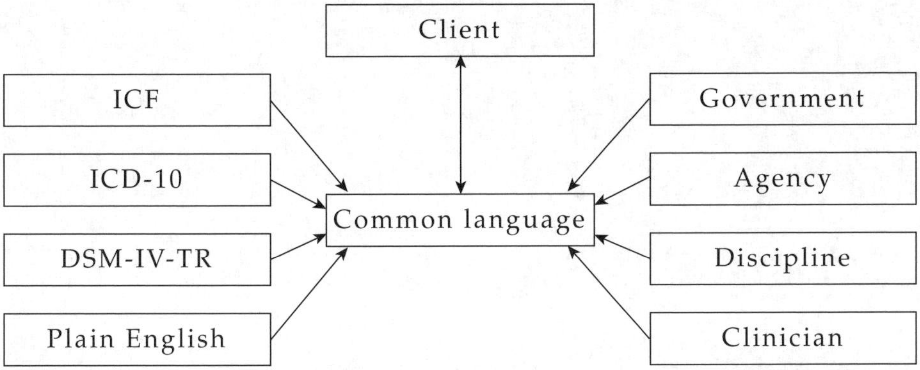

Figure 2.1 Common language: the central focus of effective clinical practice

approach and to ask lots of questions, for clarification. There must be a commitment to effective communication and the time it requires, acceptance of individual differences, flexibility, reflection in practice, and valuing the input and participation of others (clients and co-workers). Thus, whenever possible, professionals should adopt a language that is current and easily understood, that is respectful of clients and families, while being mindful of the significance and connotation of certain words. Professionals should also learn new terminology to help with interdisciplinary and interagency communication and develop an evidence-based approach. Importantly, they should keep an open mind. Finally, professionals should be aware that 'the lack of a common language across agencies has been identified as one of the critical factors in the success or failure of multi-agency collaborations' (Salmon & Rapport, 2005, p. 430).

3

Structured assessment of mental health problems in children and adolescents with intellectual disabilities

Louise A. Ellis and Stewart L. Einfeld

Introduction

Over the past decade, there has been an emergence of structured assessment tools developed specifically to assess psychopathology in children and adolescents with intellectual disabilities (ID). This chapter highlights the importance of incorporating structured instruments into clinical practice when working with young people with ID, and describes a number of the most widely used and psychometrically sound measures currently available for this population. Although limitations are identified with many of the existing instruments, the routine use of structured assessment tools may significantly improve the diagnosis of, and quality of care for, people with ID. A comprehensive multimethod approach to assessing psychopathology in individuals with ID is advocated, as well as the routine use of structured tools to monitor progress and treatment response over time.

The identification and correct diagnosis of psychopathology in young people with intellectual disabilities (ID) is complex, and can be highly challenging for even the most experienced clinician. Atypical presentations, maladaptive behaviours, communication and cognitive limitations, differential developmental trajectories, and limitations in lifestyle, as well as reliance on diagnostic criteria developed for intellectually normal individuals, can lead to under- and misdiagnosis (see Costello & Bouras, 2006, for review). The deficiency of adequate assessment measures has also contributed to the under- and misdiagnosis of psychopathology in young people with ID (Rush et al., 2004). However, over the past decade there has been an emergence of structured assessment tools specifically developed to screen for psychopathology, thus improving our ability to conduct adequate assessments.

Why structured psychometric assessment is important

The unstructured traditional diagnostic assessment has been the standard practice for making initial psychiatric diagnoses. To increase diagnostic validity and reliability, clinicians have expanded the Mental Status Examination (MSE) and the history of present and past illnesses, and are using more structured formats (Miller et al., 2001). As asserted by Frances and colleagues (1995):

> most clinicians are now imbued not only with the content of the DSM-IV sets but also with a different method of interviewing patients and eliciting psychopathology. Compared to pre-DSM-III days, clinical evaluations are now much more likely to be more semi-structured and less open-ended (p. 66).

These changes have largely reflected concerns raised in the 1980s that unstructured clinical assessments may lead to inconsistency, biases, and inaccuracies in diagnosis. Much of the discussion focused upon the dichotomy of clinical versus actuarial assessment (Dawes et al., 1989). In the clinical method, the assessor, in this case the diagnostician, 'combines or processes information in his or her head' (Dawes et al., 1989, p. 1668). The questions that the clinician asks will often be subjective, inconsistent, and perhaps even only tangentially related to the problem under consideration. On the other hand, 'in the actuarial or statistical method, the human judge is eliminated and conclusions rest solely on relations between data and the condition or event of interest' (Dawes et al., 1989, p. 1668). An actuarial assessment tool asks the same set of questions of each individual, asks them in the same way, and interprets the answers consistently.

The idea that actuarial judgment is superior to clinical judgment is not new, and was championed by Meehl and colleagues 50 years ago (Meehl, 1954; 1957; 1959). Since that time, others have joined in, and research has consistently shown that actuarial methods are more accurate or, at minimum, equally as accurate as clinical predictions (e.g., Ægisdóttir et al., 2006; Dawes et al., 1989; Garb, 1994; Grove et al., 2000; Russell, 1995; Wiggins, 1981). The most comprehensive meta-analytic investigation conducted to date (Grove et al., 2000) compared the accuracy of actuarial versus clinical predictions in 136 studies of human health and behaviour. Actuarial procedures were, on average, 10 per cent more accurate than clinical predictions, and substantially more accurate in 33 to 47 per cent of the studies examined.

Because of past concerns about the suitability and accuracy of unstructured clinical assessments, considerable effort has gone into improving psychiatric assessment procedures. The development of structured and semi-structured interviews for individuals with ID has followed the development of such interviewing schedules for intellectually normal individuals (Harris, 2006). A number of problem checklists and rating scales have also been developed to improve the reliability and validity of psychiatric evaluation for young people with ID.

Structured assessment tools for children and adolescents with intellectual disability

Several standardised assessment tools have been developed to assist in the identification of mental health problems in children and adolescents with ID. Some of these measures focus on making a specific diagnosis, whereas others are used to assess the range and severity of behavioural and emotional problems. The most widely used and psychometrically sound tools for this population, including interview schedules, behaviour checklists, and rating scales, are described below.

Interview schedules

A small number of structured and semi-structured psychiatric interview schedules have been developed specifically for children and adolescents with ID. The *Schedule of Handicaps and Behavior and Skills* (HBS-Revised) (Wing, 1982) is a semi-structured interview schedule based on parents' ratings of the abilities and behaviours of their child. The HBS can be used to assess children and adolescents with mild to profound ID. Although the stated purpose of the HBS is to provide all information that is necessary to arrive at a diagnosis and develop a prognosis, the schedule places a very heavy emphasis on questions related to autism behaviours rather than a wide range of psychiatric disorders (Aman, 1991a). Also, while there is some psychometric data available for the HBS, this schedule appears to have received little attention by researchers and clinicians in the field (Handen, 2007).

The *Structured Clinical Interview* (SCI) (Spragg, 1988) is another interview schedule designed specifically for individuals with ID. It comprises approximately 130 questions, and is intended to complement other types of clinical data by providing information in the cognitive and affective domains. However, there is limited available data on the SCI's psychometric properties, and there is little evidence of its use for either clinical or research purposes (Aman, 1991a; Handen, 2007).

A small number of interview schedules have also been designed to assess specific disorders in young people with ID. For example, the *Autism Diagnosis Interview–Revised* (ADI-R) (Lord et al., 1994) is a structured interview used with the child's primary caregiver and is designed to accompany the *Autism*

Diagnostic Observation Schedule (ADOS) (Lord et al., 1999). The ADI-R consists of 93 items applicable to any person with a mental age of two years and above. However, administration time for the ADI-R is long (up to three hours), and clinicians need extensive training in order for it to be administered reliably.

Behaviour checklists and rating scales

Behaviour checklists and rating scales have been used extensively to augment the diagnosis of psychopathology in children and adolescents with ID. Most rating scales are informant-based measures, which are particularly relevant to the assessment of young people with moderate to profound ID, where self-reporting is not possible. Some of the advantages of rating scales are: they are easy to administer; they capture perceptions of low-frequency behaviours; they provide structure for informants; and they typically have better psychometric properties than other subjective measures, such as interviews (Rush et al., 2004).

These tools allow the professional to obtain information from multiple informants (such as teachers and parents) who might otherwise not be available during the assessment (Handen, 2007). If administered routinely, they also provide a history of behaviour, which is valuable for monitoring progress and treatment response (Einfeld & Tonge, 1995). In general, there are three categories of behaviour checklists and rating scales available for the assessment of psychopathology in individuals with ID. These include: (a) instruments designed to assess a broad range of psychopathology specifically for individuals with ID; (b) instruments designed originally to assess psychopathology in typically developing individuals that have been extended to individuals with ID; and (c) instruments designed to assess specific disorders in individuals with ID.

Instruments assessing a broad spectrum of psychopathology in young people with intellectual disabilities

Aberrant behavior checklist

The *Aberrant Behavior Checklist* (ABC) (Aman & Singh, 1986) is an informant-based problem behaviour rating scale that was originally developed for institutionalised intellectually disabled individuals (aged five years and above) with moderate, severe, and profound ID. The ABC has since been revised for community use, and there are now two versions available: the original ABC, now renamed *ABC–Residential (ABC-R),* and the newer *ABC–Community version* (ABC-C) (Aman & Singh, 1994). Both versions consist of 58 items, each scored on a 4-point rating scale (0 = not a problem to 3 = problem is severe in degree). The instruments consist of five subscales: (1) Irritability, agitation, crying (15 items); (2) Lethargy, social withdrawal (16 items); (3) Stereotypic behaviour (7 items); (4) Hyperactivity, non-compliance (16 items); and, (5) Inappropriate speech (4 items).

A number of psychometric studies have shown that the ABC-R and ABC-C are reliable and valid behaviour rating scales for adolescents and adults (see Brown et al., 2002, for review). Research has also shown that these instruments may be suitable for children, though there are some potential limitations with the use of the both ABC-R and ABC-C for this population (see Rojahn & Heisel, 1991; Brown et al., 2002).

Developmental behaviour checklist

The *Developmental Behavior Checklist* (Einfeld & Tonge, 1995) was specifically developed to screen for behavioural and emotional disturbances in children and adolescents (aged 4 to 18 years) with all levels of ID. Two versions are available: a *Primary Carer Version* (DBC-P) consisting of 96 items, and a *Teacher Version* (DBC-T), consisting of 94 items. Each item is rated from zero to two (such as 0 = not true as far as you know; 2 = very true or often true). The DBC consists of five subscales: disruptive/antisocial; self-absorbed; communication disturbance; anxiety; and social relating (Einfeld & Tonge, 2002). The instrument has strong psychometric properties, with high test-retest internal consistency, adequate interrater reliability, and good predictive validity of clinically significant behaviour and emotional disturbance (Einfeld & Tonge, 1995, 2002).

The DBC has also been used widely in research on children and adolescents with ID, and the DBC-P has been translated into various languages. *The Developmental Behavior Checklist–Monitoring* (DBC-M) (Evans et al., 2003) is an additional tool that has been developed for monitoring specific behaviours. This allows for up to five behaviours to be scored daily. Using the DBC-M requires far less time than completing the full DBC versions. Thus, while the DBC-P or DBC-T is recommended for assessment purposes, the DBC-M can be used in clinical interventions with young people to map progress.

Nisonger Child Behaviour Rating Form

The *Nisonger Child Behaviour Rating Form* (NCBRF) (Aman et al., 1996) was designed for use with children (aged 3 to 16 years). The NCBRF has a parent version and a teacher version, with identical content and similar factor structures. Both versions contain 10 social competence items and 66 problem behaviour items, which are rated on four-point scales. The social competence items are distributed on two subscales: compliant/calm and adaptive/social. The problem behaviour items are distributed on six subscales: conduct problem; insecure/anxious; hyperactive; self-injury/stereotypic; self-isolated/ritualistic; and overly sensitive (parent)/irritable (teacher). The NCBRF has good psychometric properties (Aman et al., 1996; Lecavalier & Aman, 2005) and has been translated into several languages.

Reiss Scales for Children's Dual Diagnosis

The *Reiss Scales for Children's Dual Diagnosis* (Reiss & Valenti-Hein, 1994) is a 60-item measure for children (aged four years and over). The instrument is completed by informants (such as teachers and parents), and items are rated on a three-point scale from zero to two (0 = no problem; 2 = major problem). The instrument consists of 10 subscales (anger/self-control; anxiety disorder; attention deficit; autism; conduct disorder; depression; poor self-esteem; psychosis; somatoform behaviour; and withdrawn/isolated) and 10 specific behaviour problems (such as crying spells and hallucinations). Although research suggests that the total score produced by the instrument is a highly reliable and an accurate indicator of the presence or absence of psychopathology in children with ID, the results appear to be less favourable for the individual subscale scores (Reiss & Valenti-Hein, 1994).

Instruments designed for assessing psychopathology in typically developing individuals

Structured behaviour checklists and rating scales developed for typically developing individuals have also been used to evaluate psychopathology among children and adolescents with ID. Although these instruments generally have good test-retest reliability, they vary in terms of their interrater reliability, internal consistency, and validity (Harris, 2006). Examples include the *Child Behaviour Checklist*, the *Beck Depression Inventory*, the *Rutter Behavioural Scales*, the *Zung Self-Rating Anxiety Scale*, and the *Zung Self-Rating Depression Scale*. While these tools have been used with young people with mild to moderate ID, they are less likely to be used in the assessment of young people with severe or profound ID. As a general rule, the use of appropriately designed tools for young people with ID is recommended.

Instruments designed for assessing specific disorders in individuals with intellectual disabilities

Only a few rating scales have been developed to assess specific disorders in young people with ID. For example, the *Self-Report Depression Questionnaire* (SRDQ) (Reynolds & Baker, 1988) has been designed to assess depressive symptomatology in adolescents and adults with mild ID. The *Anxiety, Depression, and Mood Scale* (ADAMS) (Esbensen et al., 2003) is an informant-based rating scale used to measure symptoms related to anxiety, depression, and mania in individuals with ID (aged 10 years and over). The *Social Communica-*

tion Questionnaire (SCQ) (Berument et al., 1999) is a parent questionnaire that can be used to help evaluate communication skills and social functioning in children (aged four years and over) who may have autism or autism spectrum disorders.

Instruments designed for assessing adaptive functioning in individuals with intellectual disabilities

Information that is most useful when assessing psychopathology in young people with ID includes not only information about the presence of psychiatric problems, but also information regarding the young person's adaptive functioning (Rojahn & Tassé, 1996).

The *Vineland Adaptive Behaviour Scales* (VABS-II) (Sparrow et al., 2005) is a widely used measure of adaptive behaviour for children and adolescents with ID. The VABS assesses four domain areas: communication; daily living skills; socialisation; and motor skills. There is also a maladaptive behaviour domain that can be used to assess problem behaviours. Another popular measure of adaptive functioning is the *American Association on Mental Retardation (AAMR) Adaptive Behavior Scales (ABS)*, which consists of two versions: *School and Community* (ABS-S2) (Lambert et al., 1993) and *Residential and Community* (ABS-RC2) (Nihira et al., 1993). Norms are provided for young people with and without ID (aged 3–21 years).

Conclusion

When working with young people with ID, clinicians are recommended to use a comprehensive multimethod approach to assess psychopathology, with a combination of structured and unstructured techniques and information from several sources (such as the young person with ID, professionals, parents, carers, and teachers). The unstructured aspect allows the development of adequate rapport, and the expression and evaluation of feeling. The structured component utilises systematic questioning to ascertain the presence and severity of a range of important psychiatric symptoms. Specifically, when assessing psychopathology in young people with ID, the assessment should include: (1) clinical assessments, which include history, individual and family clinical interviews, and mental status examination of the child or adolescent; as well as (2) structured interviews, questionnaires, behaviour checklists, and rating scales (Harris, 2006). If behaviour checklists and rating scales are administered routinely, they also provide a valuable history that can be used in monitoring progress and treatment response over time (Einfeld & Tonge, 1995).

4

A paediatrician's approach to the assessment of a child with intellectual disability or autism

Joseph Macdessi

Introduction

Consultation regarding a child with intellectual disability or autism spectrum disorder (ASD) is a highly challenging process, yet one that can be systematically worked through by using an approach with three dimensions. Focusing on a purely medical approach is one dimension. The second dimension is the extent to which both the home and school domains have appropriate structure and stimulation that matches the developmental age of the child. The third dimension is an understanding of the family unit's emotional welfare. This includes how rules and emotional regulation are managed, including welfare emotions of affection and care, and the extent of emergency emotions, such as depression, anxiety, and anger. This systematic approach usually needs to be conducted over a few consultations, but if forewarned families usually respect the more thorough approach, rather than a rush to prescribe psychotropic medication.

A comprehensive assessment involves a number of challenges. The first challenge of the initial consultation is to develop a rapport with the parents or carers, and at least to secure a connection with the child with the disability. That connection relies on the paediatrician demonstrating that he or she is comfortable with the child, who may not demonstrate a perfect model of behaviour in the consultation room. The room needs to be prepared to allow the child the scope of exploration without causing any sense of apprehension or hypervigilance on the paediatrician's part. Fragile equipment needs to be secured away, play resources need to be carefully selected, and cabinets locked—all in the hope of avoiding constricting or negative instructions and pleas from all. Free-range play, with the parent guiding the child, while the paediatrician respectfully shows confidence in their relationship, goes a long way in securing rapport with the parents.

Generally, the paediatrician should try to engage with the child at an early stage, as parents want to see that the paediatrician is comfortable with their child and his or her disability. Presenting a downturned hand for the child to reach out to is a reliable introductory gesture, used in conjunction with a calm manner to make welcoming comments or ask simple questions. This enables the paediatrician to observe the child's level of engagement and communication. Even if this fails, the attempt is the part that the parents respect, and makes it easier to start speaking about the child in detail. It also establishes a connection so that the child is less anxious about subsequent consultations. The aim of the initial appointment should be for the parents or carers to leave knowing that the paediatrician has respect and empathy for them, and that a comfortable line of communication has been opened with them.

It is important that the paediatrician avoids putting pressure on the child in a way that causes distress. If this occurs, one parent can be asked to take the child outside, while the paediatrician continues the consultation with the other parent. This is usually appreciated, especially if it is apparent that the paediatrician has genuinely attempted to connect with and keep the environment as calm as possible for the child. The paediatrician should never show frustration, but rather acceptance of the developmental age of the child.

The initial assessment process

Medical history

The standard paediatric history taking and examination should be conducted. However, often a systematic examination cannot be achieved at the initial consultation, but can be a priority for the next stage of the initial assessment process. It is important to note that, when investigating a child's challenging behaviours, there are several important domains that need to be explored as possible maintaining or exacerbating factors.

Ear, nose, and throat system

Otitis media (inflammation or infection of the middle ear) is a possible exacerbant of challenging behaviours. The manifestations can be ear tugging, gouging, or banging, but can be less specific: head banging, generalised aggression, or distress. It can be difficult to examine the tympanic membranes properly if a child is unable to cooperate, and thus this simple diagnosis can easily be missed unless an obvious perforation has evolved. Baseline audiology is a must, particularly if it has been more than two years since an assessment.

Sleep problems are an important area of history taking (Cotton & Richdale, 2006). Compromised sleep, particularly during the REM phase, will lead to daytime fatigue and a lower threshold to irritability, with daily demands and easily precipitated aggression, especially in the afternoons. Establishing effective sleep patterns is possibly the most important therapeutic target for challenging behaviours. Habitual snoring is permissible, but obstructed sleep with apnoeas warrants further investigation.

It is important to clarify sleep hygiene, including mapping the pre-sleep routine (such as caffeine intake via carbonated beverages, aerobic routines, noise levels, and stimulation from TV, DVD, computer, or console games), the approach to bed time, latency to sleep time, frequency of awakenings, and the approaches to resettling. The secondary gains of nocturnal awakening (such as co-sleeping and other interactions and engagements with family members) need to be asked about, as they are potentially sources of positive reinforcement. Behavioural approaches are usually the main approach required; however, medication may be a necessary complement. The opportunity to ascertain how members of the entire family sleep and their level of daytime exhaustion follows on naturally.

The degree of work with breathing and possibility of apnoeas needs to be explored, as well as interruptions of sleep from pruritus (related to eczema) or postnasal drip (related to allergic rhinitis). A sleep diary over a seven-day period may be required, as usually sleep studies are not tolerated. Lateral airways x-rays and allergy skin testing (for allergic rhinitis exacerbants) are very helpful for determining whether surgical (tonsillo-adenoidectomy) or medical intervention (nasal inhaled corticosteroids or antihistamines) is required.

Gastrointestinal system

When taking a dietary history, the paediatrician should ask about exclusions and excesses of food types. Unless there is an obvious food allergy or intolerance, particularly in the context of family history, excluding certain food items or elimination diets is usually unnecessary. Where the child excludes food types, the history should establish whether the dietary profile is too restrictive to maintain iron, B_{12}, and folate stores. This should be formally tested at some stage, to ensure that there is no underlining microcytic or macrocytic anaemia at hand. There have been reported cases and personal experiences of correction of B_{12} deficiency allaying challenging behaviours.

Constipation also needs to be excluded as a contributor to the burden of care and mental health problems of the child (Bosch et al., 2002). Regular soft to firm bowel motions without the components of strain, pain, or PR bleeding should be an established baseline and maintained aim. It may be difficult for carers to correlate this temporarily with challenging behaviours accurately, but when it is presented to them as a plausible explanation, there is usually an agreement that it should be a shared objective. At times a diary of bowel motion consistency and habit is required. The choice of laxative or stool softener, or bulking agent, is a matter of individual prescribing choice. The trial of various options should occur until optimal management of bowel habit is established.

Neurological system

Seizure disorders may be a comorbid diagnosis in this select group of patients. Epilepsy treatment may already be established, but it is still pertinent to ascertain both the benefits and harm profile of prescribed anticonvulsant therapy, which may influence sedation, irritability, and impulsivity, and may fuel aggressive outbursts (Ring et al., 2007). There may be a balance between modifying anticonvulsant regimes and adding psychotropic medication to modify the side-effects of the anticonvulsant regime (Rutecki & Gidal, 2002). It is important to establish a strong line of communication with the co-involved neurologist in such complex clinical dilemmas.

On the other hand, the nature of the seizure itself (particularly partial complex and frontal seizures) may be a sufficient explanation of aggression (Hirsch, 2005). If seizure-related activity is a diagnosis that has not been considered, but is strongly suspected based on history, a home video recording of events is worth requesting. This has been found to be an invaluable source of information while working through the possible differential diagnoses and before resorting to specialist investigations using an EEG under anaesthetic or video telemetry.

Physical examination

In the consultation room

The physical examination of the child should concentrate on delineating dysmorphic aspects and focal neurological signs. The art of observation will yield much information, and can be done while the child is playing or sitting on the parent's lap. The types of observations that can be made are described in table 4.1.

The extent of a hands-on examination depends on the level of rapport established with the child and how confronting or imposing the examination is in respect of possible sensory-averting tendencies. This part of the examination may require the parents rather than the paediatrician to manoeuvre the child gently into position. The paediatrician may even need to make the examination into a play scenario; for example, performing a procedure such as measuring blood pressure on the parents first so that the child feels safe.

Hospital-based physical examinations

There are situations in which physical examination of the child in a consulting room is impossible or unsafe (in terms of exacerbating the child's aggression), despite repeated attempts. In such situations a planned examination in hospital under sedation may provide the opportunity for a thorough systemic examination. Options for sedation include nitrous oxide gas, clonidine, midazolam, ketamine, or chloral hydrate.

It is suggested that there be close liaison with an anaesthetist, and that this is done within the domains of a hospital. If sedation is unsuccessful, then planning for a general anaesthetic may be required. At such a strategic point,

Table 4.1 Initial consultation observations

At the time of meeting and greeting the child:
• General nutrition: appropriateness of height and weight • Dysmorphic features of head (asymmetry of shape), face, hands, and digits • Bite marks, scars, and callouses of the forearm (self-injurious behaviours) • Obvious dental caries during a smile (clue to need for formal dental assessment to exclude significant dental pathology as a source of pain) • Symmetry of facial expression (at rest or even when crying) • The nature of cry (hyponasal in adenoidal hypertrophy)
While the child walks around the room and plays during the course of history taking from the parents:
• Stability and symmetry of gait • Ability to transfer from lying to sitting to standing positions (Gower's sign) • Symmetry of limb movements (peripheral weakness or cental tonicity changes)
While sitting up in the parent's lap:
• Coordination of conjugate eye movements while encouraging the child to visually follow interesting play items (cerebellum signs) • Accuracy of the reach and the absence of resting and intentional tremor or past pointing while offering the child interesting play items (cerebellum signs)
While lying back on the parent's lap with upper garments lifted or removed:
• Neurocutaneous stigmata • Rashes (eczema as a source of irritation and possible sleep deprivation) • Excoriation marks as a clue to where pain is manifest (e.g., significant gastritis or oesophagitis can be associated with scratches localised to the epigastrium and lower sternal edge) • Presence of palmar or conjunctival pallor (iron or B_{12} deficiency secondary to restrictive diets) • Subcutaneous fat stores • Cardiac examination and anterior respiratory examination • Abdominal examination via inspection for distension (coeliac or chronic constipation) and gentle palpation faecal loading (constipation), and hepatosplenomegaly (storage disorder) • If the child is comfortable, further inspection to exclude hernias, undescended testes, and perianal fissures (chronic constipation)
While the parents carry the child or hold the child while squatting to their level:
• Abnormal spinal curvature • Neurocutaneous stigmata • Posterior respiratory examination
Leave the following to the very end or for another consultation:
• Measurement of head circumference, weight, and height • Examination of – ears (effusion and hearing impairment) – nose and symmetry of nasal air flow (adenoidal hypertrophy as a cause of obstructed/fragmented sleep patterns) – throat (tonsillar hypertrophy as a cause of obstructed/fragmented sleep patterns)

Table 4.2 Clinical presentations and investigations to be considered

Clinical presentation	*Considerations and investigations*
Child with low average to borderline delay alone	Variation from family norms
Child with mild-to-moderate or above delay with language delay or dysmorphism	• Thyroid functions tests, DNA for fragile X, karyotype and (after consultation with a geneticist) possibly transferrin isoforms and comparative genomic hybridisation (CGH) array • Specific genetic testing for clinically apparent syndromes
Boys with above	Creatinine kinase
Child with severe disability	Above plus urine metabolic screen
Developmental regression (including loss of speech skills)	Urine metabolic screen, liver function tests, serum ammonia, matched serum lactate and pyruvate, guided plasma substrate and enzyme assays, EEG, MRI and MRS, CSF neurotransmitter studies, ASOT and AntiDNAaseB, as well as fundoscopic assessment by ophthalmologist
Child with macrocephaly, microcephaly, head shape asymmetry, focal neurological signs, and neurocutaneous stigmata	MRI and MRS
Child with altered seizure pattern	EEG and MRI/MRS
Child with small head	Review newborn screening results, TORCH, maternal PKU
Child with nutritional concerns	Ferritin, folate, B_{12}, FBC and film, coeliac serology and LFT, stool microscopy and culture

as well as your examination, it may be prudent to coinvolve a dental review, venesection (if investigations required), and EEG or MRI (if also indicated).

Additional investigations

Investigative screens for disability often have a low diagnostic yield and should be tailored to the presentation (Cass et al., 2006; Moeschler, 2008). Possible considerations for additional investigations are outlined in table 4.2.

Developmental assessment

This is probably the most important component of the assessment. The aim is to ensure that the behaviours of the child and expectations of carers and other professionals are aligned with the developmental age of the child. This then provides an opportunity to assess the functionality of supports and strategies at home and school. If the child's developmental age is inaccurately rated (under or over) and the approaches of well-meaning adults are mismatched (either under or over), then there is large therapeutic target to aim for.

The best approach is to ascertain the child's abilities in activities of daily living as a reflection of cognitive abilities, including:

- vision and hearing
- fine motor, gross motor, and coordination skills
- self-care skills
- communication (verbal and nonverbal skills, use of augmentative and alternative communication systems)
- how and with whom the child plays and the scope of interests and likes.

The degree of independence, socialisation, and communication are the salient aspects of the developmental assessment that the paediatrician, carers, and other professionals need to be aligned on. In children with problems of social reciprocity or below the developmental age of two years, the paediatrician needs to consider sensory sensitivities and preoccupations in play.

Clinical developmental assessment provides a functional test of skills, and may identify specific skill deficits, such as memory, appreciation of time, emotional understanding and reciprocity, emotional and behavioural regulation, capacity for planning and future anticipation, and insight. Review of prior psychometric assessments is helpful, and may extend the paediatrician's understanding of the child's development. In most instances, previous assessments will support the paediatrician's clinical findings, observations, and formulation of the developmental profile. Where there are discrepancies, it is generally safer to rely on the clinical assessment and look for further expertise in understanding the difficulties of psychometric assessment. However, if there is a discrepancy raised with the formulation, then a multidisciplinary assessment is recommended.

Formal developmental assessments for preschool children could include multidisciplinary team observations, *Griffiths Mental Development Scales* (Griffiths, 1970), *Stanford Binet Intelligence Scales* (Roid, 2003), and *Differential Ability Scales* (Elliott, 1990). For the older child (before school entry), standard intelligence tests include the *Wechsler Preschool and Primary Scale of Intelligence* (WPPSI–III) (Wechsler, 2002) for ages 2½–7 years, or the *Wechsler Intelligence Scale for Children* (WISC–IV) (Wechsler, 2003) for ages 6–16 years. A handy office tool for developmental screening is the *Brigance Inventory of Early Development* (IED-II) (Brigance, 2004) from birth to the developmental age of seven years. The developmental assessment also provides the basis on which to make the diagnosis of developmental disorders such as ASD and attention deficit hyperactive disorder (ADHD).

The paediatrician should ensure that there is a dedicated session to developmental assessment (principally by history), and ensure that the parents truly understand the discrepancy between the child's developmental age and chronological age. However, what is often not explained well or understood by parents is that there is a *ceiling effect* of the developmental trajectory after the age of 16 years. For example, a mildly delayed child's independence and academic skills are likely to remain at the developmental age of 10–12 years old even though his or her temperament settles down in adulthood, and he or she has sufficient skills to competently fulfil most adult roles.

Psychological and psychiatric co-diagnoses

Ascertaining the mental health of the child or adolescent, as well as the rest of the family, may require separate consultation time with the parents alone. The child may have co-diagnoses such as:

- *ASD*, with delays in development of social-emotional capacity and adaptability
- *ADHD*, leading to impulsive aggression
- *depression*, leading to a miserable or irritable demeanour and in turn easily flared aggressive lashouts or
- *obsessive compulsive disorder* or *anxiety disorder*, leading to anxiety-fuelled agitation and aggression.

Some of these may be innate traits, while others may be reactive to the environment at hand.

The paediatrician needs to gauge parental exhaustion and possible concurrent depression, which is frequent, and often minimised and undertreated in this context. This consultation time also provides an opportunity to delineate the existence of comorbid depression, anxiety, and obsessive compulsive disorders. In addition, it allows the paediatrician to ascertain siblings' adjustment to the potentially stigmatising burden and challenge of living with and accepting a sibling with disability.

Parents' or siblings' psychological issues are important concomitants that may also underlie the challenging behaviours of the child with a disability. Such psychological issues can compromise the quality of family interactions through emotional withdrawal and passivity, or highly expressed emotion, such as emotional over-involvement, criticalness, or hostility. This style of emotional communication can erode the autonomy or motivation of the young person with disability, and affect supervision of play, predictable structure, and access to other relationships and the community.

School and community services perspectives

Establishing an open line of communication with the child's school is required to confirm the extent that problems are context dependent or pervasive. This also ensures that strategies are shared between parents and teachers, and may assist in achieving consistent results in containing threatening or difficult behaviours.

The paediatrician has a responsibility to raise concerns on whether the child is receiving the appropriate supports at school to match his or her needs. School visits are invaluable, either by the paediatrician directly, or through the community disability services. In more complex cases, the availability of a community case manager can serve as an interface between the office-based consultant paediatrician and other community services, such as occupational therapy for sensory profiling, speech pathology for augmentative communication strategies, and behaviour support or psychology for behavioural strategies.

Conclusion

Assessment of children or young people with intellectual disability or ASD involves a complex matrix of medical, developmental, psychological, and environmental dimensions. A well-structured, multistaged approach is essential, and several consultations are required for a comprehensive initial assessment. This relatively methodical and thorough approach is necessary before considering the role of psychotropic medication. While psychotropic medication has a definite role in the optimal management of developmental and psychiatric disorders, it should only be considered if other approaches to intervention at home and school have been duly explored.

5

Disabilities and multicultural issues

Hadia Baassiri and Louisa Carroll

Introduction

Cultural and linguistic factors add an additional layer of complexity to family coping and resilience in the context of intellectual and developmental disability. To explore this issue, this chapter gives an introduction to the concepts of culture, and cultural and linguistic diversity. It then looks at how culture interacts with disability, and how this interaction can affect access to health and mental health services. Finally, it explores cultural awareness in clinical practice, and provides a practical example of culturally skilled practice using a case study based on the experiences of a specialist cultural consultant working at a tertiary children's hospital in Sydney, Australia. In combining knowledge of the significance of culture, its interaction with concepts of disability, and the clinical implications of this for practitioners, the chapter aims to provide a framework for enhancing cultural competence in clinical practice in intellectual disability.

Culture, and cultural and linguistic diversity

Culture refers to those elements that collectively characterise a particular society or group and its way of life, encompassing factors such as customs and traditions, teaching and parenting style, beliefs and attitudes, manners, and values. Culture is influenced by both internal and external factors, both contemporaneously and over time, with a culture evolving gradually but constantly in response to the interactions it has with its circumstances and environment, and also as it is passed from one generation to the next. Cultural overlap also exists—for example, between groups that share elements of religious, linguistic, ethnic, migrational, educational, or socioeconomic experience—and it is possible for an individual or family to identify with more than one cultural group.

Cultural and linguistic diversity (CALD) refers to the variability, both within and between groups and individuals, in terms of the language they speak, and how they identify with different cultural practices. Factors such as increased personal mobility, skilled migration, family reunification programs, and politically and socially mandated asylum have seen ethnic, linguistic, and cultural diversity become increasingly common across Western developed nations. Australian society, for example, is becoming increasingly ethnoculturally diverse, with the 2006 Australian Bureau of Statistics census data (ABS, 2006) revealing that approximately 22 per cent of the Australian population identified as coming from a CALD background.

In seeking to better understand cultural and linguistic diversity, it is important to recognise that, while language can be a marker of cultural difference, culture remains distinct from language. Believing that people from one country or region only speak one language can obscure the variability that exists within groups. For example, Wong and Fuji (cited in Echemendia & Westerveld, 2006) estimated that there were 32 different cultural groups within the Asian culture. Arabic- and Latino-speaking people can also come from a broad range of countries that share a common language but differ greatly in their cultures, religious beliefs and practices, education, values, experiences, sociocultural and sociopolitical perspectives, and identities.

Culture and access to health services

The influx of immigrants and refugees entering countries such as Australia has brought a wide variety of cultural experiences, religious beliefs, values, attitudes, and perspectives about health and mental health. Competence in working in a healthcare setting with families from CALD backgrounds requires an appreciation of this diversity, alongside specific knowledge of cultural factors such as language, client attitudes, and values, culturally based remedies and beliefs about illness and disability, the cultural interface between the clinician and client, and the assumptions of normative cultural values (Flores, 2000). This can present a significant challenge to clinicians and services, who remain vastly English speaking, and who draw predominantly from the Western models of mind–body relationships in which they were raised and trained. Culturally attuned practice also requires an awareness of potential issues pertinent to the migrant experience, including factors such as acculturation, transition, socioeconomic status, experience before and after settlement, language, and education (Echemendia & Westerveld, 2006).

It is also important for clinicians to be mindful of the social and environmental influences that affect whether and how families access health services. For example, in countries like Australia, children for whom there are early concerns about development or behaviour are typically able to access a general medical practice or paediatric clinic. This enables timely developmental screening, followed by referral to more specialist assessment or early intervention services as appropriate. In contrast, health systems in many other countries do not offer this level of care; for example, in places like Afghanistan and Africa, where people have lived among wars for a long time, there is limited opportunity for children to access health screening. Thus families arriving as migrants or refugees from these regions may have no awareness that such early childhood services even exist, and so would not seek such support even where they did have concerns about their child's development.

A similar contrast can exist even within national boundaries. For example, in China, while Hong Kong retains a health service system adopted from Western culture (a legacy of its previous status as a British colony), this is not the case for health service systems on the Chinese mainland (Fung & Wong, 2005). Further, while the focus of programs for children with developmental delays in Hong Kong is modelled on British approaches to early intervention, comprehensive rehabilitation programs for children on the mainland include many Eastern influences, such as acupuncture, traditional herbal medicines, and massage. Yet further contrast exists in China between services available in the larger cities, as compared to those that can be accessed by families who live in rural areas. For the latter, services of any kind are often not available (Wong et al., 2004). This diversity in health experiences and practices can have a large impact on how families from these cultures access health and mental health services in Australia, and the expectations that they have about these services.

A variety of cultural experiences, perceptions about health, and family relations may also bear upon willingness of families to access mental health and other support services, independent of their availability. Language barriers, racism, negative stereotypes, and attitudes all contribute to CALD families' experiences of disadvantage (Cho et al., 2003; Trute & Hiebert-Murphy, 2002). There can also be a tendency to rely on informal networks, such as extended family, friends from the same culture, and religious networks, in dealing with the consequence of a disability.

Culture and disability

Having a child with developmental delay has been shown to increase family strain (Trute & Hiebert-Murphy, 2002). However, for many CALD families this can be compounded by additional psychosocial stressors, such as settlement issues, trauma, pre- and post-immigration experiences, unemployment, limited social support, and poverty. These factors influence indirectly how families are able to meet the needs of their children with a disability.

Cultural factors also affect coping more directly, in that cultural differences in the family perception and response to disability have been found to influence the level of family stress and involvement, which in turn affect long-term outcomes (Echemendia & Westerveld, 2006). A family's way of explaining and understanding their child's disability, and the meaning that they ascribe to its occurrence, will be influenced by their cultural worldview. For example, regardless of whether a biomedical cause for their child's disability is identified, some CALD families may simultaneously also hold a traditional or folk explanation for their children's difficulties, which may influence their openness to different therapeutic interventions, or their willingness to seek professional assistance (Diken, 2006).

Attitude and values in family and social life can also highlight significant differences between the model held by the predominant culture, as compared to the CALD groups within a community. Collectivism, for example, in which the responsibilities of the individual rest with the welfare, needs, and expectations of the group, can run counter to the strongly individualistic values that are embraced by many Western cultures. This has particular implications in the case of disability, where issues of dependence and interdependence are especially salient, and may lead to differences with respect to the longer-term goals for the person with a disability, as well as in the expectations that the family holds in terms of service entitlement and longer-term responsibility of care.

Cultural attitudes will also influence the life experiences and expectations for a person with a disability. Certainly, where racism, negative stereotypes, or broader negative social attitudes towards disability exist, this creates an additional level of social disadvantage that restricts access to services and opportunities, and contributes to the complexity of the emotions experienced by both the individuals and their families (Summers & Jones, 2004; Yuan, 2003).

Cultural awareness in clinical practice

Culturally sensitive practice in the developmental disability field first involves knowledge of cultural and linguistic diversity, including a general appreciation of the different ways in which culture can have an impact on access to healthcare, as well as more culture-specific awareness about disability. Clinicians then need to adjust the way they provide health and mental health services, using knowledge of the culturally mediated values, attitudes, and experiences that may apply to a given case, and through effective communication skills, and a willingness to advocate on behalf of families.

Cultural knowledge

In exploring the interaction between culture, disability, and family coping, an understanding of the family's culture of origin is important. This includes knowledge of cultural beliefs and attitudes based on factors such as gender, religion, stigma, and social norms.

Gender

The gender of the individual with a disability can have implications both in terms of coping and acceptance by the family, quality of life, and life opportunities for the individual. For example, in some regions of the Middle East, disability can be viewed as one of multiple oppressions when combined with factors such as gender and race. Abu-Habib (cited in Crabtree, 2007) described how girls with disabilities can be much more devalued within the setting of the family and the wider community than boys with the same disability. This was because in strict societies, girls with disabilities created an additional burden of care for their families, in needing to be kept aware of personal care routines and to maintain social decorum appropriate to their gender. They were also viewed as sexually vulnerable in those societies, and perceived as needing more supervision or even containment within the family home, as a means of preserving their safety. In contrast, boys with a disability were more likely to receive some vocationally based training, and also to get married (sometimes through an arranged marriage).

Another illustration of how cultural values can interact with attitudes towards disability is evidenced in a feeling reportedly common amongst fathers of boys with a disability in the United Arab Emirates. There, despite having access to a higher quality of medical care and disability support services than is available in most other countries in the Middle East, having a boy (as compared to a girl) with a disability is experienced as a greater disappointment because of the loss of expectations usually attached to sons, such as of working, and carrying on the family name (Crabtree, 2007).

Religion and spirituality

Beliefs and values associated with religious and spiritual practices can also have significant implications for how a child with a disability is managed. Blacher and Baker (2007) found that reliance on religious belief systems may incline parents toward positive reframing, providing families with a spiritual framework for understanding the disability and for providing hope. In many cultures, religious principles serve to protect people with disabilities from discrimination, and encourage others to extend care to those in need. For example, in Islam, disability is generally viewed as the will of Allah, with parents expected to deal with the situation with acceptance and grace, treating the child with a disability with the same love and attention as they do his or her siblings (El Naggar Gaad, 2001). Similarly, expressions such as *'No hay mal que por bien no venga'* (which translates as 'There is nothing bad out of which good cannot come', Zuniga, cited in Blacher & Baker, 2007, p. 151) form a part of the spiritual counsel that helps

Latino parents to accept the will of God as it relates to their child's health or disability (Flores et al., 2000).

Stigma

Issues around stigma and embarrassment are another recurring theme amongst many CALD families who have children with disabilities. Kerr and Mcintosh (cited in Wong et al., 2004) found that many Chinese families who had children with Down syndrome were concerned about the reactions of others to their child, while others described having difficulties disclosing their child's condition to other people. Similar concerns about public reactions have been noted in studies of several other CALD communities, for example, among new immigrant families from Korea (Cho et al., 2003), Middle Eastern families (El Naggar Gaad, 2001), and within many Asian communities (Kerr & Mcintosh, cited in Wong et al., 2004). In some cultures, the presence of disability can be even more stigmatising if it does not have clear physical indications.

The issue of stigma is closely tied to families' needs for their children to be accepted into their community and by peer groups. Not surprisingly, greater community acceptance of the young person with a disability has been shown to have a positive impact on parental coping and resilience. Negative public reactions are thought to indicate a lack of acceptance and limited knowledge about individuals with disabilities. This fear of stigmatisation and exclusion is illustrated by one mother's comments: 'How is the world going to see my son, being an Afghani, a refugee, and delayed? That's three negatives when you deal with a big society that doesn't look very positively upon Afghani people'. Similarly, El Naggar Gaad (2001) commented that, despite progressive Islamic precepts that teach tolerance and equality of treatment for people with a disability, the social stigma of disability remains a relatively widespread phenomenon among Middle Eastern families. As such, although discriminatory attitudes may officially draw censor, the social pressures remain such that the birth of a child with disability (including intellectual disability) is frequently accompanied by parental feelings of guilt and shame (Crabtree, 2007).

Social mores

Another important cultural consideration is the recognition that many CALD families derive from collectivist societies (Parette Jr et al., 2000). This ascribes a value system that places the needs and rights of the group ahead of those of the individual, a framework that can be at odds with the predominantly individualistic value set of Western developed nations. This collectivist orientation places emphasis on ensuring that the needs of extended family and siblings are factored into any decision-making around treatment for the child with a disability. It also assumes an ongoing obligation and commitment for the family to provide support, protection, and education for the person with a disability. In this context, the child with a disability is integrated into the family experience, navigating his or her life journey supported by a web of connections that include the family unit of parents and siblings, and also the extended family, faith, and sometimes friends from the same community (Hodapp, 1995).

Accordingly, clinicians working with CALD families should recognise that the presence of a disability can affect all family members within both the immediate and extended family (Aldwin, 1994; Parette Jr et al., 2000). Establishing a rapport with each member of the family may thus be necessary to establish compliance with medical recommendations. This can require the clinician to meet a large number of people from several generations, including grandparents, uncles, aunties, and other relatives. Families need to feel that they are integral to the treatment planning and decision-making, with this sense of involvement critical in reducing potential frustration with professionals, and improving compliance with intervention strategies (Parette Jr et al., 2000). For example, in a Western model of care, it is typical that the mother and father are seen as the family unit responsible for the child, whereas in a collectivist culture, while it may be the parents who attend for the clinic appointment, the medical advice will be further processed and evaluated among the child's extended family at home, often with particular deference to the grandparents. As such, much of the decision-making around treatment and service engagement can occur outside of the clinic setting, with influence from family members who (unless this is specifically addressed by the treating clinicians) may not have had any direct contact with the service provider.

Communication

Guidance provided by the clinician around the provision of psychosocial, education, and specific services can strengthen family coping and positive adjustment (Brinchmann, cited in Trute & Hiebert-Murphy, 2002; Ello & Donovan, 2005; Larson, 1998). Psychoeducation has also been shown to improve family engagement and involvement with treatment (Bailey Jr et al., 2009). Being able to communicate effectively, and having access to appropriate information about services and resources, increases CALD families' confidence in being able to understand and meet the needs of young people with a disability.

Barriers to effective communication include overt factors, such as language and literacy levels, as well as more subtle factors, such as the presiding normative cultural values (for example, the expected roles of the professional versus the patient during a consultation). In ensuring effective communication with CALD families, it is important for clinicians to consider each of these factors.

Engaging the services of an accredited interpreter is always recommended. Clinicians should pay attention to details such as dialect. They should also be alert to the fact that CALD families may not be aware that they can request an interpreter, or may minimise the need on the basis that at least one member of the family has an adequate command of English. For example, parents may bring one of their children along to interpret for them, or between a couple, may have the English-speaker interpreting for his or her spouse. As a clinician it is important to consider the social and power dynamics that this can engender; in using an accredited interpreter, these influences are significantly reduced.

Clinicians should aim to speak in plain English and avoid jargon, as even professional interpreters can have difficulties with highly technical language. Using appropriate body language and gesture to accompany verbal explanations can aid comprehension. The use of analogy can also be helpful for explaining concepts, provided that examples are drawn from experiences that the family can relate to.

Clinicians also need to facilitate access to information for CALD families, particularly when considering an area such as disability, where the quality and accessibility of information can be highly variable, even in English. This can be addressed by strategies such as sourcing translated psychoeducation materials, referring families on to professionals in the field who speak their preferred language, providing details of foreign-language websites, and linking families in with culturally based support groups and services. Clinicians should also be mindful that parents from CALD backgrounds may have experienced interrupted or limited access to schooling in their homelands. As a consequence, these parents may present with literacy problems of their own, even in their own language, making written psychoeducation materials of limited value. In such circumstances, use of strategies such as gestures and visual supports can be very effective in sensitively supporting better communication.

Advocacy and systemic awareness

In addition to responsiveness at the level of individual clinicians, client advocacy and a greater systemic awareness regarding cultural issues are also important. Despite the rhetoric of equity of access, CALD families are frequently at a disadvantage when it comes to connecting into care systems. Advocacy can target specific elements of this, for example, in educating families about existing disability services and how to access them, acting as an intermediary for families for whom language issues can protract and confound referral processes, and ensuring that where families are successfully referred, they are well informed as to why and how a service may be able to assist them. Ensuring that systems remain aware of the CALD family's circumstances can be a further advocatory role, putting them on more equal footing with those who are able to persist with asserting their needs more directly to service providers.

At a systemic level, culturally competent practice needs to be integrated into the model of service delivery for clients at all levels. An illustration of this can be found in a model of care at a leading Australian children's hospital, which includes a consultative clinic at a quaternary level for children who present with extremely complex developmental psychiatric issues. A multidisciplinary team with clinical expertise in disability consults with the family and their treating service team, working together to formulate an intervention plan to address the longer term support needs of the client and their family. Professional representation at this clinic includes specialist psychiatric, paediatric, behavioural, psychological, pharmacological, disability, educational, allied health, and cultural consultation, wherein the expertise of a specialist cultural clinical consultant is integral to the provision of culturally appropriate service for those families who come from a CALD background.

The following case study of Yaseen, a 15-year-old male from an Afghani background, provides an illustration of how culturally sensitive practice can enhance assessment, treatment engagement, and outcome.

Case study 5.1

Yaseen was referred to the psychiatry department of a tertiary level children's hospital in Sydney, Australia, following a spate of anger outbursts, physical and verbal aggression, and episodes of antisocial behaviour and larceny that had resulted in police involvement. At the time of referral limited information was available; however, through the course of the assessment it was revealed that he had a mild to moderate level of intellectual disability, history of speech and language impairment, short-term memory deficits, attention deficit hyperactivity disorder (ADHD), and a probable frontal lobe syndrome. Yaseen's early history included health complications around his birth, possible head injuries in early childhood, and exposure to potentially life-threatening events in wartorn Afghanistan. The family and social history was also complex, with repeated experience of war-related violence, and their eventual seeking asylum in Australia (nine years before). Yaseen was the seventh of nine children, and the only one to experience significant learning or behavioural difficulties.

Assessment and intervention

Expert consultation and reflective clinical practice were sought around culturally based issues at several points during the assessment and intervention process. The first occurred before the initial appointment with the family, as part of preparing appropriately for the assessment. Issues identified at that time included ensuring that an interpreter was arranged (Dari language) and researching factual information relevant to the social and political circumstances of the family in Afghanistan. Further reflection with respect to cultural factors followed the initial assessment, because of difficulties in engaging with the family. It transpired that there were concerns around using an interpreter from particular cultural groups, because of sensitivities stemming from the political circumstances in Afghanistan, and concerns about confidentiality and potential discomfort associated with using an interpreter who was socially from the same community as the family. There were also difficulties within the family because of differences in beliefs and expectations related to disability. There were further issues within the family around expectations and responsibility attributed to different family members; for example, Yaseen's grandparents felt that his mother was responsible for many of his behavioural and learning problems. This in turn triggered strong feelings of parental responsibility and shame, particularly around Yaseen's challenging behaviours. Finally, there were issues with establishing a clinical rapport, resulting in parental ambivalence about whether and how Yaseen's difficulties could be treated, and affecting compliance with medication and other treatment recommendations.

Intervention around the cultural issues identified incorporated a number of elements. Yaseen's family came from a Hazara ethnic background (Shiite Muslim minority) in Afghanistan, a minority that was persecuted by the Taliban. Many from this community consequently missed out on an education, which had implications for how information was communicated to the family in the clinic setting. It also meant that the family was more at ease with an interpreter from a non-Afghani background. An Iranian Dari-speaking interpreter was therefore engaged, improving both direct communication and therapeutic rapport.

A number of other issues were also addressed to improve communication with the family. First, in providing psychoeducation regarding Yaseen's diagnoses, clinicians were encouraged to avoid jargon and medical terminology, use clear descriptions in ordinary language, and use accompanying body language, gesture, and visual supports in their explanations with the family. These included putting a hand to different parts of the head when referring to different parts of the brain, as well as pointing to different areas on a picture of a brain. The use of analogy and metaphor to explain some of the more abstract concepts was also very effective (for example, in describing executive functioning, using a musical analogy relevant to background information that Yaseen's father had provided regarding his own interests and musicality). More practical issues were also addressed, for example, having the interpreter assist members of the family with writing down Yaseen's medication, dosage, and instructions in their own language. A referral was also made to a specialist transcultural mental health service, which could provide a bilingual therapist from Iranian background who spoke Dari, and who was able to provide followup to the hospital consultation with home visits to the whole family, including siblings and grandparents.

Stigma and embarrassment contributed to the family's reluctance to use an interpreter, despite the evident communication challenges. As in many CALD communities, Yaseen's parents felt judged by the way their child behaved. The family became more comfortable and more engaged after it was explained to them that Yaseen's criminal activities were not going to be discussed, but rather that the team was interested in helping the family to improve his condition.

Thus, a careful evaluation of the cultural background and concerns helped the treating clinical team better identify and respect the problems of communication, comprehension, and treatment compliance. Accommodating and integrating knowledge of the influence of cultural factors, including language, beliefs about disability, and social mores, the family became more involved in the decision-making process and more engaged with Yaseen's treatment, and a more effective partnership was established between the family and the treating clinicians.

Conclusion

To support a child with a disability effectively, integrating cultural knowledge and understanding into clinical practice provides a powerful mechanism through which family acceptance, coping, and resilience can be enhanced. The capacity to work with cultural and linguistic diversity is increasingly a requirement of all professionals working in health and mental health services, highlighting the need for clinicians to develop skills in cultural competence that will enable them to provide culturally sensitive and effective services for clients regardless of their cultural background. Cultural competence incorporates an awareness of cultural diversity and its impact, as well as specific knowledge about the values, beliefs, and other cultural practices of clients. This requires attention to issues such as language spoken, as well as knowledge of factors such as religious practices, beliefs and value systems, political issues, and social structures.

Beyond knowledge, cultural competence also requires sensitivity and attunement to the interaction between client and service provision, encompassing an awareness of the clinician's own culture and values, and the influence that this has in professional interactions. This is critical because, irrespective of the quality of the technical clinical knowledge and recommendations offered, best practice is based on partnership, and the overall success of a clinical consultation relies on maintaining a level of engagement and commitment with the family. At a systemic level, cultural competence includes acknowledgment of the discrepancies that can exist between what is recognised as best practice and what is implemented in service systems, and requires an active commitment from practitioners to client advocacy.

Part 2

Focus on family and carers

6

Breaking the news of diagnosis: Facilitating adjustment and acceptance

Natalie Silove

Introduction

Johnny has autism. This is a lifelong developmental disability with no cure. While autism may present differently at different ages, and Johnny may develop new skills, the gap between Johnny and a typically developing child will most likely increase with age. In addition, Johnny has an intellectual disability, which not uncommonly occurs with autism. This combination makes it likely that Johnny will need support class placements and, even with that, it is unlikely that he will live independently as an adult.

The time of diagnosis is described as a crisis event, an experience a family never forgets (Ptacek & Eberhardt, 1996). It is the critical time when parents are told that their special child is likely to have a lifelong disability with an unknown prognosis, and when they realise that their lives will be changed on a permanent basis. Families' memories of being told that their child has a disability are often very vivid and important many years later (Woolley et al., 1989). Parents report mixed emotional responses to receiving a diagnosis, including fear, confusion, isolation, loss, grief, shame, anger, despair, exhaustion, relief, hope, protectiveness, and love. It is suggested that the manner in which the bad news is presented influences a family's ability to cope and adapt as well as the family members' perception, acceptance, and subsequent care of the child. This places a significant burden of care on the professional breaking the bad news to do this in as constructive and supportive a way as possible.

Fortunately, the debate has gone beyond whether or not professionals should inform a family about a diagnosis or a prognosis, but is focused on how best to deliver the information and support the family subsequently. Ignoring parents or withholding prognostic information from them may lead to false hope and a sense of anger, betrayal, and distrust. A central tenet of physician–parent communication is that parents need information to make treatment decisions for their child (Meert et al., 2008).

How does one then balance the need to provide a clear diagnostic formulation and management plan, while not devastating parents who wish to hear the 'truth', but are likely to not be ready to accept it yet? Interestingly, but not surprisingly, the 'guidelines' on the 'how' have been formulated by observing experienced clinicians and gaining parental feedback. This is one opportunity to strengthen the strong partnership of mutual respect and collaboration in the care of the child and adolescent.

Models and frameworks

Descriptive academic terms have been ascribed to these clinical practices. For example, the *perspective-display series* (Maynard, 1991) describes a situation in which professionals first invite clients to display their opinion on the problem, and then deliver the diagnostic findings as a confirmation of the clients' displayed perspective. In another strategy, termed the *incomplete syllogism*, the clinician presents a series of related, general, and particular premises that point to an implied diagnostic conclusion, allowing the recipients themselves to deduce the upshot (Maynard, 1995). In a 'negotiating stance', professionals were found to 'accommodate the distance between a professional's and a parent's point of view, modifying the label to conform to parental wishes, and modulating levels of optimism and pessimism' (Abrams & Goodman, 1998, p. 96). Some of the dilemmas and issues will be discussed to allow the reader to formulate an individual opinion and style. Current practice accepts that the *family-centred care model* is one to strive towards. This encompasses exchanging complete and unbiased information between families and professionals in a supportive manner, recognising and honouring cultural diversity, strengths, and individuality within and across families, and recognising and respecting different methods of coping (Shelton & Stepanek, 1994; 1995).

Bartolo (2002) discussed the dilemma of the delivery of bad news in terms of two poles: *realism versus hopefulness*. While there is a need for a degree of realism, it could always be framed in the light of hopefulness. Without some hope it would be difficult for carers to be proactive and find a reason to invest the emotional and financial time and energy that is required in caring for a child with a disability to maximise his or her potential. The realism pole focused on the child's deficits, while the hopefulness focused on the parental coping process and supporting the child's progress. Realism focused on the honesty of the diagnosis and the limitation of the prognosis, while hopefulness focused on the compassion and the potential. The skill of the professional lies in the ability to be able to convey the information in the most hopeful and realistic way, constantly reflecting back on how the parents are feeling and whether the information conveyed is consistent with their perspective of their child.

Bartolo (2002) also described three major types of frameworks: that is, parent-friendly frame; defocusing bad news; and hopeful formulation of the disability.

The *parent-friendly framework* incorporated empathising with parents, relating positively to the child, reassuring parents that they were already addressing the needs of the child, aligning parents through a perspective-display-series frame, and allowing parents time to seek clarification. He emphasised the need for professionals to present 'one story' to parents and not to disagree in front of them. This would be just as important in a multidisciplinary team as in private practice, where families may see professionals in different locations at different times. It would necessitate professionals discussing opinions before feeding back to parents to avoid confusion, particularly if one professional was aware the family had consulted with another who has specialist knowledge.

The *hopeful formulation frame* focuses on stating the positive achievements first (such as 'This is what Johnny can do and demonstrated for us today'), hedging conclusions (for example, 'This is a baseline from which to work and we will monitor progress'), and focusing on relevant support strategies (such as 'What are we going to do about the situation or the management plan?').

The *defocusing frame* avoided labelling the disability, and focused on the child's individual improvement and special education provisions. This is considered a contentious point of view, as many service and funding providers depend on a diagnosis to assess relevant services and financial support for the child. For example, on the one hand, a diagnosis of Rett syndrome clearly defines a high level of support required and a long-term prognosis, while a diagnosis of autism spectrum disorder (ASD) is less clearly defined and the prognosis much more variable.

There is little argument that labelling developmental disorders for research purposes is important and valuable, and that labels can be helpful to define the scope of support and describe the areas where an individual is having difficulty. However, there may be many more children who have very high functional needs, who do not clearly fit into any specific diagnostic category, and who therefore may miss out on the necessary funding and support. This is a different argument, which requires further discussion with governments and organisations to include a needs-based assessment as part of their funding criteria and not rely solely on labels. Furthermore, there is often a perception that labels will lead to bullying and disadvantage a child socially and educationally. Unknown long-term consequences (as when obtaining life insurance or disability cover) may be an issue for some. It is therefore necessary that parents and professionals engage in a process of negotiation over the need to ascribe a label to a child and the meaning of such a diagnostic label.

Abrams and Goodman (1998) noted that professionals use euphemisms to soften and mask the truth. Terms such as 'developmental delay', 'slow', and 'immature' are less direct, concrete, graphic, and offensive than the term 'mental retardation'. Second, professionals cover their own uncertainty and discomfort, and wish to mitigate the truth, by hedging. Language that is indirect, vague, and uncertain serves both to manage professional uncertainty and to minimise the impact of the diagnosis. Hedges used to approximate a condition (such as 'sort of', 'kind of', and 'a little bit') help shrink the distance between normative expectations and the abnormal condition of the child (Prince et al., 1982). Abrams and Goodman (1998) write:

> Professionals can preserve parental self-esteem and allay distress through a process of negotiation. The concept of negotiation describes the socially constructed nature of encounters in which participants are able to forge a mutual understanding through language. Thus, the meaning of the encounter and the understanding of the information the parents maintain are interactionally and not individually based. The encounter is seen as a bargaining process in which each participant must adjust his or her line of action in terms of what they can expect to attain under the circumstances and in accord with how the others are developing their lines of action. The content of the information is not static and discrete, but fluid and continuous, subject to modulation, change, and adjustment to accommodate such contextual features as goodness of fit between the child and the diagnostic category and parents' emotional needs. By fine-tuning the diagnostic feedback as conversation progresses, professionals and parents can keep the interpretation circulating around a mutually acceptable set-point (p. 88).

This view point rings true, balancing up and down the fine line between realism and hopefulness.

What parents want

Reviewing the research describing parental experiences with diagnosis delivery has identified a number of common factors that increase and decrease parental satisfaction. Parents have expressed similar preferences on how the interaction could be improved. Boyd (2001) noted that overwhelmingly parents wanted health care professionals to demonstrate empathy, sensitivity, and caring when delivering bad news. Parents find it helpful when they are allowed to show their feelings in a safe and nonjudgmental environment. Parents should be allowed time to process the information and their feelings, and have the normalcy of the emotions they are experiencing acknowledged. A box of tissues in the consulting room never goes astray!

Parents appreciate having time to talk and ask questions without feeling rushed, but this is a difficult atmosphere to create when there is a busy waiting room. Gestures such as requesting not to be interrupted, and not taking phone calls or answering mobile phones, impart a feeling of concern, a sense that the professional is listening to the parental concerns. Parents also value privacy. Bad news should always be delivered in a location that is private, comfortable, and quiet, with attention paid to minimising interruptions and distractions. Families strongly agree that bad news about their child should be delivered in person, with both parents, and preferably the child, present. This provides support for both parents, and also removes the burden of one parent having to impart the bad news to the other, and being in a position not to be able to answer questions effectively. It also allows the parents to begin the grieving process at the same time.

It is always best that the news be delivered by the professional that the parents have come to know and trust. It may be that the information and diagnosis are conveyed by the experienced consultant, rather than a junior member of staff who may feel insecure or uncomfortable in such a difficult situation. When receiving bad news, parents prefer that the health care professionals attending the meeting are known to them. It is important that all the relevant information is collected before the meeting and is readily available. If the bad news is conveyed as a team, there should be consistency and agreement about what information each professional will present.

Parents appreciate the timely provision of current, accurate, and straightforward information about their child's diagnosis, prognosis, treatment, care, and future expectations. The news should be presented in language that is easy to understand and jargon free. A professional interpreter should be available for translating information when families are not fluent in the language of the individuals delivering the news. It is preferable to provide written information on the day, so that parents can have something tangible to read and reflect on after the meeting. This written information should include additional sources of information for families, including support groups that can offer emotional support and practical advice. Parents value an individualised approach, where their cultural and unique needs and aspirations are respected. Guidelines that have been published include the delivery of news about Down syndrome to parents (Cunningham et al., 1984). This model service is outlined in table 6.1.

Professional training and guidelines

Research has indicated that parental dissatisfaction with disclosure remains high (Skotko, 2005). It cannot solely be relied on that disclosure is an innate

Table 6.1 Model service for delivering news about Down syndrome to parents

Procedure for model service
• Consultant paediatrician and specialist health visitor to convey diagnosis • Disclosure given as soon as possible • Discussion takes place with both parents together • Interview located in a private place with no other professionals present • Infant is present • Parents given news directly • Parents given as much time as they wish to ask questions • The specialist health visitor sees parents again as soon as they want • Parents provided a private place immediately after the interview • Follow-up interview arranged 24 hours after the disclosure

Adapted from Cunningham et al., 1984

skill of professionals, and that experience, sound knowledge about the chronic disorder, empathy, and sensitivity are sufficient. There is a need to teach medical students and registrars basic skills and principles to increase their confidence in delivering bad news in a manner with which parents feel comfortable and let parents feel confident that their child is receiving the best treatment. A study by Horwitz and Ellis (2007) in the UK noted that most registrars did report receiving training in delivering bad news, and their perceived level of confidence in this skill was high. However, this form of self-assessment is often inaccurate, with weaker students and often male students frequently overestimating their skills, while stronger students, and often females, underrate themselves. Multisource feedback has therefore become the preferred method in the UK.

Many methods of teaching how to disclose diagnostic information have been applied in clinical practice. One method is the use of interactional skills training, which has an impact on a clinician's skill in communicating with patients. This training, however, should be delivered at undergraduate and postgraduate levels to ensure skills maintenance (Perkins & Sanson-Fisher, 1996). However, teaching communication skills is only one aspect to be addressed. The challenge is far broader than the clinician-to-child-and-family interaction, as the diagnostic assessment often occurs in multiple settings with multiple professionals and agencies. Therefore, there is a need to develop guidelines that negotiate the boundaries between assessments and agencies to facilitate the process for children and their families.

Providing specific training and guidelines has been found to be welcomed by professionals and parents in the field of disability. Such an example is 'Informing families of their child's disability: National best practice guidelines' (National Federation of Voluntary Bodies, 2007), which was developed in Ireland as part of the Informing Families Project. The practice guidelines were initiated in response to feedback from parents that the news of their child's disability had been conveyed insensitively or in inappropriate environments, and that the experience of being told the news had caused additional distress at the time of disclosure. Similarly, feedback from professionals to delivering the news indicated that they felt there was an absence of training and clear guidance available to support those undertaking the sensitive and challenging task of giving families the news that their child has a disability.

An important finding of the Informing Families Project was that a broad range of professional disciplines were involved from mainstream health settings and disability specific services. This meant that clear planning and ownership of tasks within the disclosure and support process, interdisciplinary training, and a structured cross-sectoral approach to the dissemination of the best practice were necessary. Parents and professionals indicated a clear need for continuity of care to be provided within service settings (where more than one medical or social care team was involved in providing the diagnosis), across settings (where families are discharged from hospital settings into the community), or when waiting referral to early services. Parents and professionals identified a need to provide continuity of care and a coordinated team approach to avoid:

- the distressing vacuum following discharge and before reaching early services
- the mixed messages that were often received when internal teams did not communicate effectively.

The central aims of the Informing Families Project were to develop evidence-based national best practice guidelines, and education and training on appropriate procedures to inform families of their child's disability. The guiding principles included:

- family-centred disclosure
- respect for child and family
- sensitive and empathetic communication
- appropriate, accurate information
- positive, realistic messages and hope
- team approach and planning
- focused and supported implementation of best practice.

Followup support

Long-term followup and support is an important component of care to facilitate individual and family adjustment to living with a disability (Bailey et al., 2009). Families require a written plan of action and a road map as to how they may proceed to address the medical, physical intervention, educational, emotional, financial, and community supports. Most often this is provided in a comprehensive written report at the conclusion of the diagnostic and assessment process, which includes a date for a followup appointment to discuss the report and any other issues that may arise. Ongoing support includes:

- providing ongoing access to accurate and understandable information
- facilitating support from professionals and other parents
- active surveillance of child health development and behaviour
- general and targeted interventions mutually determined by parents and professionals
- scheduled visits at times of known increased stress, such as transition periods to high school, or to adult services.

A contact person, or case worker, should be identified for parents to contact if further information or support is required. Parents and carers deserve evidence-based information and practical support to allow empowerment to adjust to living life with their child's chronic disorder, and fulfil their hopes and the dreams for their child.

Conclusion

The following scenario incorporates best practice in delivering bad news to parents about their child with a disability:

> We have enjoyed meeting you and getting to know Johnny today. We were really pleased that he managed to settle in this unfamiliar environment and was able to enjoy some of the toys and activities that were presented to him. We do share your concerns regarding his development, particularly your concern about his delayed language and play skills. Based on the information you have provided, the reports from his therapists, and our observations and testing today, Johnny's development is different to that of other children his age.
>
> The combination of difficulties in the area of communication with others, in the way he is socialising and preferring his own company, and finds comfort in familiarity and routine, is consistent with what we see in the autism spectrum disorders. Johnny would meet the DSM-IV criteria for a diagnosis of autistic disorder. All individuals on the spectrum have impairments in communication, socialisation and behaviour, but they are all also very individual and unique, with their own set of skills and personalities.
>
> There were a number of encouraging features that Johnny displayed today. He did show interest in some of the activities we presented to him, allowed us to direct some of his play, and did not tantrum too much when we removed his trains. This suggests that, with time and perseverance, he will engage in therapy with his speech pathologist and special educator. Even

though Johnny took very little notice and did not initiate with us, he is very aware that you are his parents and frequently approached you for assistance, which is also very encouraging.

The Griffiths Mental Development Scale today has documented a moderate global developmental delay. This is the term that we will be using in his report, as it is required in order for him to access appropriate services. This assessment should be viewed as a baseline of Johnny's skills, and we know that he has at least demonstrated these skills, but it is not at this point in time indicative of his potential. This will become much clearer with time.

We will continue to monitor Johnny's development very closely and continually review the most appropriate support, intervention, and educational placements for him. Anita will continue to assist you to navigate your way through the maze of public and private services until we have established the best service providers for Johnny, but please do not hesitate to contact us if you need any further assistance.

7

Children with developmental disability: Is providing care a burden?

Jacqueline Small

Introduction

> I tried to teach him everything, to just say one word, or how to shower … going to all the meetings … I tried my best with everything, in the end, he just stopped learning … He kept trying to hurt me … after that I gave up (Mother of a 17-year-old male with autism and intellectual disability).

It is clear that carers of children with severe disability have a role that is far in excess of usual parenting responsibilities. Further, the care provided for the person with a disability is not always by the parents. Both the ageing carer population and the increasing survival of children born with significant disability are having an impact on the role of carers in our community. The burden of chronic conditions in adolescence is also increasing, as larger numbers of chronically ill children survive beyond the age of 10 years.

It was quite clear to the Carer Payment (child) Review Taskforce (FaHCSIA, 2008) that the role of carers of children with severe disability or medical conditions was substantially greater than the usual parenting role. Although it is difficult to define 'usual' parenting, the fundamental nature of parenting is the provision of a level of care that decreases over time and is replaced by monitoring, supervision, and finally, independence as the child becomes more competent. Parents who are carers of children and adolescents with significant disability may not have the same decrease in their caring and supervisory roles. This is also coupled with increases in personal responsibility for judgments and decisions about the child's or adolescent's care, disability, or medical condition. But what do we know about who is providing the care, and what are the extra care needs at different levels of impairment or with different types of disability? What factors determine whether the extra care is considered to be a burden or stressful by the carers? What factors influence the parents' ability to cope with extra care demands, and what lessons do these have for service providers?

Children should live in a family home

Current Australian and international policy is that children with a disability should remain with their family. The NSW Department of Ageing, Disability and Home Care states in its *Supporting Children and Young People with a Disability* (DADHC, 2004) policy document that its vision is 'to enable them [children and young people with a disability] to live as part of a family and community so that they have opportunities to reach their full potential at all stages of their lives' (p. 3). The American Association of Intellectual and Developmental Disability states in its *Inclusion Position Statement* (AAIDD, 2002b) that 'children should live in a family home' (Position section, ¶ 1) and in its *Family Support Position Statement* (AAIDD, 2002a) that 'Federal, state and local governments must recognize the important role played by parents when they keep their children with mental retardation and related disabilities at home' (Fiscal and other public policies must support families section, ¶ 5).

The consequences of providing care to children with a significant disability

In order for children or an older person with a disability to remain or to choose to live at home, substantial support from family and friends may be needed. To describe this sort of care as 'informal' is somewhat if a misnomer, as there is nothing casual about taking primary responsibility for another person's welfare. An Australian Bureau of Statistics (ABS) survey in 1998 (Australian Institute of Health and Welfare (AIHW), 2004) revealed that 60 per cent of care recipients always needed assistance with one to four activities of daily living, and a further 24 per cent always needed assistance with five to nine activities of daily living. In addition, the ABS survey revealed the following information about carers in Australia:

- 70 per cent of primary carers were women
- over 50 per cent of primary carers spend 20 or more hours per week in the caring role, and over 33 per cent spend 40 hours or more per week in an unpaid carers role
- 75 per cent of primary carers had spent at least five years in the caring role and 40 per cent had been caring for at least 10 years

- carers had a lower labour force participation rate (39 per cent) than people who were not carers (68 per cent), and for carers in paid employment, the caring role can have a significant impact on their work; for example, reduction in work hours after commencing, time off to meet care needs (ABS, 2005), and declining job transfers or paid jobs (Trute & Hiebert-Murphy, 2002)
- 46 per cent of people with severe to profound restriction received assistance only from family and/or friends, 48 per cent received assistance from family and friends, supplemented by formal services, and 3 per cent received assistance only from formal services (AIHW, 2004).

Substantial financial costs are born by carers as a result of both income limitation and increased costs associated with the child's or adolescent's disability. Estimates have been made that the costs of disability correspond to 29 per cent of equivalised household disposable income. However, when a more extensive disability variable was used to do the calculations, the estimate increased to just over 37 per cent of disposable income (AIHW, 2004). Where there is someone in the household with a disability, the costs of disability represent a substantial percentage of disposable income, poverty rates are higher, and hardship is more prevalent (Emerson, 2003b; Saunders, 2006). In 2005, Access Economics researched the economic value of informal care for people with disability or chronic illness and the frail aged. They found that if all informal care were replaced with formal care, the cost was estimated at $30.5 billion annually (Access Economics, 2005).

The extra care required for children with different levels of impairment

Intellectual disability is a disability characterised by significant limitations both in intellectual functioning and in adaptive behaviour (AAIDD, 2009). *Intelligence* involves the ability to reason, plan, solve problems, think abstractly, comprehend complex ideas, learn quickly, and learn from experience (AAIDD, 2009). *Adaptive behaviour* represents the 'conceptual, social, and practical skills that people have learned to be able to function in their everyday lives' (AAIDD, 2009; Key concepts in the AAIDD system section, ¶ 3). These skills may include reading, money skills, the ability to follow rules, maintenance of personal care, preparation of meals, housekeeping skills, and occupational skills. Significant limitations in adaptive behaviour have an impact on an individual's daily life and affect his or her ability to respond to a particular situation or environment. The 'supports approach' of the AAIDD evaluates the specific needs of the individual, then suggests strategies and services to optimise individual functioning. The supports approach also recognises that individual needs and circumstances will change over time.

Results of an international study conducted by Haveman and colleagues (2000) suggested that time demands and expressed need for services were higher for children diagnosed with severe intellectual disability and comorbid conditions (such as epilepsy, cerebral palsy, heart failure, and vision impairment). If the child has additional severe physical impairments or health problems, he or she may require daily exercises to prevent contractures, regular interventions for constipation (such as stool softeners, bowel stimulants, and occasionally enemas), daily administration of medications, and gastrostomy tube feeding (involving complex preparation of formulae and use of an electrical pump for long periods of time) in order to maintain nutrition (Cooley, 2004). Carers may be required to attend frequent appointments with doctors, therapists, and other professionals, and may experience repeated hospitalisation of their child. Wallander and Noojin (1995) found that mothers of children with disabilities reported a wide range of problems in parenting their child. They found that almost half of the mothers' concerns centred on their child and how they were functioning.

The impact of different types of disability on care needs and carer stress

> My day begins with that adrenaline pump and muscle clench I always feel when I hear him first stir in the morning. Perhaps you can imagine a 6 foot 100 kg three-year-old going through that terrible time when they want your constant attention, except he isn't a toddler you can pick up and put down somewhere safe while you take a break or catch your breath. The things most people take for granted, like taking a shower, talking to a friend on the phone, or simply doing the housework, I cannot do without first making sure that he is entertained or that someone else is caring for him. My subconscious is always focusing on him no matter what I am doing. That kind of vigilance is exhausting.
>
> Extract from a letter of a mother of an 18-year-old male with intellectual disability

High care needs because of impairments in adaptive behaviours do not necessarily predict high stress levels for carers. Higher rates of maladaptive behaviours, not age, intelligence, mental age, or other variables, were the strongest predictors of increased stress in parents of children with genetic aetiologies in studies of intellectual disability (Hodapp, 1997). However, while other studies have also failed to find an association between the child's level of intellectual disability and parenting stress (Hassall et al., 2005; Walker et al., 1992), some studies have found that there is a relationship between parenting stress and level of intellectual disability (Minnes, 1998; Eisenhower et al., 2005). Generally it seems that specific characteristics associated with the disability are more important correlates of parental stress (Minnes, 1988). These include the child's communication skills (Frey et al., 1989) and particularly the child's behavioural difficulties (Quine & Pahl, 1991).

Challenging behaviour has been found by others to predict family stress levels and the ability to maintain the child with a disability in the family home. A survey of mothers of 103 young adults with severe intellectual disability identified that behaviour and/or mental health problems significantly predicted the mother's perceived negative impact of the young adult on the family, as did better young adult health and the mother's higher educational attainment (McIntyre et al., 2002). Other researchers have also confirmed that parents perceive the psychiatric or behavioural problems of their child to be an extra burden, making it more difficult to raise and manage such a child, and that as a result, they tend to seek support from services (Maes et al., 2003).

The impact of caring for a child with intellectual disability varies throughout life. The impact may vary from the period of anticipatory care, to diagnosis with potential lasting effects of disclosure, through the period of struggle to maintain a 'normal life' in the face of extra care demands, to the time of 'letting go' as the child reaches adulthood (Grant et al., 2003). It has been noted in the literature that the adolescent period is one of the most critical phases in the lives of people with intellectual disabilities. There is a view that this phase is marked by greater parental malaise and increased levels of parental stress influenced by significant life transitions (Baxter et al., 1995).

Explanations for the relationship between adolescence and increased parental stress are diverse. For the most part, the major disruption in service provision and the uncertainties this invokes are typical explanations, as are concerns over the developmental progress of the child and its social implications (Thorin et al., 1996; Heslop et al., 2002). This is reported to hold true even where the mother had viewed the early years of parenting as similar to those of her friends, a 'life as ordinary'. However, the social content and events of the middle years of parenting prompt a realisation that carers' lives and, for some cases, their sense of self, are undergoing considerable change (Todd & Jones, 2005).

There are suggestions that the underlying cause of the intellectual disability may predict parental stress. Studies have suggested that a diagnosis of fragile X syndrome creates more challenges to maternal psychological well-being than a diagnosis of Down syndrome (DS), and that the combination of fragile X syndrome and autism can be particularly challenging (Lewis et al., 2006). Even by the preschool years, mothers of children with autism may show an elevated risk for high stress, and this stress parallels behavioural difficulties (Noh et al., 1989). However, not all of the maternal stress can be explained on the basis of behavioural problems (Eisenhower et al., 2005). Furthermore, the lower personal well-being, or stress, of care-givers of children with autism, and more reported maladaptive behaviours, may persist through to the time the child reaches adulthood, regardless of cultural group (Blacher

& McIntyre, 2006). In some cases, other factors can influence the response of parents. In contrast to correlates with the DS group, stress levels of fathers of children with other types of intellectual disability seemed to be more influenced by such demographic variables as the child's gender and their own level of education (Ricci & Hodapp, 2003).

The relationship between children's care needs and carer stress and coping

Persistent, constant demands for care and support can be exhausting for carers, who are sometimes referred to as 'perpetual parents' (Grant et al., 2003). The Australian Institute of Health and Welfare (AIHW), in its report *Carers in Australia* (AIHW, 2004), found that many factors influence the caring experience of carers. These factors include: personal circumstances and characteristics of the carer and care receiver; the nature and strength of the relationship; living arrangements; and the level of support available from formal services and social networks. The financial, emotional, and physical hardships, always being 'on call' even when a child is school aged and attends an educational facility, time pressures associated with caring, and responding to the demands of education staff for care-related assistance in school life, combine to place intense pressure on carers. In addition, the AIHW (2004) reported that 'the physical and psychological demands of the caring role itself can lead to adverse health outcomes for carers' (p. 23). Caring can increase levels of fatigue, worry or depression, and have an adverse impact on well-being. Parents who care for their disabled children often report ineffective coping and feel overwhelmed by their responsibilities (Johnson, 2000).

The interaction between informal support networks and the degree of disability in the child for the carer was highlighted by a population-based survey conducted by Leonard and colleagues (1993). They found that one-third of their sample of caregivers of children with disabilities reported that they needed more help managing the care or could not manage much longer when the children were more severely impaired and functionally dependent. The mothers in this survey reported that they were in poorer physical and mental health, had greater demands on their time and finances, and received less emotional support from family and friends.

However, the relationship between stress and level of care needs is not at all straightforward, with some studies clearly implicating psychological processes in the response of the carer to high care demands. In the parenting domain, self-efficacy has been shown to have an impact on parental behaviours and parenting stress (Harty et al., 2007), as has expressed emotion towards the child (Datta et al., 2002), parental locus of control, and parenting satisfaction (Hassall et al., 2005). Hassall and colleagues (2005) demonstrated that when child behaviour difficulties were added to parental locus of control and parenting satisfaction, only a further 5 per cent of the variance in parenting stress was added to that accounted for by the first two variables—self-efficacy and expressed emotion—that accounted for 54 per cent.

Cognitive appraisal has also been shown to be an important factor in parental stress, and that positive and negative appraisals are independent (Leonard et al., 1993). Further, the appraisal that parents hold of the family impact of childhood disability is formed early in the life of the child with the disability, and tends to remain unchanged through to the preadolescent years of the child. Identifying parents who are at risk of high levels of stress while the child is young provides an important opportunity for preventative child mental health services (Trute & Hiebert-Murphy, 2002).

The complexity of the journey through identification of disability, diagnosis, and day-to-day living presents huge challenges for parents. *Straddling behaviour* embodies the parents' precarious balancing on three levels of parental functioning:

1. Living with one foot in the present and one foot in the past (as in diagnosis)
2. The dilemma of trying to view the child as 'normal' when in fact, as evidenced by the parents' activities to secure special services, he or she is not 'normal'
3. Dealing simultaneously with the child's issues and feelings, and the parents' issues and feelings (Johnson, 2000).

However, it is important to acknowledge that, while some parents experience high care demands, and at times overwhelming stress levels, many parents do not. Researchers have increasingly adopted the view that families with a disabled child are not generally characterised by high levels of pathology, and that families may employ various strategies to adapt successfully to the demands posed by the child (Stoneman, 1997, Kenny & McGilloway, 2007).

Lessons for service providers

Children with significant intellectual or developmental difficulties are usually cared for by parents, particularly their mother, at home. While this is often associated with significant employment and financial costs, in many cases it is not associated with significant psychological distress. However, it is clear that some child and carer characteristics are likely to lead to increased stress, which may eventually result in breakdown of the family situation. These characteristics include substantially increased care needs of the child or adolescent, the presence of challenging behaviour and substantial communication limitations, especially from certain diagnoses, such as autism, impaired parental locus of control, and perceived parental efficacy. Further, it is likely that the trajectory of increasing carer stress and negative appraisals are initiated early in the life of the child.

Thus, the provision of intervention and support services directed towards challenging behaviour and communication impairments is a priority. Services to address these issues should be available from the early preschool years. Identification of those carers with psychological responses which have been shown to be associated with increased stress might enable counselling (with an emphasis on increasing the sense of parental control) to be offered. The service system should be designed to be responsive to parental needs rather than being a bureaucracy that offers services far too late to meet the needs of the child or adolescent, carers, and family.

8

Promoting parent readiness for change: A motivational interviewing approach

Lesley Whatson and Wendy Grice

Introduction

In recent years, there have been many successful efforts made to treat behaviour disturbance in children with intellectual disability by improving the parent–child relationship through parent education. Indeed, there are a number of well-evidenced programs designed specifically for the parents of children with intellectual disability. Social learning theory underpins the more successful of these programs. In many cases, teaching parents key strategies, such as how to reward desirable behavior and not reward the unwanted, has the effect of reducing and preventing problem behaviour. While some families are highly motivated to participate in parent training and seem eager to apply the skills and strategies learned, others appear more reticent. Typically, parent training programs do not address how to engage reluctant parents who may not be ready for change, and present as resistant. So, what should a clinician do? Engagement and participation are essential to successful treatment. Therefore, assessing parental readiness for change and enhancing parent education with strategies that improve motivation would seem useful.

There is a large body of evidence to support the notion that parenting children with intellectual disability and behavioural disturbance is both complex and difficult (Hudson et al., 2003). Research confirms an interrelationship between child behaviour, parent behaviour, and parental stress. Parents regularly report that increased stress is primarily a result of the extent of child challenging behaviour, rather than the intellectual disability or reduced adaptive skills (Baker et al., 2003; Hastings & Beck, 2004; Beck et al., 2004; Plant & Sanders, 2007). The stress brought about by child behaviour in turn influences parenting behaviour, which further shapes child behaviour. A higher level of parental stress is a key risk factor for the development of additional challenging behaviours and the exacerbation of existing difficulties (Baker et al., 2003). The relationship that exists between parental stress, parenting behaviour, and child behaviour is a potentially problematic one (Baker & Feinfield, 2007; Hastings & Beck, 2004). The imperative then is to interrupt this cycle by engaging the parent and intervening to break the cycle.

Parental stressors

While many families are extremely resilient and adapt well to the demands of parenting a child with an intellectual disability, a child with accompanying social and emotional disturbance generates increased parental stress, which is often chronic and persists over many years (Beck et al., 2004). Parental worry and strain have great potential to shape parenting behaviour and influence family relationships (Woolfson & Grant, 2006). Stress can lead to the development of unhelpful parenting behaviours, such as rigid, coercive approaches that include punishment, or permissive parenting strategies that make few demands on the child and leave the parent with little control. Other parenting behaviours that typically lead to exacerbation of challenging behaviour include inconsistent discipline practices across the parenting team, a lack of inclusion of the child in family activities, and a lack of supervision. Stress may make it more difficult for parents to develop a warm, positive relationship with their child and encourage him or her towards independence.

The emergence of challenging behaviour, in addition to an intellectual disability, appears to fuel parental concerns about the impact of the child on siblings and other family members, family cohesion, and the family's sense of the child as a member of their 'unit' (Llewellyn et al., 1999). Yet, attaining an adequate family quality of life is essential, as it underpins the mental health and well-being of children.

For some families, stressors directly associated with the extent of the challenging behaviour will be additional to others, such as marital conflict, a lack of extended family involvement, inadequate availability of advice and support, financial difficulties, and parental psychopathology (such as anxiety, depression, and substance abuse). For some parents, their experiences of being parented, the pressure of parenting without a partner, changing family roles and relationships, cultural expectations, difficulties coordinating services, poor health, problem behaviour in siblings, and social isolation also influence their hopefulness regarding change and willingness to engage in intervention (Sanders et al., 2004).

Intervening to assist parents to change their behaviour can positively influence patterns and sequences of parent–child interactions that include or lead to behavioural difficulties (Rhodes, 2003). Relationships within a family, most importantly that between the child and parent, have a critical influence on the social, physical, and psychological development of the child.

Parental engagement

Strategies underpinned by social learning theory and designed to improve the parent–child relationship have become the cornerstone in treating children with intellectual disability, and behavioural and emotional disturbance. One well-evidenced approach is parent education aimed at increasing parent skills and knowledge, and enhancing self-belief (Sanders et al., 2004). These substantial, evidence-based programs are widely used. However, despite the many successes of these programs, there are some parents and children who do not benefit. There is little information at hand regarding the engagement and subsequent involvement of families with children with an intellectual disability and behaviour disturbance. However, it is known that in other childhood populations, such as families with children with conduct problems, initial engagement is frequently difficult, and intervention dropout rates of between 25 and 50 per cent have been found (Scott & Dadds, 2009).

Why are some parents more difficult to engage than others? Why do some parents appear so resistant? The clinician may attribute a lack of compliance with recommendations to a number of factors, including:

- a lack of parental participation in formulating the treatment plan; that is, the recommendations do not reflect the key priorities and concerns of the family or have not been developed in collaboration with the family
- parental doubt regarding the benefits and usefulness of the recommendations for the child
- difficulty with the recommendations because they are poorly matched to the child's developmental level
- reluctance to engage in services that involve outsiders knowing the family's business
- the family's negative experiences with services in the past, related to their child with intellectual disability, or their own social history
- a lack of insight about the future; that is, a poor understanding of the risks associated with maintaining the current situation without action or intervention
- situational barriers; for example, the competing needs of siblings, work commitments of parents, parental use of alcohol and other drugs, and lack of physical resources
- a mismatch between the intervention and parental beliefs and values (Hutchings & Lane, 2006).

Importantly, a lack of collaboration around describing the child and family's difficulties, goal setting, and formulating interventions often leads to parental reservations regarding the plan. Patterson and colleagues (1990) suggest four factors that are likely to influence a parent's reluctance to engage in treatment:

- the parent's experience of interacting with their child; for example, some parents come to training with a history of many unsuccessful 'discipline confrontations'

- pre-existing parental anxiety, depression, or other form of psychopathology
- contextual factors, such as social disadvantage
- the skill and intensity of the therapist's attempts to teach the parents.

Understanding and managing parental reactions

There are a number of typical responses a parent might make when he or she is asked to change behaviour as part of intervention: resistance; helplessness, and hopelessness; panic and anxiety; agreement without commitment; or relief and a decision to change. It is imperative that the clinician attempt to understand the parental response, because the consequences of non-engagement and non-participation are significant. These include:

- the family not receiving the necessary intervention
- a more entrenched pattern of child behaviour
- maintenance of the cycle of unhelpful parenting, challenging behaviour, and stress
- a change in the clinician's behaviour, and subsequent reduction in the clinician's effectiveness (Patterson & Chamberlain, 1994).

It is necessary therefore, to have a planned approach to managing the process of initial engagement, and subsequent involvement of the family, as both are necessary for effective change.

Most intervention programs do not describe strategies for use when parents prove difficult to engage or when parents disregard the proposed intervention. So, what does a clinician do when he or she cannot get past the front door or treatment isn't utilised? Social learning theory remains most effective in parent training intervention, but ideas drawn from motivational interviewing practices may enrich the clinician's ability to help bring about change in families who are stuck. Motivational interviewing is well suited to addressing the barriers described above, as well as a range of other issues the clinician may encounter when working with parents (Miller & Rollnick, 2002). Understanding the theoretical foundation of parent training is essential to good practice; this will be addressed below.

Social learning theory states that attending to moment-to-moment interactions is critical: if children receive an immediate reward for their behaviour, such as getting parental attention or approval, then they are more likely to do the behaviour again, whereas if they are ignored or penalised for unwanted behaviour, then they are less likely to do it. To date, this has been the primary evidence-based approach (Scott & Dadds, 2009).

Patterson (1982) identified two main processes operating in families with children with disruptive behaviour. First, parents model unwanted behaviour, so the child learns it too. Second, family process involves *reinforcement traps*; for example, a parent makes a request of a child, the child protests with unwanted behaviour such as aggression, and the parent then backs off. Thus, the child is learning that aggression can be useful in avoiding having to do something unpleasant and is more likely to do it again. Then, as the parent gets more and more angry and aggressive, and in this way gets the child to obey, they too are learning that aggression works (Scott & Dadds, 2009). In another common reinforcement trap, the more a child engages in undesirable behaviours, the less he or she will get rewarded for positive behaviours (Sanders et al., 2003). Many efficacious behavioural interventions have focused on this issue, including parent education programs (Scott & Dadds, 2009).

What is parent education?

Research evidence verifies that parent education is useful in assisting the development of effective strategies for managing a variety of child behavioural difficulties. Positive effects of parent education have been noted and replicated many times across studies, investigators, and countries (Sanders, 1999). Parent education programs typically aim to do more than ameliorate the behavioural disturbance. Program intent often includes positive change to parental behaviour, knowledge, attitudes, and self-efficacy; improvement in satisfaction of parents in their parenting roles; promotion of the child's cognitive development, pro-social behaviour and health; promotion of the well-being of family members; enhancement of family relationships; and a reduction in the risk of out-of-home placement (Kaminski et al., 2008). Thus for the clinician, increasing parental warmth and rewards for wanted behaviour, and setting clear limits and consequences for unwanted behaviour, are essential. It is desirable to promote positive behaviour first, so that the overall relationship improves before punishments are given (Sanders et al., 2004).

Assessing parental perceptions and readiness for change

It is imperative that any attempt to involve a family in parent education is preceded by a careful assessment. Behavioural disturbance is usually not the result of a single cause, and requires a thorough clinical assessment. For the child, this requires the clinician to include in his or her assessment the child's temperament, cognitive and emotional functioning, developmental and medical history, and behaviour. Assessment of parental and family factors is also essential, such as routines and living patterns, current strategies used to manage challenging behaviour, the goals of the family, access to and use of support services, parental problems, parental availability, cultural factors, the parent–child interaction, and the potential contextual fit of the parent education program. Matching assessment findings to the training approach is critical. Similarly, goal setting and the measurement of outcomes should be reflective of the whole family, as well as the child (Wiese et al., 2005). Several well-evidenced parent education programs, designed specifically for the families of children with an intellectual disability, describe a robust process of initial assessment and ongoing monitoring (Sanders, 1999; Hudson et al., 2003; Sanders et al., 2004).

It is important that the clinician asks the parents about their *beliefs* regarding parenting, their *hopes* for intervention, the *importance* of making the change, their *readiness to change,* and their *confidence* in making the change (Manchester, 2007). In order to do this, it is often useful to design a series of self-report measures, so that parents can rate their readiness for change or to comply with (jointly developed) treatment recommendations. Parental responses can be made on a Likert scale, or 'change ruler', using a visual representation of a ruler marked from zero to ten. Parents can be asked to show their *readiness to change* on the ruler, with zero being 'very ambivalent about making changes', and ten being 'ready for change'. The next step in the plan is based on the family's readiness for change.

The clinician may assess *importance* of changing by asking, 'On the scale, how important is it for Natalie to sleep in her own bed?' Helping the parent list the pros and cons of the change can be an effective way of helping them identify the importance of the change and any barriers to change. *Confidence* can be assessed by asking, 'If you decided tomorrow that you were going to teach Natalie to sleep in her own bed, how confident are you that you could achieve this goal?' Using the scale can help the parent share more detail about readiness for change, confidence, and importance. If the parent is, for example, a 3 on a 10 point ruler, the parent is saying that he or she thinks it is a *bit important* to increase the daughter's sleeping behaviour. The clinician could then ask, 'And why are you at a 3 and not at a 1 or 2?' An alternate question could be, 'What would it take to move to a 4 on the scale?' These questions help parents state what is important to them about the change, and suggests strategies they could use to achieve the change.

In the example above, a rating of 3 is a sign that the parent is not ready for change. The clinician can acknowledge the parent's uncertainty and accept the lack of readiness to change. This does not mean, however, that the clinician does nothing. Rather, the clinician helps the parent to explore *discrepancy* between desired goals and current behaviour (sleeping in the parent's bed versus sleeping in the child's own bed). The goal for the parent is to state the need to change in order to achieve the goal. This is known as *evoking change talk,* which is designed to increase the likelihood that the parent will act on what has been discussed (Manchester, 2007).

What might a successful intervention in parenting look like?

Hutchings and Lane (2006) identified a number of actions that are important in 'engaging multi-stressed, hard-to-reach families who have many other difficulties in their lives and feel blamed for their child's problems and abandoned by authorities/services' (p. 481). These actions include:

a Building a collaborative alliance with parents
b Mobilising parents' resources and working in a way that is compatible with their beliefs and values
c Empowering families to solve their own problems by building on existing strengths
d Accepting parents' goals at face value, tailoring tasks and suggestions to them, and collaborating in exploring material that is relevant to them
e Conveying an attitude of hope and possibility without minimising the problem or the pain that accompanies it; that is, encouraging parents to focus on the present and future possibilities instead of past problems.

A transtheoretical model of the *stages of change* (see figure 8.1), developed by Prochaska and DiClemente (1986), is a framework for understanding how people change behaviour and the theory underpinning *motivational interviewing* (DiClemente & Velasquez, 2002). The process begins at a stage of *pre-contemplation,* in which the family is not ready to change behaviour. Parents might have no problem recognising this, and could appear, for example, resistant, reluctant, rebellious, or resigned. Readiness for change then moves toward *contemplation,* a stage during which the family is aware that a problem exists but is ambivalent about the need for change. From here, the family members move into *preparation and planning for action* in the near future. *Action* is where changes are made. *Maintenance* involves the family integrating changes and working to prevent 'slipping' or relapse. If a slip or relapse occurs, the family is assisted to identify the problem, evoke *change talk,* and move on in a way that maintains parental confidence in their ability to make change.

Motivational interviewing is designed specifically to help clinicians work with people who are less ready to change (Miller & Rollnick, 2002). It can be used alongside parent training when engagement is proving difficult, or when parents actively resist proposed courses of action. Miller and Rollnick (2002) defined it as 'a client-centred, directive method for enhancing intrinsic motivation to change by exploring and resolving ambivalence' (p. 25).

There are a number of principles involved in motivational interviewing, as motivation is an interpersonal process open to influence and change. When using the motivational interviewing approach, clinicians move away from labelling and blaming parents, and move toward understanding the process of change. The clinician no longer considers parental denial, resistance, or lack of motivation (Prochaska et al., 1994). When a clinician has identified a parent's stage of change, feedback can be provided to increase the parent's understanding of the need or potential for change. Parents, rather than the clinician, should identify the need for change and talk about how this change might happen. Motivational interviewing assists the parent's decision to change by facilitating reflective conversations. Clinicians facilitate reflective discussion by:

- expressing empathy
- exposing discrepancies between the parents' current reality and their desired goals

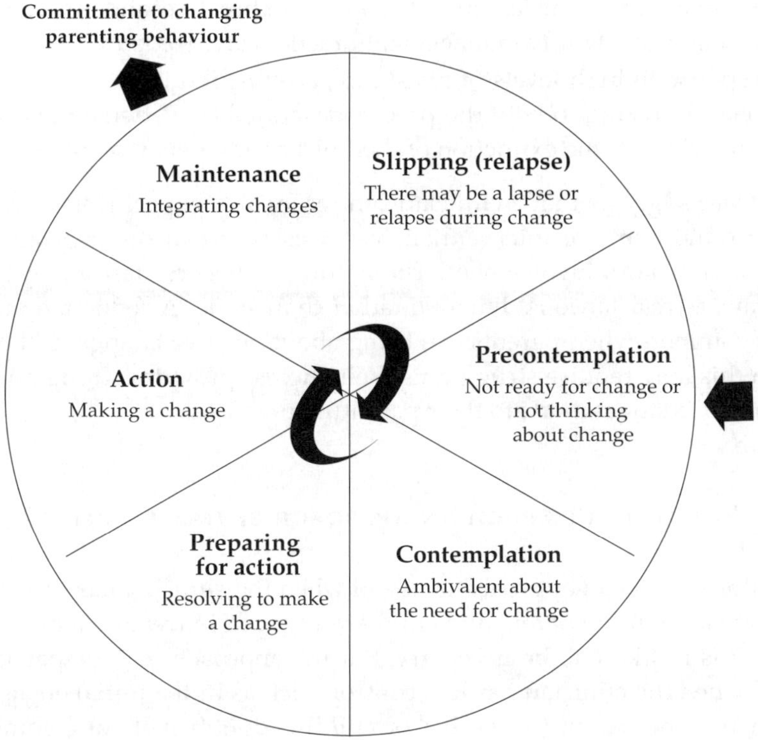

Figure 8.1 Stages of change

Source: adapted from Prochaska and DiClemente, 1986

- avoiding arguments
- noticing resistance and viewing it as feedback that they need to change their strategies
- supporting parents' belief in their ability to change or create change (Miller & Rollnick, 2002).

Using the motivational interviewing approach, the clinician acts as a partner in the process of change, not as an expert who tells parents about the necessity of change. Change talk is contrasted with *resistance talk*. The clinician is likely to elicit resistance by arguing for change, assuming the expert role, criticising, shaming or blaming, and labelling (Manchester, 2007).

One significant outcome of parental resistance is that it changes the behaviour of the clinician. Evidence suggests that these changes are likely to include:

- a shift in the focus of the clinician's involvement *away* from social learning, *towards* managing the family
- a subsequent increase in the number of sessions provided by the clinician in order to address social learning while managing resistance
- a change in the clinician's efforts to teach and confront the parent. Sometimes the clinician will increase his or her efforts to teach and confront, hoping to force change (the outcome usually being further resistance); at

other times, the clinician may become nondirective and unclear about what changes to family management practices are needed
- in response to high levels of resistance, a reduction in the interest of the clinician in trying to help the parent, described by Patterson and Chamberlain (1994) as 'the extinction of therapist caring behaviours' (p. 68).

Evidence suggests that a clinician can reasonably expect resistance at the initial to midpoints of intervention, yet resistance can occur at any point during a clinician's involvement. The nature of this resistance may change over time, as resistance is dynamic rather than static. A reduction of resistance is common when parents can bring about positive change in the child, though this may require struggle, as their success provides strong reinforcement of any changes made to their parenting practices.

When should such an approach be implemented?

Typically, this type of approach is useful when the clinician has little control of the situation. If the parent and child are engaged in treatment and participating, it is unlikely to be necessary. But the approach may be particularly helpful when the clinician has less control, such as in the initial engagement phase when the parent (or teacher or child) is doubtful about commencing treatment or accepting a view suggested by test results, or when a parent is dropping out of treatment because the clinician is getting increasingly coercive (as when trying desperately to get the parent to turn up on time or at all (Scott & Dadds, 2009). For example, take the situation where both parents come in, each having had a busy week and feeling unable to implement the program, and when they gave it a try it didn't work anyway. If this pattern is repeated, it is time for the clinician to reflect and then go back and really listen to what the parents are trying to tell him or her.

The following case study demonstrates the potential usefulness of the *stages of change model* (see figure 8.1) in conceptualising readiness for change. It also shows how *motivational interviewing (MI)* techniques can be used to alleviate difficulties in engaging a parent in behaviour change. The case study is an example of working with a parent in the *contemplation stage*.

Case study 8.1
Pulling it together

Background

Stephanie is the mother of a 10-year-old girl. She reports being overwhelmed by her daughter's behaviours, which include aggression towards others, minor property damage, and sleep disturbance. Stephanie has had contact with several agencies over most of her child's life. This involvement has included parent training, which she says was not helpful. Stephanie says she found it difficult to remember the appointments for training, difficult to understand the course content, and difficult to use anything she learned at home.

In response to a recent request for help with her daughter's behaviour, Stephanie was allocated a clinician, and sat with her for several meetings, providing information about her daughter and her behaviour. A month later, she was left with a copy of a lengthy behaviour assessment report, and had difficulty understanding the relevance of the material to her day-to-day problems. In post-assessment planning, the clinician advised Stephanie that intervention should focus initially on social skills training. This was a mismatch with Stephanie's beliefs about her daughter's behaviour. Stephanie has little confidence in her ability to bring about change, and has little hope about the future being different.

Parental reactions and signs of resistance

- Passive agreement and acquiescence: 'Sure, leave the report, I'll read it when I have time.'
- Disengagement: 'Too tired, maybe another time.'
- Avoidance: Not home when clinician visits; reschedules appointments into the future: child sick, work commitment, and holidays.
- Changing the focus: 'I forgot that appointment'; 'I couldn't get there'; 'I had to work'; or, 'No, I haven't gone through the report, but let me tell you about his new teacher'.

Clinician roadblocks to listening

- Providing solutions: 'Social skills training has helped with a lot of other clients like your daughter. I would strongly recommend we start there.'
- The goals of the clinician were at odds with Stephanie's goals. The clinician reported to the clinical supervisor: 'The visit went quite well. All the assessment items were covered with no problems'; 'I gave her the report and she seemed happy. I'll give her a call next week and get started; she is obviously ready.'
- Assumptions and labelling: 'Mum tends to be unreliable'; 'Mum won't take data'.

How might a motivational interviewing approach help?

Using an MI approach, the clinician might express empathy; that is, discuss issues with Stephanie without judgment or criticism. In doing this, the clinician would check Stephanie's understanding, beliefs, and concerns using counselling microskills, such as reflective listening and summarising of Stephanie's experience of parenting her daughter. Statements and questions that the clinician might have usefully used include:

- 'You must be very tired after having your daughter tossing about in your bed last night, but you're here this morning. I'm thinking that perhaps, when you decide something is really important, you're willing to make a huge effort.'
- 'So what makes you think that it might be time for a change?'

The clinician would consider if there were any potential discrepancies between Stephanie's values and her parenting behaviour; for example, wanting her child to have good sleep habits, but allowing her to sleep in Stephanie's bed. When discrepancies become apparent, feedback about these differences can motivate a change in behaviour. In this instance, the clinician would not confront or accuse Stephanie of exacerbating the problem, but would help her move forward.

Resistance to change is seen as ambivalence in the contemplative stage. Ambivalence can help a clinician understand the mother's hopes and fears, and suggest how best to work with them. Here, the clinician would explore the pros and cons of change. She might explore the parent's best hope for change (goals) by asking questions such as, 'If you were 100 per cent successful in making the changes you want, what would be different? What would your life look like six months from now?'

For the clinician, working to evoke change talk and build self-efficacy would remain a priority. Exploring Stephanie's strengths and resources, as well as amplifying past successes, would support Stephanie's self-belief. For example, Stephanie's clinician might comment, 'I can see you've had a lot on this week', in response to Stephanie's news that she hasn't had time to read the report. Changing a parent's perception of her or his own performance and capacities from negative to positive is critical in this process.

Conclusion

Parental readiness for engagement in treatment can be promoted by using a motivational interviewing (MI) approach. This requires the clinician to act as a partner in the process of change. When a parent is ready to become involved in parent training, there is great potential for a number of desirable outcomes, including the development of effective behaviour support strategies, positive changes to parental behaviour, the promotion of the child's development, enhancement of family relationships, and an improvement in the well-being of all family members.

9

Cognitive behaviour therapy for carers of children with intellectual disability and challenging behaviour: Two cases

Cal Paterson

Background

There is an established link between challenging behaviour in children with intellectual disability and parent stress. Two cases are presented in which a brief course of manualised cognitive behaviour therapy (CBT) to reduce parent stress led to a reduction in each child's reported challenging behaviour.

Introduction

When responding to a referral for behaviour support for a child with an intellectual disability and challenging behaviour, it can be difficult for the clinician to know where to start. Clinicians are often confronted with a range of carer issues concurrent with the child's behaviour, including parental or other interpersonal conflict (Nicoll et al., 2004), financial hardship, social isolation, challenging behaviours in siblings (Strohm, 2002), and longer-term emotional or interpersonal impacts of the child's initial diagnosis on family members (Poehlmann et al., 2005). Evidence has emerged that the impact of child challenging behaviour on parents is greater when the child has an intellectual disability (Baker et al., 2003). This challenging behaviour, in combination with these other issues, may thus have a range of impacts on the parents.

Emerson and colleagues' (1988) definition of challenging behaviour hints at the nature of these impacts. They define challenging behaviours as 'behaviours of such intensity, frequency or duration that the physical safety of the person or others is placed in serious jeopardy, or behaviour which seriously limits the person's access to ordinary settings, activities, services, and experiences' (p. 16). Two impacts implied by such a definition are physical injury to carers, and social isolation for both the child and the carer. Traditionally, carer stress or distress is appraised by the clinician as a potential barrier to intervention, or perhaps as a basis for giving priority to one referral over another. Given the association between child challenging behaviour and carer stress, there may be merit in the clinician directly treating carer stress, alongside the child's behaviour.

Much of what a child with a disability brings to his or her family is undoubtedly positive (e.g., Taunt & Hastings, 2002; Nicoll et al., 2004). Yet there is now ample evidence that caring for a child with intellectual disability and challenging behaviour, while being rewarding, can also lead to stress, depression, or other psychosocial difficulties for the parent, as well as the child, often persisting throughout and even beyond the child's lifespan (Hauser-Cram et al., 2001; Nicoll et al., 2004). A correlation between behaviour problems in children with intellectual disabilities and parental distress has been established for over 30 years (e.g., Dorner, 1975; Quine & Pahl, 1985; Tew & Lawrence, 1975). However, correlation does not demonstrate causation. What, then, is the nature of the link between child challenging behaviour and parental stress or distress? Recent findings by Beck and colleagues (2004) add to the growing empirical evidence supporting the anecdotal reports of clinicians that the presence of challenging behaviour in children with intellectual disability positively predicts parental stress (e.g., Tomanik et al., 2004; Hastings, 2002).

While there is both intuitive and empirical support for the notion that challenging behaviour is stressful for carers, evidence to support the reciprocal hypothesis that carer stress leads to child challenging behaviour remains sparse. According to Hastings and Beck (2004), while 'in general terms' such an effect is likely, and there is evidence for such an effect in non-disability literature, 'there are few studies within the intellectual disability literature to offer direct support for a relationship between parental stress and parenting behaviour' (p. 1338). Hastings (2002) has nevertheless provided a model for an 'interrelation' of child behaviour problems, parental stress, and parenting behaviour. The model, reproduced in figure 9.1, depicts his proposal that 'parents and children reciprocally affect each other, children's behaviour problems lead to stress in parents, and parents under stress adopt certain parenting behaviours that tend to reinforce the child's behaviour problems' (p. 151). Woolfson and Grant (2006) have contributed preliminary empirical evidence in support of Hastings' model, concluding that the impact of challenging behaviour on parental stress is mediated by parenting style.

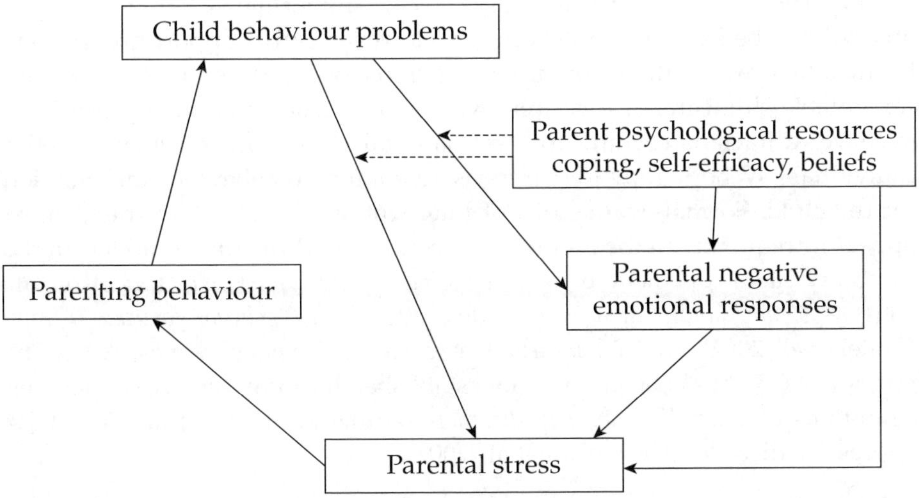

Figure 9.1 Model illustrating key variables affecting the relationship between child behaviour problems and parent stress

Source: Hastings, 2002. Copyright 2002 ASSID. Reprinted with permission

Hastings' model allows for three possible points of intervention for clinicians seeking to assist a family with a child with intellectual disability and challenging behaviour. These points of intervention are (a) the child's behaviour per se; (b) parental stress; and (c) parenting style. Efficacious interventions directly targeting the first of these, the *child's behaviour,* will not be canvassed in detail here. The dominant paradigm for such interventions currently appears to be a combination of positive behaviour support strategies (Koegel et al., 1996; McVilly, 2002) and psychoactive medications (McVilly, 2002). The role that parents play in these interventions is typically as program implementers. The third potential intervention point, *parenting style,* is most commonly addressed as a subset of any comprehensive positive behaviour support program under the label of *parent training* (e.g., McVilly, 2002; Plant & Sanders, 2007). *Parental stress* is not directly targeted in most behaviour support programs, simply because the child, not the parent, is seen as the client. Parental stress or distress is typically addressed indirectly if at all. This may occur during social gatherings, support planning meetings, or parent training and education sessions. Case workers or clinicians may find themselves becoming involved in counselling-style conversations with parents seeking an understanding and uncritical ear to talk to about their day-to-day challenges. There is yet to be a formal exploration of the efficacy of this *incidental counselling* in alleviating parent stress or distress.

Parent stress may also be more directly alleviated with attendance at carer support groups, or through specific clinical interventions. The benefits of carer support groups are well documented (e.g., Adamson, 1972; Gavidia-Payne & Hudson, 2002; Greaves, 1997; Hastings & Beck, 2004; Hawkins &

Singer, 1989; Pegram, 1989; Wikler et al., 1984; Zimmerman & Popynick, 2003), and will not be explored in detail here. However, carer support groups may be unsuitable where there are difficulties transporting the child, or arranging for suitable childcare, or for carers who find interpersonal interaction itself aversive. Clinicians seeking to treat parental stress directly may consider individual psychotherapy for carers as an adjunct to behaviour intervention for the child. Formal evaluations of interventions for carers in this context appear infrequently in the literature. Recommended treatment models in the disability literature include *cognitive-behaviour therapy (CBT)* (Nicoll et al., 2004), *systemic family therapy* (Rhodes, 2003), *brief solution-focused therapy* (Bratel et al., 2002), and *rational-emotive behaviour therapy* (Greaves, 1997). The efficacy of CBT has been empirically established for individuals experiencing symptoms of *generalised anxiety disorder* (Barlow et al., 2002) and/or major depressive disorder (Craighead et al., 2002).

Present study

The model by Hastings (2002, see figure 9.1) can be amended to indicate two key avenues for intervention via CBT, one cognitive (stressful automatic thoughts) and the other behavioural (personal resources and coping strategies). Figure 9.2 shows an amended version of Hastings' model, with CBT intervention points indicated in bold. This amended model also depicts a rationale for providing individual intervention to carers as an indirect means of addressing parenting practices, and thereby the child's challenging behaviour. If carer stress can be reduced through increased personal and social resources, and reduced stressful automatic thoughts, then the interrelated issues of parenting style and child challenging behaviour might also be positively affected. Any resulting improvement in challenging behaviour would, in turn, have an additional positive impact on parental stress.

Method

Design

A case series design was used to observe the effect of an intervention to reduce parental stress on (a) parental stress; and (b) child challenging behaviour for one male and one female parent. The intervention incorporated cognitive-behavioural therapy (CBT) strategies into a nine-week program of individual counselling for stress-related behaviours and cognitions. Parental stress and child challenging behaviour were monitored before the commencement of the treatment sessions (collection of pretreatment data), as well as weekly over the nine weeks of sessional treatment (before each session), then finally at a six-month followup. A brief assessment interview was conducted immediately following the collection of pretreatment data, to ensure that potential risks (such as suicidality and substance misuse) were identified and monitored where necessary. Parents were interviewed again after the

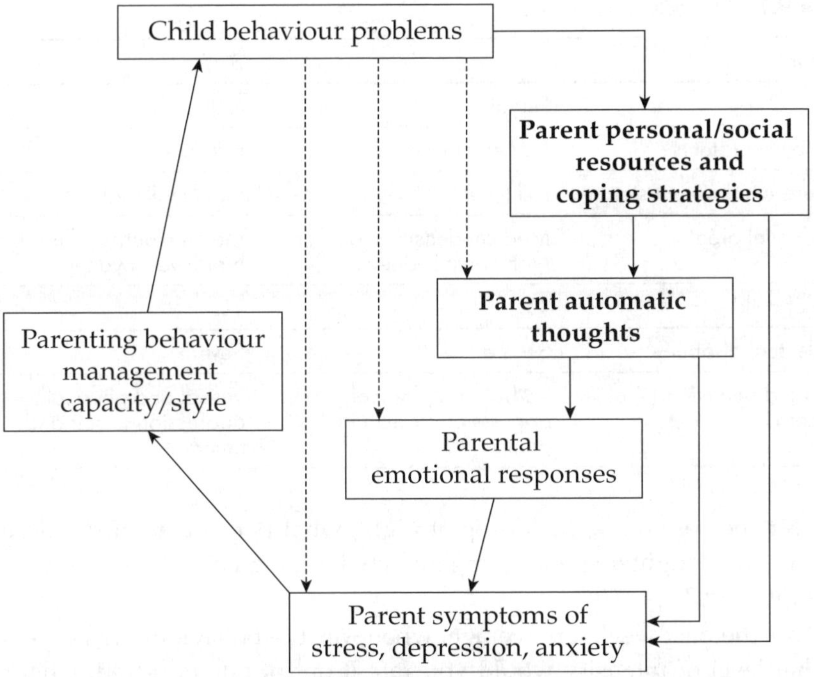

Figure 9.2 Reconceptualised model of relationships between child behaviour problems and parental stress (potential new intervention points are identified in bold)

collection of final followup data (six months post treatment), to obtain anecdotal information about their experience of the relationship between stress and parenting style, and changes in the frequency or severity of child challenging behaviour.

Participants

Two parents (one mother, and one unrelated father) participated in the treatment program. Ethical approval for the study was provided by the Macquarie University Ethics Committee (Human Research). Participants were recruited via an advertisement placed in the newsletter of the New South Wales Association of Psychologists in Developmental Disabilities, and potential participants were asked to contact the researcher by telephone for information about the study. The parents gave written consent to participate in the study, and the demographic characteristics of the two cases are provided in table 9.1. The parents did not know each other, and did not meet at any time during the research study. Both parents reported that their children had received behaviour intervention from disability services in the past, but neither was receiving behaviour intervention services at the time of the study.

Measures

Each parent was asked to rate his or her child's challenging behaviour according to the following questions:

Table 9.1 Characteristics of cases

Parent	*A*	*B*
Sex	Female	Male
Employment status	Not employed	Full-time
Spouse employment status	Full-time	Not employed
Residential area	Medium-density suburban Northwest Sydney	Medium-density suburban Northwest Sydney
Age of child	15	11
Intellectual disability	Severe	Severe
Reported behaviour(s) of concern	Verbal and physical aggression to self and others	Verbal and physical aggression to self and others

1 'Over the past week, including at night, what percentage of the time did your son/daughter spend doing any challenging behaviour, regardless of its intensity?'
2 'Over the past week, on average, whenever the behaviour was occurring, what level of intensity would you rate it out of one hundred, where one hundred is the most intense you can imagine it being, and zero is no behaviour at all?'

Parental stress, depression, and anxiety were then measured using the 21-item version of the *Depression, Anxiety and Stress Scale (DASS)* (Lovibond & Lovibond, 1995).

Development of intervention workbook

To ensure a degree of uniformity for parents, specific psychotherapeutic tasks were gathered into a workbook. Elements for the workbook were selected by examining common elements of generic CBT self-help workbooks (e.g., Barlow & Rapee, 1997; Copeland, 1993; Greenberger & Padesky, 1995), as well as other resources describing the array of CBT techniques available (Leahy, 2003; Giarratano, 2004). From these, techniques were selected that enhanced social and family connections, individual coping strategies, and cognitions, yet required minimal time investment by the parent. The aims of the workbook were to: (a) assist both parent and researcher by providing a consistent, time-limited agenda for tasks to be carried out during and between therapy sessions, with supporting information where necessary; and (b) form a lasting resource for the parent to retain and refer back to after sessions had finished. The elements of the program are summarised in table 9.2.

The workbook comprised an introduction followed by nine sections, each corresponding to a weekly one-hour session focusing on a different CBT

Table 9.2 Elements of the treatment program

Week	*Session topic*
1	Introduction to the workbook and development of joint definition of challenging behaviour
2	Development of joint understanding of interrelatedness of CB, parent stress, and parenting style
3	Motivational interviewing and goal setting
4	Planning for enhancing support network, and pleasant activity scheduling
5	Relaxation via diaphragmatic breathing, progressive muscle relaxation, and visualisation
6	Feelings identification
7	Identifying automatic thoughts
8	Challenging automatic thoughts
9	Review and relapse prevention

element or coping strategy. The sections contained self-administered exercises, narrative explanations of concepts (such as principles of controlled breathing), and record forms (such as thought monitoring forms). Each component of the workbook was labelled to indicate if it were a collaborative exercise, or to be carried out by the parent between sessions. All notes and entries were made by the parent or therapist directly into the workbook, which formed a single record of all work done during and between sessions, and which could be reviewed if necessary by the parent during times of future need.

Results

Participation in treatment

Both parents completed all tasks, and were able to demonstrate proficiency in the skills involved in the treatment program. Both parents completed the nine program elements over a 10-week period. In each case, intervention was interrupted approximately midway through the nine weeks, resulting in a mid-program gap of one week. Because of time constraints, followup data was collected six months after completion of intervention for parent A, and four months after completion for parent B.

Feedback from parents during follow-up interview

Both parents reported during the followup interviews that they were continuing to refer to the workbook, and continuing to use more than one, but not all, of the strategies in it. Both parents felt the intervention was beneficial for them, but only parent A reported a decrease in her child's challenging behaviour, while parent B reported an overall increase in behaviour severity. Both parents commented that they found behaviour incidents less stressful, although parent B reported ongoing concern about the challenging behaviour overall and the impact of the behaviour on his family.

Quantitative results

All of the raw scores for both parents are presented in table 9.3. Challenging behaviour product scores were generated by multiplying frequency rating by severity rating. Between-parent Pearson correlations of $r = 0.675$, $r = -0.690$, and $r = 0.563$ were obtained for weekly DASS (total) score, weekly challenging behaviour frequency rating, and weekly challenging behaviour severity rating respectively. A Pearson correlation of $r = 0.191$ was obtained for challenging behaviour frequency and challenging behaviour severity using data from both parents. Pearson correlations were calculated for mean parent ratings of child challenging behaviour and mean DASS scores. The coefficients thus generated are presented in table 9.4.

Observed effects of intervention

Changes in parent stress (DASS total) and challenging behaviour (product) are summarised in figure 9.3. This figure depicts mean scores for the measures of parent stress and challenging behaviour over time.

Discussion

Challenging behaviour ratings

The low correlation between parent ratings of challenging behaviour frequency and severity indicated that the parents responded to these two

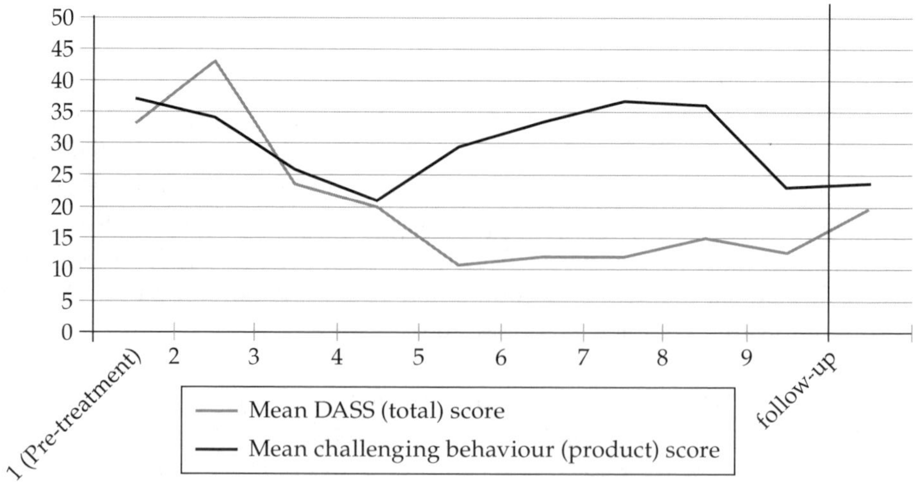

Figure 9.3 Trends on mean DASS total scores and challenging behaviour score products during and after intervention. While challenging behaviour appeared to fluctuate, DASS scores decreased, becoming more independent of challenging behaviour level

Table 9.3 Raw scores obtained for both parents on DASS and challenging behaviour ratings

		Week									
Measure	*Parent*	*1 (pre-treatment)*	*2*	*3*	*4*	*5*	*6*	*7*	*8*	*9*	*Followup*
DASS (depression)	A	17	16	7	7	0	0	0	0	1	4
	B	10	16	9	7	7	9	8	11	8	7
DASS (anxiety)	A	9	13	6	4	1	0	0	2	2	6
	B	5	11	6	3	3	4	7	5	4	6
DASS (stress)	A	15	17	10	9	1	1	1	3	3	7
	B	10	13	9	10	9	10	9	10	8	9
DASS (total)	A	41	46	23	20	2	1	1	4	5	17
	B	25	40	24	20	19	23	24	26	20	22
Challenging behaviour (frequency)	A	70%	80%	90%	70%	45%	45%	45%	60%	60%	40%
	B	30%	40%	40%	50%	55%	58%	60%	55%	40%	50%
Challenging behaviour (severity)	A	80%	60%	35%	35%	8%	8%	8%	8%	40%	45%
	B	60%	50%	50%	35%	50%	63%	70%	55%	55%	60%
Challenging behaviour (product)	A	0.56	0.48	0.32	0.25	0.03	0.03	0.03	0.05	0.24	0.18
	B	0.18	0.20	0.20	0.18	0.28	0.37	0.42	0.30	0.22	0.30

Table 9.4 Pearson correlation matrix of stress and behaviour level measures

	DASS scores			
	Total	*Depression*	*Anxiety*	*Stress*
Challenging behaviour				
Frequency	0.365	0.351	0.308	0.408
Severity	–0.076	0.009	–0.005	0.174
Product	0.197	0.285	0.183	0.107

questions in an orthogonal way. The moderate correlation between DASS scores and behaviour severity may have reflected the subjective nature of this behaviour rating, while the near-zero correlation between DASS scores and behaviour frequency may indicate that frequency ratings provide more objective information about the status of challenging behaviour. This has implications for clinicians, who are often forced to rely solely on parent report when monitoring challenging behaviour over time. With careful question wording, orthogonal estimates of frequency and severity can be obtained, with frequency rating providing a more subjective indication of the parent's experience of the behaviour, and severity rating providing a more objective indication of the challenging behaviour.

Interpretability of results

Both parents were highly motivated to participate in treatment, despite both also indicating that they felt their children were in greater need of intervention. The 'n=2' design of this study precludes all but the most tentative inferences being made about the wider population. Nevertheless, some of the results obtained bear interpretation at a broader level. In particular, the moderate correlations between child challenging behaviour severity ratings and parental DASS scores align data from the current study with data from other studies that confirm this link, thus allowing the results to be interpreted somewhat more broadly.

Parent stress and child challenging behaviour

Two key trends may be observed in the results, best reflected in figure 9.3. First, overall parent stress appears to have steadily reduced over the course of the intervention and remained low at followup. Second, although child challenging behaviour fluctuated during the intervention in a way that does not suggest any particular pattern (for example, the behaviour did not reduce over time), there appears to have been a progressive dissociation between the parent's stress level and the child's challenging behaviour. During early sessions, stress and behaviour appeared to have moved in unison, while this link appeared to have diminished in later sessions and at followup. This trend was also reflected in the comments of both parents that they were experiencing less subjective distress during behaviour incidents as a result of participation in treatment. Parent B commented during the followup interview that 'even if the behaviour got worse, it does not affect me as much as it used to'. Even where the child challenging behaviour remained elevated, the reduced degree to which parents' emotional states were 'at the mercy' of the child's behaviour was itself an important treatment outcome.

Conclusion

The relationship between child challenging behaviour, parent stress, and parenting style proposed by Hastings (2002) continues to be an important and useful model for clinicians working with families. Further research is needed to verify the causal link between parental stress and child challenging behaviour, and the present study provides a model for such research to be carried out with a larger sample. Regardless of the precise mechanism of the interrelationship between parental stress and child challenging behaviour, the association between these two phenomena means clinicians may target either one of them, in order to improve both. Where clinicians are struggling to address the behaviour, they may opt instead to target parental stress, in the knowledge that this may be an indirect avenue to behavioural intervention. If challenging behaviour and parental stress are reciprocally causal, then it is important that clinical intervention for the parent is given at least equal attention as the behaviours of the child.

Acknowledgments

The author would like to thank Dr John Franklin at the Macquarie University Department of Psychology for his assistance in preparing the chapter, and Professor Richard Hastings, Intellectual and Developmental Disabilities Unit, School of Psychology, University of Wales Bangor for kindly providing permission to refer to and reproduce his model of parental stress.

10

Brothers and sisters with a disability: Rewarding or challenging?

Jacqueline Small

Introduction

The recognition by members of a family that their child has a disability highlights the beginning of a journey that may bring both challenges and rewards. Siblings as well as parents face adjustment and adaptation to having a child with a disability in the family (Mulroy et al., 2008). Increasingly over recent years, families, services, and the community have recognised, and to some degree responded to, the impact on a child of having a brother or sister with a disability in the family. While in some cases the whole family copes and manages very well, in others the experiences and feelings aroused by the demands of caring for a child with a disability in the family may have adverse effects that may lead to significant mental health problems.

While it is unlikely that any one particular circumstance evokes either entirely positive or entirely negative experiences for siblings, at times the negatives experiences may overwhelm. One only need listen to the stories of siblings to start to develop some understanding of the impact of having a brother or sister with a significant developmental or intellectual disability. But what do we know of the experiences of siblings of children with a disability? What factors can improve adaptation to having a brother or sister with a disability? What current models of service are there to support siblings of children with a disability?

The impact of a child with a disability on siblings

> I felt completely isolated. I thought I couldn't share any of that part of my life with my friends. They didn't understand and I felt alienated from them. Other kids never had the same responsibility (Megan) (Strohm, 2002, p. 19).

Research has indicated that, while the majority of siblings are well adjusted to having a child with a disability in the family, a small number of siblings are at risk of developing significant adjustment difficulties (Rossiter & Sharpe, 2001; Sharpe & Rossiter, 2002) for reasons such as often missing out on parental time and attention, and being excluded from family discussion. There is increasing recognition of the significant impact that siblings can have on each other's development, and the potential stress and role confusion that siblings may experience when there is childhood disability in the family (Prizant et al., 1997). There is some evidence that a sibling may even experience advantage, in terms of both sibling relationships and of slightly better health and lessened depressive symptoms, if there is a child with disability in the family (Hodapp & Urbano, 2007).

Studies have investigated adjustment in siblings of children with particular diagnoses, such as autism (Sharpe & Rossiter, 2002; Rodriguez et al., 1993; Fisman et al., 1996) and Down syndrome (DS) (Cuskelly & Gunn, 2006), and shown that maladjustment is not inevitable. Further, positive appraisals in multiple areas, including parental perceptions of externalising and internalising behaviours, parental perceptions of sibling competence, and sibling perceptions of their own competence and self-worth, have been demonstrated (Cuskelly & Gunn, 2006). However, studies have demonstrated elevated risk of internalising problems in siblings of children with autism when these are specifically sought. There is often a difference in prevalence of problems in self-reported data compared to data in which the study participants are examined or interviewed.

In a study by Ross and Cuskelly (2006), 40 per cent of non-disabled siblings had scores for internalising problems on the Child Behavior Checklist (Achenbach, 1991), which placed them in the borderline or clinical range. In another study, Orsmond and Seltzer (2007a) compared adult siblings of people with Down syndrome or autism spectrum disorder (ASD). It was found that siblings of people with ASD had 'less contact with their brother or sister, reported lower levels of positive affect in their relationship, felt more pessimistic about their brother or sister's future, and were more likely to report that their relationships with their parents had been affected' (Orsmond & Seltzer, 2007a, p. 682).

Population-based studies can overcome some selection biases associated with self-referral. The parents of 186 Western Australian children with Down syndrome and 141 Australian girls and women with Rett syndrome were surveyed. The majority of parents reported both disadvantages and benefits for siblings, with some impact of place of residence, socioeconomic status, and size of family. Major disadvantages for siblings from the study centred on parental and personal time constraints, relationships and socialising, restrictions, parental emotion, and the burden of helping. Major benefits were related to personality characteristics; for example, siblings were more accepting of differences, more caring and compassionate, and more mature than in families without a child with disability (Mulroy et al., 2008).

Feelings experienced by siblings of a child with disabilities

Strohm (2002) identified that siblings of a child with disabilities may experience a variety of negative feelings, including:

- isolation: feeling that they have no one to talk to, an awareness that friends' lives are different and a sense of being alone
- that they have limited information about disability, which leads to the creation of fantasy explanations, reliance on a limited use of diagnostic terms by parents, and facing the impact of parents' grief
- fear of failure, disappointing the parents, adding to parents' burden, all of which may lead to becoming super helpful
- being affected by society's message that the child with a disability is somehow 'special', therefore they are made to feel that they are lucky to be normal
- the impact of the reaction of others (such as pity, avoidance, derogatory terms), which may lead to overly protective behaviour towards the child with a disability, but at the same time give them feelings of conflicting loyalties
- inward-turned feelings, particularly in the presence of high levels of parent distress, (Fisman et al., 1996)
- a sense of unfairness, that life revolves around the child with special needs, whose needs must always be put first
- feelings of abandonment or neglect
- frustration at the practical impact on the family of having a sibling with disabilities
- feeling of being abandoned because the subsequent child with a disability requires a lot of time and attention
- confusion resulting from the message that having a child of disability in the family should be a positive experience.

Benderix and Sivberg (2007) conducted a thematic analysis of interviews with 14 siblings of children with autism and intellectual disability. The analysis resulted in seven content categories, including precocious responsibility, feeling sorry, feeling exposed to frightening behaviour, empathetic feelings, hoping that a group home will be a relief, physical violence making siblings feel unsafe and anxious, and relations with friends being affected negatively. The conclusion was that these siblings' experiences revealed stressful life conditions.

An earlier study by Bagenholm and Gillberg (1991) involved interviewing 60 siblings and mothers of children with autism, intellectual disability, and typically developing children. Siblings of children with a developmental disability, and especially siblings of children with autism, were more concerned about the future than siblings of typically developing children. The siblings of children with autism and developmental disability also felt lonely more often, and many of them had peer problems. They often regarded their siblings as a burden and tended to have only one sibling. Siblings often did not know why their brother or sister with disability was different from other children. There were more behaviour disturbances in the siblings of disabled children, and mothers with a child with autism reported more 'stressful events'. Between the three groups there were no differences as regards the personality of the mothers and the self-concept of the children (Bagenholm & Gillberg, 1991).

Sibling awareness of disability

> He was playing with my hat and then went very quiet under the dinner table. There was such a panic in the house—it was Christmas lunch. I never let my brother play with anything of mine after that—it was an obsession—in case it caused another seizure (Tara) (Strohm, 2002, p. 22).

From a very young age, children may have different experiences associated with the disability of their brother or sister, with certain factors potentially leading to increased vulnerability among young siblings. Their egocentrism may lead to greater misunderstanding of their brother's or sister's condition and its impact on the family (Lobato, 1993). Parents may be particularly confused about how and when to share information about the child's condition with young siblings (Lobato et al., 2000). In some cases, some of the very young siblings initially want to be similar, and attempt to imitate their brothers and sisters, particularly if he or she is also physically disabled. However, even before they are two years old, children are able to recognise that their older brothers and sisters are different, and often imitate the parents' behaviour towards the older child (Hames, 1998).

A longitudinal study by Hames (1998) described the changing understanding of younger siblings aged between 4½ months and 6½ years. Some siblings in the study copied their older sibling (such as by responding to questions with 'ahah', asking for splints for Christmas), while others wanted their older sibling to be like them. Some siblings copied their parents' behaviour towards their older brother or sister. Before the age of two years, some siblings had already stopped trying to persuade their brother or sister to be like themselves; for example, a 21-month-old girl ceased setting a place at dinner for her sister, who had a feeding tube. Hames (1998) found that by the age of two or three years, depending on the physical disabilities of the older child, siblings were no longer trying to be like their older brothers and sisters, but more often like their parents. Siblings with brothers and sisters with profound learning and physical disabilities very quickly become aware that they were different (Hames, 1998).

It may not be possible to explain the abstract and less visible features of a disability to children under the age of seven years, but by 11 years, children are able to understand the irrevocability of learning disabilities (Lewis, 1995). Therefore, clinicians should expand efforts to reach out to the siblings of children with disabilities, especially during adolescence, a stage of life during which the sibling may be particularly sensitive to the social stigma of a brother's or sister's disability. It is suggested that supporting and educating siblings about mental illness and disability issues may help them develop a deeper understanding of their brother's or sister's experience, which in turn may foster a closer relationship (Greenberg et al., 1999).

Factors that predict sibling involvement

There are a variety of factors that influence how much involvement a sibling may have in the life of their brother or sister with a disability. These factors may include:

- expectations of parents that the sibling will be involved once they are no longer able to support their son or daughter with a disability (Orsmond & Seltzer, 2007b; Begun, 1989)
- the gender of the sibling: sisters tend to provide more emotional support than brothers (Greenberg et al., 1999)
- the relative age of the brother or sister with disability (Hodapp & Urbano, 2007; Rodriguez et al., 1993)
- the existence of behaviour problems (Seltzer et al., 1997)
- the demands and constraints of the adult years, which involve responsibilities of work and parenting as well as the degree of closeness with the family of origin (Greenberg et al., 1999; Horwitz et al., 1992).

Another factor that pushes the sibling towards the caregiving role is feeling closely connected with the family. Life course research suggests that continuity in family relationships over time, and thus the quality of family-of-origin relationships, forms a template for sibling relationships in adulthood (Cicirelli, 1995). Thus, sibling involvement with the brother or sister with a disability may be sustained by family values that emphasise closeness across the generations and over time. Greenberg and colleagues (1999) suggested that if siblings were willing to take on at least some responsibility, the cost to the public would be reduced, and the continuity of family-based support would be maintained.

Factors that influence sibling response

> When I was a kid I would be playing outside all day and when I got hurt or had my feelings hurt I felt like I couldn't go to my parents. They had so much work to do with my sister as it was, I took care of myself (Strohm, 2002, p. 33).

The well-being of the sibling and the nature of his or her response to the brother or sister with a disability may also be influenced by 'external' factors, such as parents' marital satisfaction (Rodriguez et al., 1993). Although marital satisfaction, lack of parental depression, a cohesive family, and a warm non-conflictual sibling relationship were protective for some siblings, this has not been found to be a straightforward association. In a study by Fisman and colleagues (1996), it was the parent distress factor (composed of parental stress and depression scores) that mediated the relationship between quality of sibling adjustment and parental reports of internalising and externalising behaviour problems in the healthy (non-disabled) sibling. The findings stressed the importance of a transactional mechanism rather than identification of single-risk or protective factors in predicting sibling adjustment (Fisman et al., 1996). Furthermore, when the level of environmental stress became overwhelming, factors that were previously operative no longer served to be protective (Garmezy, 1984).

Other researchers suggest that the levels of risk and resilience factors in a family were better predictors of sibling adjustment than siblings' own experiences of stress and coping resources. This highlights the importance of familial and parental contributions to the sibling adjustment process. More specifically, socioeconomic status, past attendance at a sibling support group, parent stress, family time and routines, family problem-solving and communication, and family hardiness predicted sibling adjustment difficulties. Finally, siblings' perceived intensity of daily uplifts significantly predicted sibling prosocial behaviour (Giallo & Gavidia-Payne, 2006).

While stress may be generated in part by the difficult temperament of the child with the disability, the sense of failure that is engendered in the caregiver (generally the mother), and the internal psychological distress, may be the mechanisms connecting chronic family stress and behaviour problems of the healthy (non-disabled) sibling (Fisman et al., 1996). The variability in sibling outcomes may be related to a variety of potential moderating and mediating factors. These factors include genetic predispositions (Orsmond & Seltzer, 2007b) and the problem-solving approach used by the sibling, with the siblings being closer when the sibling used more problem-focused coping strategies (Orsmond & Seltzer, 2007b). However, it is unlikely in healthy siblings of children with autism that they convey specific characteristics related to the genetic risk associated with autism (Pilowsky et al., 2007).

Available supports and services

> To know of other children my age who were 'normal' but had disabled sibs, to be able to meet them, write to them, talk with them, share with them, especially as we grew up and faced different challenges (Strohm, 2002, p. 181).

The perception by siblings that they are well supported may serve to reduce the risk of internalising or externalising problems (Sharpe & Rossiter, 2002). Further, it is important to recognise positive family bonds, which encourage sustained involvement of family members in the care of adults with a disability (Greenberg et al., 1999). Once adjustment disorders have been identified, counselling for the family and for siblings may be recommended to help them deal with their feelings and problems (Benderix & Sivberg, 2007). However, several studies have shown that accessing professional support, such as medical and educational services, can have a negative impact on families of children with a disability (Giallo & Gavidia-Payne, 2006), perhaps underscoring the importance of parents' sense of self-efficacy and control.

Increasingly, services are responding to the growing awareness that supporting the family of a child with a disability is likely to contribute to improved quality of life for the person with a disability and reducing the risk factors for poor mental health outcomes. It is worthwhile engaging the sibling in discussions about the disability, and respecting the difficulties they experience, as well as the significant contributions they make towards their sibling's welfare. Many organisations now offer siblings activities (for examples see <http://www.siblingsaustralia.org.au/ds_nsw.asp> and additional sources of support listed in table 10.1), which include both recreational and fun elements in the

Table 10.1 Sources of support for siblings

Details
Facebook for siblings of children with Down syndrome Example: <http://www.dsansw.org.au/index.php?pg=444>
Email chat groups Example: <http://www.siblingsaustralia.org.au/young_sibs.asp>
Books Example: <http://www.amazon.com/s/ref=nb_ss_b?url=search-alias%3Dstripbooks&field-keywords=siblings+disability&x=15&y=14>
Movies Example: <http://www.theblackballoonmovie.com/>
Telephone helpline Example: <http://www.nas.org.uk/nas/jsp/polopoly.jsp?d=124&a=3989>[1]
Camps Example: <http://www.cooinda.org.au/Sibling_Activities.html>
Other online information Examples: <http://www.youngcarers.net.au/> <http://www.reachout.com.au/default.asp?ti=2626> <http://www.healthinsite.gov.au/topics/Siblings> <http://www.acd.org.au/siblings/index.htm, http://www.youngcarersnsw.asn.au/>

1 In Australia, the national organisation (Siblings Australia) is already mentioned. Siblings Australia lists some state-based services on its website.

program. Goals that are typical of the programs include connecting with other siblings, realising that their circumstances aren't unique, developing coping skills for stressful situations, and exploration of strengths of both the sibling and the child with a disability.

Of concern, however, is the limited analysis that participation in siblings groups has received. There is some evidence that participants enjoy and report benefit from attending group programs (D'Arcy et al., 2005). Evidence also indicates that sibling knowledge, sibling sense of connectedness with other children in similar family circumstances, and sibling global functioning are increased through participation in groups, and that negative emotional or behavioural outcomes are unlikely (Lobato & Kao, 2005).

Conclusion

Given the available evidence, professionals working with families need to consider the impact of disability on siblings as well as the identified child and his or her parents. Given that family contexts play a critical role in determining sibling adjustment difficulties, interventions that focus on supporting the whole family, in addition to directly supporting siblings, may be most effective. In particular, interventions aimed at helping parents to manage stress, improve parenting skills, strengthen family communication and problem-solving skills, as well as maintain family routines, may be useful. Strengthening sibling, parent, and overall family functioning may also improve the ability to cope with and meet the needs of the person with a disability (Giallo & Gavidia-Payne, 2006).

11

Understanding and responding to challenging behaviour: Valuable contributions from attachment theory

Anders Hansson

The role of attachment in the development and maintenance of challenging behaviour in children and adolescents with intellectual disabilities has to date received little attention from traditional positive behaviour support approaches. However, emerging thinking and research within attachment theory is offering a perspective that focuses on socioemotional relationships and the importance of security and safety when understanding why some children and adolescents with an intellectual disability engage in challenging behaviour. This chapter explores and elaborates on how this new perspective can complement the current traditional positive behaviour support framework by conceptualising and responding to challenging behaviour more effectively.

Introduction

When responding to challenging behaviour among children with disability, traditional interventions have come from behavioural approaches grounded in learning theory, such as applied behaviour analysis and the positive behaviour support paradigm. Surprisingly little attention has been given to the child's pattern of attachment, and the role it has in the development of challenging behaviour. It is argued that the more practitioners learn about the bio-psycho-social concept, the better equipped they are in developing effective treatment options that consider not only the child with the disability but their dyadic relationships with others and the contexts in which these interactions are occurring. Therefore, emerging research in the area of intellectual disability (ID) and the role of attachment in the occurrence of challenging behaviour (e.g., Janssen et al., 2002; Sterkenburg et al., 2008) may have a significant impact on how to design and deliver future interventions.

To various degrees, people of all ages, with or without a disability, depend on others for safety, security, and emotional support, especially at times of distress and discomfort, but also when developing social and intimate relationships. Interestingly, the central goal of most disability services has been to foster independence (Clegg & Sheard, 2002). Clegg and Sheard (2002) proposed that *attachment theory* provided a conceptual base for a shift from this position because it theorised emotional development, not as a move to independence, but as a move from immature to mature dependence. More specifically, they refer to challenging behaviour as being a separation protest in individuals, noting that treating separation protest with behavioural intervention or medication does not address the problem, which is embedded in key relationships.

Similarly, Pickover (2002) argued that traditional behavioural approaches address the behaviour but may miss the importance that children place on maintaining their attachment systems. Sterkenburg and colleagues (2008) offered some incentive for this trend to change. These researchers found that providing attachment-based therapy combined with traditional behaviour intervention, as opposed to traditional behaviour intervention alone, decreased challenging behaviour and resulted in significantly more adaptive target behaviours.

Theoretical underpinnings of traditional behaviour approaches

Emerson (2001) defined *challenging behaviour* as 'culturally abnormal behaviours of such intensity, frequency, or duration that the physical safety of the person or others is likely to be placed in serious jeopardy, or behaviour which is likely to seriously limit the use of, or result in the person being denied access to ordinary community facilities' (p. 3). Positive behaviour support practices are arguably the most widely applied behaviour intervention approaches in disability services today. This approach uses educational methods to expand individuals' behaviour repertoires, and emphasises the importance of adapting their living environments to, first, enhance their quality of life and, second, to minimise their challenging behaviour (Carr et al., 2002). Underpinning this process is the comprehensive behavioural assessment, which investigates the past contexts and the current context in which the individual lives, works, and plays, his or her life experiences and life history (developmental history, educational history with successes and failures), and family history, with any losses and tragedies identified (Willis & LaVigna, 1996).

Theoretical underpinnings for attachment-based intervention approaches

Bowlby (1982) defined *attachment* as 'the disposition of the child to seek proximity to and contact with a specific figure and to do so in certain situations, notably when frightened, tired or ill' (p. 371). He argued that children need a reliable ongoing attachment to primary caregivers, and that they suffer grievously, even irreparably, if the attachment is interrupted or lost. In later writings, he elaborated that a successful attachment allows for security, whereas anxiety and jealousy develop from poor attachments, as does anger, grief, and depression (Bowlby, 1988).

Ainsworth and Wittig (cited in Bretherton, 1992) demonstrated Bowlby's theory scientifically in the *strange situation procedure*. They were able to categorise the responses of toddlers to their mothers in three attachment patterns, referred to *insecure-avoidant* (A); *secure* (B); and *insecure-ambivalent* (C). This experiment also contributed the concept of the attachment figure as a *secure base* from which an infant can explore the world. The concept of *maternal sensitivity* to infant signals and its role in the development of infant–mother attachment patterns was another contribution of Ainsworth (cited in Bretherton, 1992). Main and Solomon (1990) classified a fourth group of children as *disorganised* (D), as they appeared to lack a coherent coping strategy for several seconds upon the attachment figure's return during the strange situation procedure, before resuming either of the ABC classification attachment patterns.

Disorganised attachment is common in individuals with an ID, as they are more vulnerable to stress and use less effective coping strategies (Janssen et al., 2002). These researchers have proposed a stress-attachment model of the development of challenging behaviour in children with ID. The model infers that when individuals with an ID face a situation that they perceive as stressful (as when faced with the risk of getting hurt, losing out or not being able to cope with demanding tasks), fail to find a behavioural solution to the situation, and cannot use an attachment figure as a secure base, their physiological arousal builds up. Depending on the individuals' attachment patterns, this arousal may lead to a range of behavioural symptoms, such as aggressive behaviours, self-soothing behaviours, withdrawal, dissociative symptoms, and in severe cases, self-injurious behaviours (De Schipper et al., 2006).

In her *dynamic-maturational model (DMM) of attachment patterns*, Crittenden (1999; 2000a; 2000b) proposed that attachment should be conceptualised as promoting safety rather than security. Crittenden emphasised the interaction between culture, maturation, and context when trying to understand the organisation, function, and development of attachment patterns in the face of threat and danger. Crittenden further proposed that separation and loss were special categories of danger, the primary organiser of human behaviour (Crittenden, 2008). She explained that:

> children who experience danger are expected to develop strategies that reduce the sorts of danger that they have experienced. When the danger is lack of parental response, adaptive strategies will elicit parental attention, even if this involves angry or risk-taking behaviour; when danger is parent hostility, adaptive strategies will reduce it (Crittenden, 1999, p. 146).

Clinical considerations

Resilience is an important determinant for successful adjustment to having given birth to a child with a developmental delay. For many parents, the initial experience may have been difficult, even traumatic, but they are still able to adjust and assume successfully the role of attachment figures for their child. Other families struggle to overcome grief and loss issues associated with the birth of their child with a developmental delay. Combined with inadequacies in the child's innate signalling system, this hinders the dyadic process of communication and adjustment around the infant's safety and comfort that is so important for the development of an attuned relationship. For some parents, the grief and loss issues may be so severe that they disclaim their baby (Bunce & Rickards, 2004). Hence, early screening for possible developmental delays or impairments and subsequent intervention for those children and families identified is vital.

Parenting is arguably the most important job in life. Still, relatively little attention is given to education and training in preparation for this role. Having a child with a developmental delay further complicates this role. Initially the parents may be able to cope, but as the child grows and becomes stronger, what was considered a tantrum could become so intense and so severe that the safety of the child and others are at risk.

For many families, parent-education programs such as the *Triple P–Positive Parenting Program* (Sanders et al., 2003), *Signposts for Building Better Behaviour* (Hudson et al., 2008), and the *Apex Behaviour Management Program* (Hartog, cited in Wiese et al., 2005) may meet their needs. Other families may require specialised support from a clinical team, particularly if the child has complex needs and behaviours, or if there are complex family issues present. The key task is to build parental confidence in managing the child's behaviour by involving both parents early on and encouraging them to work as a team. At the same time, to assist this process, other supports should be in place for parents, such as counselling, access to respite, sibling support, education around communication, socialisation, and engaging their child in play activities.

An important aspect of working with families is for clinicians to demonstrate empathy and an awareness of the families' unique situations. This allows for the development of connectedness and trust. Everybody has his or her own individual attachment history that affects emotional well-being and interpersonal relationships socioemotionally and behaviourally. This is subsequently reflected in the individual's ability to deal with challenging situations with confidence. Becoming aware of this through self-reflection and in clinical supervision will allow clinicians to prepare themselves to work closely with children and families, even under difficult circumstances. Similarly, at the intervention level, it is equally important to support parents and carers to become mindful of this and the ways that they can affect behavioural change through their positive interactions with the child or adolescent (Singh et al., 2006); in other words, the ways in which parents can offer a secure base from which their child or adolescent with ID can explore the world.

Arguably, for many mothers the attachment figure role is assumed with relative confidence from the time of the birth of their child or even earlier, during pregnancy. For others this may not be the case, because of their own attachment history and the context into which the child is born (such as disrupted family environment, difficulties in parenting, drug and alcohol use, postnatal depression or other mental illness, or being unable to cope with their child being born with a disability). In these cases, multiple variables may be present and interrelated, requiring a more complex and multifaceted intervention approach.

Some children with an intellectual disability who display challenging behaviour have experienced trauma and abuse. Emotional abuse, neglect, sexual abuse, physical abuse, and exposure to domestic violence can interfere with the development of the child's attachment. Exposure to such traumatic events leads to losses in core capacities for self-regulation and interpersonal relatedness (Cook et al., 2005). In more severe cases, the child is likely to meet the DSM-IV-TR (American Psychiatric Association, 2000) criteria for reactive attachment disorder.

Intervention approaches

Psychotherapy and psychoeduction are currently the two most frequently used treatment models for biological families with attachment disorders. Foster and adoptive families, on the other hand, need assistance to repair the child's negative internal representations by responding to their child's cues (Cornell & Hamrin, 2008). The psychoeducational model fits well with the positive behaviour support framework, as it focuses on increasing parental knowledge of child development, self-care, and relationship building. The psychotherapeutic model focuses on the child–parent attachment relationship, and includes such approaches as *dyadic developmental psychotherapy* (see Becker-Weidman, 2006) and *parent–child interaction therapy* (Bagner & Eyberg, 2007).

It is useful to view the family as a system within which there are a set of dyads (such as mother–child and father–child). Kozlowska and Hanney (2002) noted that observing children interacting with their parents, and recognising the strategies children use within this dyadic relationship, provides valuable information about how the dyad has related in the past. This assists clinicians to formulate questions and hypotheses about attachment patterns and to plan family interventions. Video recording the parent–child interactions may prove a useful way of capturing these dyadic interactions. The *Marte Meo approach* utilises this technology as part of the therapeutic process (see Aarts, 2008).

Within the positive behaviour support framework, the *multi-element support plan* (LaVigna & Willis, 1995) is the result of a comprehensive behavioural assessment. The plan has two major sections. The *proactive strategies* are designed to produce behavioural change over time, and the *reactive strategies* are designed to manage the challenging behaviour at the time it occurs (for an extensive elaboration on this treatment model, see LaVigna & Willis, 1995).

Challenging behaviours are broadly noted as being communicative in nature; that is, the child is trying to tell us something through behavioural means. Ineffective communication from others is also likely to confuse and/or frustrate the child and subsequently create a context in which he or she does not feel safe. Hence, a primary objective for the clinician is to develop communication strategies that are clear, concise, and presented in a format that the child or adolescent with a disability can understand (for example, using visual supports or augmentative and alternative communication systems), and that therefore should make them feel safer and more secure.

These communication strategies would also assist the child's communication partners to become more consistent and therefore promote the dyadic relationship. However, there are other aspects of communication that have an impact on behaviour, particularly nonverbal body language, facial expression, and tone of voice. The psychological messages embedded in communication from others can affect the responses of the child or adolescent with an ID. For example, being greeted with a warm, friendly smile in a relaxed manner is more likely to bring calmness and a sense of security to the child or adolescent than being greeted with a facial expression that suggests fear, anxiety, or dislike. The clinician needs to be aware of this when developing interaction guidelines for parents and carers. These interaction guidelines should model secure base behaviours through sensitive responding: being clear and concise while being available, calm, empathic, consistent, reassuring, and predictable.

Many individuals with a disability, and particularly those with autism spectrum disorder (ASD), have significant sensory needs. They may be hypersensitive or hyposensitive to certain stimuli in their physical environments (such as excessive noise, heat, lights, touch, and taste). Considering this, some environments can be quite stressful and frightening to the person, for example, crowded and noisy shopping centres, flickering lights, hot vehicles, noisy playgrounds or classrooms, and clothing materials (Schaaf & Miller, 2005). To identify these needs, the clinician (usually an occupational therapist) conducts a sensory processing assessment and develops a sensory profile for the child. This profile guides parents and carers in meeting the child's identified sensory needs and thereby presumably becoming better positioned to be the child's secure base.

Realistically, the world is not always a safe place, and from time to time, the individual with ID will be exposed to contexts, environments, and people that he or she may find frightening and stressful. Finding the balance between allowing the individual the freedom to explore and participate in life, at the same time as protecting him or her from undue risks, can be challenging for parents and carers. Clinicians can support parents and carers by conducting risk assessments and developing risk management strategies for known and anticipated dangers.

The focus on positive programming within positive behaviour support approaches is to assist the person systematically to develop skills and competencies that will contribute to social integration (LaVigna et al., 1989). Of particular interest are the areas that often cause greatest concern and distress to the individual with ID, such as problem-solving, changing circumstances, and relationships, and dealing with strong emotions. Programs that aim to improve the individual's social skills, assertiveness, and anger management and stress management skills should prevent the person from displaying challenging behaviour. However, as a caveat, it is important to note that an insecure attachment style may compound learning difficulties for children with intellectual disabilities, as they have fewer protective factors and resources to overcome the stress of an insecure attachment (Rosenstein & Horowitz, 1996). Hence, it is important that the learning environment is safe and positive, with lots of encouragement and positive connotations provided by the 'teachers'.

In order to illustrate some of the experiences of individuals with developmental disabilities and their families, a hypothetical example is outlined below. This case study emphasises the common threads or themes that are identified by using a set of attachment lenses to explore the attachment patterns in individuals with ID and their families (such as abandonment, danger, and security).

Case study 11.1
Peter

Peter is a 13-year-old boy with a *mild intellectual disability* (ID) and *autism spectrum disorder* (ASD). A year ago, Peter's parents relinquished their care for him by deciding to not pick him up after an overnight respite stay. They stated that they could no longer manage Peter at home safely, because of his aggressive behaviour, particularly towards his mum and little brother. Peter was temporarily accommodated in the respite centre.

Initially Peter easily became anxious, and hit staff and other respite clients. In particular, his anxiety and aggressive behaviours increased when new staff or agency staff were working with him. However, with targeted intervention Peter's behaviour has settled and decreased significantly since being away from home.

Peter visits his family home on the weekend, but the parents still have difficulties managing his behaviour. Peter's relationship with his family is tense, and his parents are feeling guilty and anxious for having relinquished their care for him. They have expressed that they would like him to start having overnight stays at home on the weekend, but feel ambivalent about how they are going to cope. Peter has also expressed that he wants to move home again.

From an attachment theory perspective, the long-term goal for the clinical team supporting Peter would be to reunite him with his family and repair the disrupted attachments to his parents and little brother. The short-term goal would be to assess Peter's immediate support needs and to develop a secure base for him. If Peter feels safe, he is less likely to become anxious and subsequently less likely to become aggressive.

Having an ASD means that Peter is not likely to cope well with changes in his environment and lack of consistency in communication messages. Consequently, Peter is likely to respond well to behaviour intervention that provides him with consistent routines and a high level of predictability. Assessments may also provide information about his sensory and communication needs. An important aspect of the intervention would be to teach the parents strategies on how to communicate effectively with Peter and how to support him with his emotional regulation. The *Behaviour Support Plan* (LaVigna & Willis, 1995) would be the guiding tool for achieving this, in conjunction with a direct teaching approach, such as the *Stepping Stones Triple P* (Sanders et al., 2003).

Conclusion

Attachment theory provides an additional set of lenses through which to view the child's challenging behaviour. It allows for a better understanding of the child's attachment history and any contributing factors, such as disrupted interpersonal relationships, grief and loss issues, and possible experiences of trauma and/or abuse. Consequently, the clinician will be in a better position to respond to the child's socioemotional needs. That said, further research with this population is essential to provide a stronger evidence base for this new approach, and to inform future direction for clinical services.

Acknowledgment

The author would like to acknowledge Frances Roberts, Manager, Statewide Behaviour Intervention Service, for reviewing this chapter.

12

Challenging behaviour and change in intellectual disabilities: Family therapy, families, and the wider system

Paul Rhodes and Lesley Whatson

Introduction

Clinical intervention for challenging behaviour in intellectual disability has come a long way since institutionalisation and a reliance on psychopharmacology and restrictive behavioural practices. Positive programming provides an ethical and contextual approach to community integration, forming a critical set of skills for any clinician working with this population. One of the limitations of this approach, however, is that systemic constraints to intervention are not sufficiently explained. They are often relegated to mediation analysis, without a sophisticated account of how to negotiate complex interactional and relational obstacles to effective behavioural work. This chapter aims to provide a detailed a account of family therapy's approach to developmental disability, with the aim of identifying a variety of potential directions for intervention when behavioural approaches fail to be effective.

Positive behaviour support: an introduction

For the past 20 years *applied behaviour analysis*, or *positive programming* (LaVigna et al., 1989; Horner & Carr, 1997) has played a critical role in the process of deinstitutionalisation of people with intellectual disabilities. Positive programming provides a means for understanding challenging behaviour, as a form of communication, and a signal of limited life opportunities. It provides the clinical tools to examine behaviour in these terms and provide appropriate interventions, rather than relying solely on restrictive practices and psychopharmacological intervention. From this perspective, problematic behaviours are seen as functional. That is, behaviours can be a means by which an individual has his or her specific needs met (when there are no communicative alternatives) or an indication of when there is a poor match between an individual and his or her current environment.

In practical terms, the outcomes of an effective behavioural intervention are varied, and may include:

- development of opportunities and routines that match the age-appropriate needs and capacities of an individual
- design of augmentative communication systems to allow the individual to better understand his or her environment and exercise come control
- introduction of coping strategies and carefully designed reactive strategies to improve the safety of caregivers
- acquisition of a wider range of adaptive skills for daily life.

The limitations of positive programming

One of the limitations of the positive programming approach is that it offers no comprehensive answer to the problems that are caused by complex relationship problems in the family and wider service system (Rhodes, 2003). While the *behaviour assessment guide* (Willis et al., 1993) offers a sophisticated tool for the conceptualisation of challenging behaviour, it fails to conceptualise adequately problems requiring mediation. Parents, caregivers, and service providers are seen as the implementers of behavioural and ecological programs, despite the potential for a range of significant personal, professional, and relational issues to interfere with their capacity to carry out this role. Issues of grief, insecure attachment, marital conflict, chronic stress, or neglect may not be considered adequately when working in the family context. In addition, issues of post-traumatic stress, burnout, team dysfunction, and poor management may not be adequately considered when working in the service context.

The conceptualisation of challenging behaviour will be further discussed from a variety of lenses that are primarily from the field of family therapy. These lenses can provide a theoretical backdrop to allow for a more sophisticated understanding of mediation analysis in developmental disabilities.

Challenging behaviour from a systemic perspective

Systemic family therapy, also known as *Milan systemic family therapy*, was pioneered by Selvini-Palazzoli and colleagues (1978) in response to the predominance of individual psychoanalytic therapy for children. They postulated that problems experienced by children could be understood as intrapersonal rather than intrapsychic problems. They considered the child's behaviour as one step in a family's dance of interactions, rather than the problem itself. In particular, they emphasised the concept of homeostasis; that is, the idea that families become stuck in rigid patterns of interaction in response to stressful life events and lifecycle transitions. These patterns are predictable, escalate over time, and help to mediate against the conflict, stress, or intimacy that might arise during the process of adaptive change.

One of the most eloquent applications of the principle of homeostasis in developmental disability is presented by Birch (1986). He proposed the concept of *timelessness* as an alternative to homeostasis. He suggested that members of the family unit can become lost travellers in the family lifecycle, becoming enchanted by certain beliefs that restrain change for prolonged periods of time, even as the person with intellectual disability approaches adulthood. Beliefs such as 'a mother is the only person who can care for a child with developmental disability' can have a significant and traumatic effect on the independence of the whole family, not just the person with the disability. This is similar to Todd and Shearn's (1996) notion of 'perpetual' or 'captive' parents who can lose touch with what was once a 'normal' life.

Goldberg and colleagues (1995) provided an additional lens to understand the potential of an extended duration of homeostasis in developmental disability. They described how interactions, in some cases, could be governed by complex grief reactions concerning the loss of the perfect child, the loss of one's own independence, and the interconnectedness of these losses with those from the parental family of origin. Family therapy becomes highly emotive in these cases, aiming to facilitate a grieving process that allows for a more normative family lifecycle to proceed.

These concepts provide some clear hypotheses that can be useful when considering possible constraints to effective behavioural intervention. From a behavioural perspective, parents are considered to be potential mediators of behavioural change, employing alternative communication techniques, redesigning routines, and teaching new skills, all of which may enhance the self-determination of the person with an intellectual disability. However, an exclusive reliance on a behavioural approach will not apply to families who are stuck in rigid patterns of interactions with one another. In this situation, a great deal of systemic intervention will need to be employed first.

Another way to articulate this point is to raise the distinction between a *communicative* and a *homeostatic* function of challenging behaviour (Rhodes, 2003). *Positive programming* postulates a communicative function of challenging behaviour, arguing that an analysis of the meaning of a challenging behaviour leads to a clearer understanding of the communicative intent behind the behaviour (such as a request for escape from aversive stimuli, boredom in the face of poor productivity, or seeking personal interaction). Alternatively, *systemic therapy* postulates that a challenging behaviour serves a homeostatic function for the person with an intellectual disability; that is, the challenging behaviour serves as a symbol of the need for significant changes in the person's relationships, and the rules and affect that govern them.

In a clinical example, the meaning of a person's challenging behaviour can be hypothesised from two angles. From a positive programming point of view, a challenging behaviour might mean, 'I'm bored; I want to do something that is interesting, makes me feel valued and helps me feel like my 20-year-old peers'. However, from a systemic therapy interpretation, the behaviour may have a different meaning, such as, 'If I became more independent my mother and father might separate because they have drifted apart so much over the past 20 years'. In the first case, the assumption is that the person actually thinks or feels this particular statement, but in the second, it is a symbolic meaning or a way for the clinician to reframe and understand the direction of treatment.

Challenging behaviour from a structural perspective

Structural family therapy was developed by Minuchin (1974), and like systemic therapy, was a direct reaction to the predominance of individual therapy for children. While Selvini-Palazzoli and colleagues (1978) focused on patterns of interaction, Minuchin was interested in hierarchy. In particular, he believed that a strong but flexible parenting team was critical to the health of the family, providing the boundaries and emotional security to facilitate emotional growth in children. Problems were seen to arise when parents entered into coalitions with their children, triangulating the child between them as a means of managing marital conflict or fears of intimacy.

Harris (1982) is one of the few clinicians to apply this model to intellectual disability. She postulated four types of structural deficits for behaviourists to consider when planning interventions. In one category, for example, a mother and child with a disability may be over-involved, with a father who appears distant and an older sibling. In another, a sibling might be parentified in support of the mother, while the father remains distant and uninvolved in family life. In both cases, Harris advised behaviourists to invite the father to serve as an expert consultant, valued for his objectivity, with the aim of supporting his wife to manage the behaviour, and in the second case, relieve the sibling of the parentified role.

Challenging behaviour from solution-focused and narrative perspectives

In the 1980s, de Shazer (1982) made a significant break from the systemic and structural models by proposing a *solution-focused approach* to family therapy. In particular, he was concerned that therapists were inadvertently pathologising clients, looking for dysfunction and deficits at the expense of solutions based on the amplification of pre-existing strengths. De Shazer believed that families needed support to recognise times when they had been successful in overcoming problems, both in the present and the past, experiences that could be garnered for the development of improved family life in the future. His model was revolutionary, in that it rejected notions of aetiology, seeing the cause of a problem as less critical. This view was an even more significant break with the tradition of psychoanalysis. Coles (2001) further argued that this was a crucial position if clinicians were to avoid seeing families as disabled themselves. Stainton and Besser (1998) conducted a qualitative study that seemed to support this notion. They asked families the question, 'What could the positive impact of intellectual disability be on your family?', and found that parents reported an increase in closeness, enhanced spirituality, and an increased involvement with the community. These findings suggested that one of the restrictions to effective behavioural intervention can sometimes be the clinician's own perspective of family functioning. Families have many strengths that need to be recognised and actively mobilised for successful outcomes.

Narrative therapy was developed by White and Epston (White, 1989; White & Epston, 1990). It has many conceptual similarities with solution-focused therapy, particularly when it comes to the rejection of the functionality of presenting problems. It differs, however, in that it is heavily influenced by social contructionism. As such, narrative therapy pays particular attention to the effect that dominant and oppressive societal stories can have in the development of problems in families. Goddard and colleagues (2000) and Gray (2001) argued that professionals can be complicit in the promulgation of these stories, with the emphasis on maternal enmeshment or chronic grief serving more as a means of control than an accurate account of the family's lived experience.

This can be particularly relevant when working with clients with intellectual disability who are violent to their parents and siblings. Fiddell (2000) raised the idea that there were parallels between the effects of this behaviour and domestic violence. Therapeutic practices that propose that family dysfunction is responsible for a client's challenging behaviour may have an abusive effect, amplifying parental guilt and self-blame and increasing the cycle of violence and disempowerment that can often prevail.

Narrative therapy, like solution-focused therapy, suggests that the position of the clinician needs to be evaluated when it comes to identifying impediments to the effective amelioration of challenging behaviour. From this perspective, clinicians need to be reflective about their own inadvertent participation in the subjugation of families, developing wariness about how the expert role may serve to obscure subtle abuses of power.

Integration of behavioural and family therapy approaches

The application of family therapy to understanding challenging behaviour in developmental disabilities demonstrates that the field has the potential to redress the balance between the comprehensive behavioural and ecological technologies available, and the limited consideration of mediation analysis. The aim of this chapter, of course, is not to argue for family therapy as an alternative to applied behaviour analysis, as no amount of systemic intervention could teach a client to communicate in a more adaptive manner or learn valued skills for independent living. Rather, the aim is to propose integration of approaches, where family therapy deals with constraints to change that improve the efficacy of the positive programming approach. A more comprehensive description of an integrative model for systemic and behavioural assessment and intervention can be found in Rhodes (2003), who described four stages of intervention:

1 Behavioural assessment following the *behaviour assessment guide* (Willis et al., 1993)
2 *Milan systemic family assessment and intervention* with the aim of isolating the homeostatic function of the behaviour (Selvini-Palazzoli et al., 1978)
3 *Amplification of small deviations in interactions* using solution-focused and narrative questions; facilitating morphogenesis, and further change from stuck patterns (Rhodes, 2008)
4 *Behavioural intervention,* including the development of a multi-element treatment plan underpinned by the principles of positive behaviour support.

What about the wider system?

One of the limitations of a pure family therapy approach to mediation analysis is its failure to consider the wider system. The sometimes overwhelming demands of caring for a child or adult with developmental disabilities mean that families are dependent on interactions and relationships with professional staff in schools, respite services, group homes, recreational facilities, case workers, and the wider governmental bureaucracies. Relationships within these services, and between them and the family, can sometimes become fraught, adding to the complexity of the clinician's role when considering interpersonal restraints to effective behavioural intervention. Problems are likely to arise during family lifecycle stages, when changes in one setting are at odds with those in another (Baum, 2006), leading to conflicting needs, beliefs, and expectations.

Imber-Black (1987) provided a rich set of systemic hypotheses to explore when considering patterns in the interactions between families and professional organisations. She suggested, for example, that problematic interactions could escalate in both complementary and symmetrical ways. In the first case, a family's helplessness can be matched with the professional's tendency to offer more and more help, until a myriad of unmanageable and sometimes unnecessary services become involved. This cycle needs to be broken by taking a proper account of the natural resources within the family, encouraging the use of these resources, and employing them in a collaborative planning process with professionals to ensure specific outcomes are achieved. A solution-focused perspective may be useful in these situations, as described earlier. In symmetrical patterns, values held by the family concerning the care of the client may be at odds with the service, leading to fierce struggles, blaming, and the eventual isolation of the family. Intervention needs to take conflicting values into account, focus on mediation, and, where necessary, challenge certain beliefs. Problems can, of course, be a great deal more complicated than those between two parties. Individuals within families and organisations can develop coalitions with one another, leading to triangulation, and a host of complex and restrictive interactions.

One of the most important tools that can be employed in these situations is a *sociogram* (Moreno, 1934), that can be used to map carefully all of the stakeholders involved. This allows clinicians to develop multiple hypotheses regarding potential to shift the presenting issue using systemic, structural, solution-focussed, and narrative lenses. The sociogram should include a genogram of the family as well as pictorial representations of other services. These services can be represented in a similar way to family genograms, where managers can be placed at the top, with staff and clients below. Relational markers, including close, conflictual, distant, enmeshed, and breached, can also be used to identify potential relationships (McGoldrick & Gerson, 1986). Hypothesising is best done with peers in a group situation, as it allows for the brainstorming of possible interpersonal restraints based on current information. It can also promote neutrality on the part of the clinician, reveal gaps in the system to guide further assessment, and eventually support the development of strategic plans to respond directly to the relational needs of the system.

Potential issues in group homes

In many situations the clinician may encounter obstacles to behavioural intervention in the group home setting alone. Clients may no longer be living in the home setting, necessitating a specific focus on this unique professional system. Group homes can sometimes be problematic, because of the blurred boundaries between the professional and personal roles of staff. Some may have been employed for many years, developing attachments with the client, who has few external sources of support. The high level of stress involved in responding to severe challenging behaviour may also affect interactions, causing breaches in attachment, the development of coalitions among staff, the erosion of authoritative leadership, or escalating symmetrical patterns of interaction between staff and behavioural consultants who present as if they know best.

Smyly (2006) provided an important overview of her work with group homes in her application of the systemic organisational approach of Campbell and colleagues (1994). Smyly was critical of the expert consultant role, and suggested that clinicians needed to engage group home staff in reflective conversations that allowed them to develop new ways of making sense of a client's challenging behaviour. Staff within a group home may be more likely to implement new strategies if they feel there has been a respectful collaboration, one that contextualises behaviour in terms of the lifecycle of the house itself, and one that assists them to find their own solutions, rather than the strategies being imposed from above. This principle is highly consistent with the solution-focused and narrative approaches described earlier. Rhodes (2000) suggested a variety of strategies that could be used by clinicians to assist in the process of group home consultation. These included:

- meeting with all staff at the same time for consultations rather than joining shifts where multiple perspectives are not possible
- spending time engaging with each staff member, including a review of his or her philosophy for working with intellectual disability and understanding of challenging behaviour
- assessing the onset of challenging behaviour with the staff using a detailed timeline of significant events in the house, including changes to staffing and residents, and difficulties with other clients
- using a sociogram to help staff review patterns of the effects of these events and on interactions that include the challenging behaviour
- gradually assisting staff to develop a new understanding of the meaning of the behaviour (as with the homeostatic function)
- conducting a behavioural assessment following the principles of the *behaviour assessment guide* (Willis et al., 1993). Many clinicians use this guide to develop a comprehensive written report that is then given to staff. It can be more useful to co-construct the intervention, based on the facilitated insights and ideas of the team with the written record representing this collaboration.

Conclusion

Family therapy has reached a degree of maturity in the field of generic child and adolescent mental health. There is growing evidence for the efficacy of family therapy (Carr, 2004), and an acceptance that it offers a rich set of skills that are fundamental to clinical practice in family settings. The field of intellectual disability has been relatively slow to respond to these developments (Rhodes, 2002), relying to a large degree on the behavioural approach and to a lesser degree on person-centred (Carr, 2004) and cognitive behavioural approaches (Dagnan et al., 2007). The aim of this chapter has been to advocate for the integration of family therapy with traditional behaviour modification approaches, not as an alternative to positive behaviour support, but as an augmentation that allows clinicians to respond more effectively to interactional and systemic constraints. Milan systemic, structural, solution-focused, and narrative models all provide a host of principles and strategies suited to this purpose.

13

Parents' perspectives

Louisa Carroll, Kate Tye, Karen Ollerenshaw, Yasemin Eris, and Judy Brewer

Introduction

Louisa Carroll

It has been both humbling and inspiring to edit this section, in which several parents share their stories. These powerful narratives are a testament to how the experiences of raising a child with a disability can bring out the extraordinary strength, love, persistence, and courage that these children need. These accounts also illustrate the extent to which professionals can work in partnership with parents, to help children with a disability grow.

Three of the narratives are about raising a young person with *Smith-Magenis syndrome (SMS)*. This is in part a chance event, but it reflects how biology and genetics are often the most important drivers of specific and very severe difficulties of development and behaviour. Society can be too ready to assume that it is the parents who are the cause of a child's challenging behaviour, and to attribute blame and censure accordingly. Communities have a duty to support such children and families with special needs, and yet so often they fail to understand the reality, let alone help.

While each of the stories reflects a different perspective and a different stage in the parenting journey, collectively, the works reveal some unifying themes. They are a reminder of the significance for families of their early contact with professionals regarding their child's difficulties, and the power of emotion that can be attached to the diagnostic experience even years after the event. They also capture the sense of relief and reassurance that stems from having a clear medical diagnosis, providing explanation for behavioural challenges and developmental differences that may previously have been carried by the parents as feelings of personal responsibility, guilt, or doubt. In particular, the third story highlights how improved information and understanding from an early age of the child with an extraordinary parent can promote developmental competencies and bring about more positive outcomes despite the evident biological differences. Support groups for particular behavioural phenotypes (such as SMS), which provide internet networks and information for parents and professionals, clearly also contribute to a platform of understanding for many children with a disability.

Another significant theme of this collection of stories is the importance and influence of emotional attachment and attunement of parents listening to their instincts, hearing the messages held within behaviours, and knowing, accommodating, and supporting their children's strengths, interests, and reactions. Patience is a really important part of this process—and the notion that in focusing and building on small steps, children's achievements over time can surpass expectations.

All the stories highlight the critical role that parents play as advocates for their children, and how instrumental this is in 'making things happen' and bringing about positive change. Each of the women who share their stories here are in their own ways heroes, and leaders in the critical challenge to communities to care for all children in society. In particular, the last of the stories in this section, by Judy Brewer, mother of a young man with autism, provides a compelling call to arms for advocacy for all children with an intellectual disability or autism spectrum disorder. Her leadership role on a national scale in advocating for services is truly inspiring, and a powerful demonstration of how a single voice can make a real difference. Many such advocates are needed to gain adequate community and political understanding and support for these families.

Finally, these stories can be placed in a broader social context. Families, generally, seem to be finding that bringing up children is getting harder and harder, with the increasing expectations of economic efficiency, and the demographic changes of modern society. This is illustrated in the dramatic increase in children presenting to emergency health services with psychiatric problems, being placed in care or in juvenile detention, or ending up as homeless youth; families who reach a crisis point and, in finding it all too hard, feel compelled to give up care of the children they love. There needs to be recognition that the clarion cry of individual freedom and responsibility, and economic self-sufficiency, are not possible for everyone in our society, and can undermine demands for much-needed community support services, knowledge, and skills.

These pressures of parenting are particularly salient for those raising children with the additional challenges of a disability. Expecting these individual families to carry the full burden of care is a fraught strategy, particularly for parents who are often already driven to desperation, and overwhelmed by their sense of responsibility for the future of their child. This makes the achievements of the following writers all the more remarkable, in having so successfully advocated for their children and thereby found access to a minimum of sufficient services.

The long road to diagnosis

Kate Tye

My husband Peter and I have a daughter, Emma-Raey, aged 19 years, who has Smith-Magenis syndrome. This is the story of our long road to diagnosis.

The long road

From the very beginning, Emma-Raey has had a somewhat difficult journey. She was born at 38 weeks after a 17½ hour labour with forceps delivery. At six weeks of age she experienced strange stiffening episodes, and before her first birthday she had suffered nine ear infections and perforations. She screamed often as a baby, and would not take to solid foods, continuing to breastfeed until she was 13 months old. She also had major difficulties with sleeping, and where the controlled crying technique is usually effective in teaching babies to self-settle, for Emma-Raey this only produced self-injurious hand-biting and further distress. We didn't know it then, but the specialist sleeping service that we went to when she was just 14 months old was to be just the first in a long line of professionals we would take Emma-Raey to see, on our 13-year journey to diagnosis.

By the time she was about 18 months of age, we recognised that Emma-Raey had significant developmental delays. Our paediatrician was sufficiently concerned to refer her to a child psychiatrist. After asking some questions (such as 'Does she line things up?' and 'Does she make eye contact?'), the child psychiatrist made a diagnosis of autism. Shortly after, we were referred to another paediatrician, who was renowned for helping with difficult 'toddler' behaviours. He pronounced Emma-Raey to be an 'enigma'—I think he was right! The paediatrician felt that we needed further psychiatric support, and referred us on to yet another specialist, whose area of interest was in developmental disabilities. We began a myriad of drugs to help Emma-Raey's lack of sleeping and challenging behaviours.

Meanwhile, Emma-Raey had started with early intervention services for children with special needs. From around three years of age she attended school, initially at a specialist autism school, then later in autism satellite classes, and support classes for children with intellectual disability. For high school she moved across to a special school for children with intellectual disabilities. Emma-Raey also continued to have an array of medical issues, including allergic rhinitis, bouts of vomiting, and high fevers requiring hospital stays.

It was during the late primary school years that Emma-Raey came under the care of an eminent psychiatrist at what is now The Children's Hospital at

Westmead, Sydney. At the time she was the youngest patient for whom he had ever prescribed lithium, and he would go on to look after Emma-Raey for about 10 years. It was this psychiatrist who, in July 2001, suggested that Emma-Raey should have a blood test to see if she had a chromosomal abnormality affecting chromosome 17: Smith-Magenis syndrome (SMS). One of his colleagues had written a paper on this syndrome, which is characterised by a recognisable pattern of physical, behavioural, and developmental features. The features reminded him of Emma-Raey. Although the exact incidence is not known, it is estimated that SMS occurs in one out of 25 000 births. At this stage, in Australia, only about 30 cases of SMS have been diagnosed. Three weeks after the blood test we were stunned to find out that Emma-Raey did indeed have Smith-Magenis syndrome. Some pieces of the puzzle began to be explained.

In March 2002, after a further nine-month wait, we were finally able to meet with a geneticist. She ordered the Baseline at Diagnosis comprehensive testing, which included a whole range of clinical evaluations. She told us about a website for parents and professionals with an interest in SMS. She also informed us of an upcoming conference in Denver that May, and about two other Australian families who were going. After a six-week scramble to fund raise, and a gift of two seats by Qantas, we were finally on our way. I think that conference was something of an awakening for us. There were 400 other delegates, including about 50 children and adults with SMS. Our eyes were on stalks as we watched these people doing all these bizarre things that we had been living with for 13 years. We felt as though Emma-Raey was finally normal there, among her own population.

After the diagnosis

Attending that first conference inspired us, and in 2003 we were fortunate to have the opportunity to tell our story at a seminar held at The Children's Hospital at Westmead. This was followed by a SMS camp at Camp Breakaway, on the central coast of New South Wales, where 21 families from all around Australia came together for the first time for respite and networking. We formed an Australian support group to replicate the warmth and support we had felt at the conference in Denver.

After another five years, Emma-Raey now attends a five-day-a-week community participation program in our local area. She has made a successful transition from school to work, and is well supported by the professional staff at the day program. We are currently preparing ourselves for residential placement for her in the future, knowing that we cannot parent this most difficult child on our own. We recently underwent a lengthy, unsuccessful transition to a group home, which fell through because of an incompatibility with the existing residents. This was an agonising investment of time and emotional energy both for Emma-Raey and the family. We are now awaiting another offer, and at least are more aware of what is involved for a successful transition for Emma-Raey.

The diagnosis of SMS puts an enormous amount of stress on our whole family, and has a huge impact on our emotional well-being. In addition to Emma-Raey, Peter and I have two sons, Bryce (17 years) and Kieren (12 years). I am thrilled to say they are healthy boys, good buddies, and extreme sportsmen. However, Bryce has suffered depression because of the impact of Emma-Raey's behaviours. Both boys have to fight off her violent attacks, and frequently witness their sister self-injure.

Both Peter and I also suffer from depression. The constancy of the battle of parenting Emma-Raey has really worn me down, and there are times when I feel at the end of the line in terms of my parenting capabilities. Even the task of getting Emma-Raey to cooperate and get ready for the day's activities can incur hours of mental, emotional, and physical strain. I also continue to feel a profound sense of loss of the 'what could have been?' for Emma-Raey: her education, career, and all the little steps along the way of her life's journey. There is the loss of my dream too, in particular, of the mother–daughter relationship I so craved, having lost my own mother as a young girl.

The future

I hope that our long road to diagnosis will not be repeated for other families. SMS was only reported in the 1980s, so I understand it was difficult to diagnose a child born in 1988 with such a rare condition. I am nonetheless sure there will be other children who have SMS who were misdiagnosed as on the 'fringe of autism'.

Looking to the future, I have taken on a professional role through which I will continue to lobby governments, both state and federal, for supported accommodation places that are in critical shortage for our adults with a disability. I look forward to an increased awareness of SMS and other disabilities in our community. I look forward to a time when we do not have to beg for services that are our children's human rights. I look forward to a safe, comfortable, stable place where my daughter can live. As for now, I can truly say I have done everything I could and needed to do for Emma-Raey.

Jay's story: a day in the life

Karen Ollerenshaw

My son Jay has Smith-Magenis syndrome (SMS). What this means for him is that he has a mild to moderate intellectual disability, moderate hearing impairment, severe sleeping disorder, and a severe behavioural disorder similar to autism. I first wrote this story about three years ago when he was 12, to speak at the inaugural Australian Smith-Magenis Syndrome Conference. As I went to update it this year, I realised that in many ways not a lot has changed.

A day in the life of Jay and our family

A typical day for Jay starts at 5 a.m., usually after two or three night-time awakenings. His first stop is the kitchen for a 'snack' of two bananas and eight slices of bread. Jay's appetite tends to be limited only by what he can get his hands on, so I've kept the other bananas and the rest of the loaf of bread stored away. He can spread his own honey or jam, but it's not only on his bread—so if we don't get up to supervise him we will wake to find honey dripping down the kitchen cupboards and into the drawers.

Jay then moves on to have a bath, which he loves because of the sensation of running water on his body. We again have the option of either supervising him, or else waking to the sound of water pouring out of the bathroom and onto the carpet. Having gone with the latter today, I busy myself with mopping up the bathroom, while Jay moves back into the kitchen for snack number two.

By now it's about 8 a.m. Tuna and baked beans are on the menu, and also on the kitchen floor, mixed with blood where Jay has cut himself opening the tins. Jay's siblings are now also awake, and taking Sam's cereal and Tiahn's toast provides Jay with his entertainment for the next half-hour. Our next challenge is to get dressed for school, which Sam and Tiahn manage fine, but which Jay takes as his cue to get back in the bath.

The phone rings. It is a school offering me a day's work (I am a casual teacher), and I immediately accept, as I know we need the money to pay for things like getting the TV fixed, or replacing the video or computer that are not working on account of Jay. Just as I am about to take down the details for the job, Jay with his moderate hearing loss realises I am on the phone and comes bounding out of the bath dripping wet, yelling at me in his gruff SMS voice and with that look in his eye, 'Get off!', 'Hang up!' . He then hangs up the phone, and runs over and reefs the cord out of the wall. Suffice to say the telephone has always been something of a trigger for Jay.

I then see Jay's taxi pulling into the driveway. As usual, Jay is still in the nude at this point, so I help him to get dressed and take his medication. When it comes to his shoes, I find he has again tied his shoelaces into knots on top of knots. I had undone yesterday's knots earlier so that we wouldn't be late for school, but he has managed to do them up again. Fortunately I have learnt to keep well stocked with laces, so I am able to cut the old ones out and replace them with new ones.

Finally ready for school, Jay compliantly gets into his taxi. This feels too good to be true, and sure enough, as I am about to breath a sigh of relief, Jay announces, 'Not going to school today', and proceeds to take off his shoes and throw them, just missing the driver and the other children in the taxi. He looks like he is starting to calm down, then, all of a sudden, he undoes his seatbelt, climbs over two other children, and runs up the street stripping off his clothes as he goes.

As I chase Jay up the street, I resolve that I am not going to get him to school today, and if I do, he will only get suspended for his behaviour. So, with the other children with disabilities now distraught, I send his taxi off without him. Feeling on edge and in tears, I then secretly use the phone to cancel my own day's work, while my nine-year-old, Sam, takes his little sister inside and gets her ready for school.

The part that really breaks my heart is that afterwards, Sam meekly comes up to me and says, 'Mum, do you want me to stay home and help you with Jay?' I put on a brave face and say that I will be okay, but wonder how on earth I am going to get through the day. Jay has in the meantime gone to his room, put on 'play clothes', and is sitting happily at the Play Station. I begrudgingly marvel at the power of not going to school as a motivation for independent dressing skills. Surprisingly, that particular day didn't end up being too bad, but if you can imagine repeating that for days or sometimes weeks on end, you will have some sense of the incredible stress that having a child with Smith-Magenis syndrome can put onto families.

Jay, his family, and the future

A few years have since passed, and Jay is now turning 15. He is 170 centimetres tall and weighs over 70 kilograms. He is much bigger than me, and because of his size and strength he is now more difficult to manage. Some of Jay's behaviours have improved, however, he still has major meltdowns over all sorts of random things. One description that has always stayed in my mind is that he is 'predictably unpredictable'. Just when we think he is settled and in a good mood, he can change and explode over something silly, while other times when we think he will not cope with something, he can be wonderfully behaved.

We remain sleep deprived, stressed, and overworked as carers, and it feels like we experience every emotion possible. There is fear of the future and what will happen to Jay, and hate of not being able to fix things, and of people who don't even try to understand. There is also grief, grieving for the child that Jay might have been had he had one tiny extra piece of chromosome 17, and grieving every time I see other children his age reaching milestones that he will never reach. Even his siblings reaching milestones or overtaking him causes mixed feelings for me. But there is also joy. The joy of every small achievement or watching Jay laugh or play on a good day; all the funny things he says; when he hugs me with all his might; gives me the sloppiest kiss ever, and tells me that he wants to marry me. In short, parenting Jay has been busy, funny, happy, exhausting, frustrating, emotional, and scary, but never, ever dull.

We love Jay. Part of our life is accepting that our life is crazy and that we will never know what will happen next. I have learned to speak up, to ask for help, have had to actively seek out the best care and education for my child, and be the squeakiest wheel around. Most of all, as a family we have learned to accept Jay and the challenges that he brings, and to love him unconditionally, just as he does us.

A story about my journey so far with Smith-Magenis syndrome

Yasemin Eris

If there's one date that's permanently etched in my memory, it is 17 August 2007. I'll never forget that date. That was the day we found out that Leyla had Smith-Magenis syndrome (SMS). Her paediatrician had called me the afternoon before, and I could tell from his voice there was something wrong. I remember thinking, 'This must be bad', and 'Please just tell me if she's going to die'. But of course he couldn't tell me anything over the phone, just that I needed to come in to see him. I wanted to go in straight away, but the earliest we could see him was the next morning. I didn't sleep at all that night—my head was sick with the worry.

I went to the appointment with my sister. I didn't even tell my husband; I couldn't. When the paediatrician told me that the Leyla had SMS, I just thought to myself, 'No way!' I was in complete denial: she hasn't got that; she must have something else. I can remember the doctor telling us how the diagnosis helped to explain the pattern of difficulties we were seeing for Leyla. But all I could think was, 'You must have got it wrong. Can we get her re-tested?' I remember looking at my sister with tears in my eyes, and seeing her looking back at me, her eyes filled with tears too. This isn't happening; this isn't real.

We went home and called the family. Everyone came home immediately, and we googled 'Smith-Magenis syndrome' on the internet. It was only when we started reading, when everything we read was describing Leyla perfectly, that I knew it was true. The period after that is a bit of a blur for me. I know I cried—for two, three, four weeks, maybe more. But at some point something inside me clicked and I said to myself, 'You have to stop crying and get on with it. You have to stop this and help her.'

What helped me to cope in those early days was to have a clear purpose. I wanted to know anything and everything that I could. I wanted to be prepared. I took Leyla to see specialist after specialist, and we checked her eyes, ears, kidneys, and cholesterol. She had grommets inserted, and we started with physiotherapy and speech therapy. That sense of doing something, of taking action rather than being victim, really helped me get through that initial difficult period.

I also learnt early on to trust my own judgment with Leyla. I remember going to a special service to learn about how to manage sleeping difficulties with babies, where they taught us about controlled crying. I know this works for some children, but for Leyla, leaving her in the bed and walking out was not a good thing. It totally stressed her out, and it didn't seem to help with her sleeping at all. After she'd vomited 15 times in one night because of her distress, I realised that I needed to accept my expertise as her mum, and listen to my instincts more. I had to teach her things the way she wanted to be taught to incorporate how she learned into how I handled things. I needed to be responsive to her needs, and Leyla's needs were for affection and adult attention.

So, rather than leaving her alone to cry, I started staying with Leyla to help her settle, and would hold her hand through the night. At first, I slept alongside her cot, and would let go of her hand just before she awoke at 5 a.m. Then gradually, I started slipping away earlier and earlier, 4 a.m., 3 a.m., 2 a.m., to return to my room. Sometimes she would wake up and cry for me, and I would go in to soothe her. As she learnt to understand more language, I could explain, 'Mummy's not going to come back in now'; 'Mummy will come in when you hear the birds'. Her problems of deferring demands also reflect her lack of understanding of time. I guess it also helped that she was in a bed that she couldn't get out of by herself. It took us nearly a year of hard work to get there, but now Leyla can get through the night without me there. I know she often wakes up, because I can hear her talking to herself, but she knows not to call for me until the birds start singing, which is usually around 6 a.m.

There are many things that I say to myself when times are difficult. When we're grappling with a new challenge or new strategy, I'll tell myself, 'It's going to work', 'I know I'm doing the right thing', and I think about it working, and how beneficial that will be. Like her sleeping, for example—it was hard, but I knew how positive it would be for her to be sleeping properly, and also how positive and beneficial her sleeping well would be for the whole family.

I guess the other thing that has really helped us to cope as a family is to maintain Leyla's routine. She needs to be in bed by 7:30 p.m., and then it's a real family effort to keep things quiet so that she's not disturbed. It's a bit of an adjustment, and sometimes I worry how it affects her baby brother. I hope that by learning to be considerate of Leyla now, when he's so little, her brother will then grow up to be compassionate and understanding of other children who are sick or have disabilities.

We do still take holidays and break the routine sometimes. For example, we went camping for a week last year, sleeping in tents, and we're about to go up north for a week-long holiday on the Gold Coast. We prepare for this by knowing that it's going to be unsettling for Leyla and expecting that. We also know, and expect, that it will take her a couple of weeks to get back to normal once we get home. But it's also important to us as a family that we don't stop doing everything that we used to do just because of Leyla's difficulties. So, it's harder than it would be, but we still do it, and we still enjoy it.

As for other thoughts I would share with families facing our situation? I guess: be patient, *really patient*; take it slow. Try not to get upset when they're upset; be two steps ahead of them and be the strongest person you can be to handle them. There will be times when you want to have a tantrum yourself. You'll have times where you're going to tear your hair out and that's okay. Don't let yourself think it's the end of the world—it gets better. Don't let yourself believe that your child can't do things. Keep hope.

Leyla has many different problems that need different approaches. My husband and I learned key word sign language (Makaton), which helped promote her language development. She now understands most single instructions, and has short functional sentences such as 'I love you Mummy'. Leyla also had low muscle tone, which has improved with swimming lessons. She loves peek-a-boo, cuddles, rough and tumble play with adults, breaking eggs and mixing cakes, and painting at the mainstream preschool she attends two days a week.

Leyla has limited social skills with other children, but likes to have attention and be around others. She has learned to cuddle her toy baby as part of teaching her to be calm and gentle with her baby brother. What some would call attention deficit hyperactivity disorder (ADHD), I see as attention and affection hunger, and it is important to always respond to her needs. This makes it very time demanding and exhausting caring for Leyla.

I've also learnt to be prepared. I've done lots of reading and research, and I'm really aware of what might be coming: behaviours such as twirling around, head banging, hurting herself, putting things into her ears, and so on. I know that being a teenager will be hard. But knowing that these things might be coming helps me prepare. As soon as I see a behaviour beginning, I can intervene really early to try to stop it. She used to bite at her fingers, really hard sometimes, leaving blisters and bleeding. I had to be very strict with her, let her know that I didn't like it, and wouldn't tolerate it. Even then, it took me nearly a year to get her to stop altogether—but she did! I also cut her nails really short every second day so she wouldn't have the opportunity to pull at or bite them—because I know this can be a problem behaviour for some kids with SMS.

Another thing is to be firm, consistent, and persistent. I remember Leyla went through a phase where she was playing with her poo: it was a terrible month! Every morning I would come into her room and I could smell it straight away. Cleaning it all up was pretty awful, and I could sometimes feel myself becoming frustrated and upset with it all. But again, I got in early. I reminded myself to take it easy; calm down; she's going to stop it; I know she is. Believing this was the first step to making it happen. Again, I got to thinking about Leyla's strengths. I knew she loved attention and affection, and I knew she was quite good at seeing how I was feeling. So I made it very clear when I went into her room on those mornings that it was not okay—so that she knew that I wasn't happy and that she was doing something wrong. I made sure she knew that I was upset: 'We don't do that, Leyla; that's yucky.' After a while, when I went in, she would make a sad face and question 'Mummy?' Then I knew that she knew that I was upset, and she didn't like that. A few days later I went into her room in the morning, Leyla turned to me and smiled, 'Mummy look, clean hands'. I was really proud of Leyla that day and so pleased, not only because she had stopped playing with her poo, but also because it was a good lesson for her, helping her to learn some self-control.

But my most important advice or suggestion would be to have help—*accept help*. Having a child with SMS is hard, *very hard*. Your child will need you 24 hours a day—so you too will need a lot of support. That's where my family has been fantastic. They have been wonderfully supportive, both emotionally and just in helping out with things. They will drop everything and come to help, and have always been there for me. My mother is my everything. I can't imagine if I was trying to do this on my own.

And of the future? Thinking about the future can still be hard. The not-knowing is difficult. I try to hope for the best—but I know, because of the way she is, it's not going to be normal (whatever normal is!). I do still cry sometimes, and wonder 'Why me? Why my child?' But I know it's not going to change anything. Every parent has those normal dreams—you want your child to go to uni, get married, and have children. I try to be realistic. But I also want to stay positive, and sometimes that means trying not to think or worry about the future too much, and just take it one step at a time. This makes it much easier to deal with. At the moment, we are only looking as far ahead as school; we want Leyla to start at a normal school.

I'm hoping Leyla will keep doing as well as she is now. If she keeps doing this well, I know she'll be all right, and I'll be okay too. I make goals I know she can achieve, and when she achieves those, I set higher ones. It's always small steps, small steps forward. But she's already surprising me; she's surprising everyone—for example, with how well she sleeps. She's already achieved so much more than we dared to hope 12 months ago, and this gives me optimism and hope.

And for me? I've come to believe that there's a reason for everything—for experiencing this. I know that having Leyla has brought out strengths in me, such as my determination and resilience. I didn't think I was this strong before. I know now that I'm a strong person, and a patient person, you have to be, and that's something that Leyla has taught me. I'm also a very loving person, and Leyla really needs that love and attention from me—she thrives on it. She loves to be hugged and kissed, and that's something I can do that makes her feel good. She knows that I love her so much, and that demonstrating this to her is a way to make her happy.

There have been other rewards, too. Leyla loves you unconditionally, no matter what happens. She's very affectionate. Her difficulties have helped me realise that you should be grateful for your health. You don't really think about that side of things until you're faced with it. So yes, I feel grateful—I thank God everyday for her. Some mornings when I wake up, I guess I can struggle a little; it's 5 o'clock in the morning, she's awake, and I'm grumpy and thinking about how difficult it all is. But then I go into her room, and there's this child there, smiling at me, reaching out to hug me, and saying, 'Mummy, I love you'. It floods me with tears when she tells me that, because I never thought I'd hear her say it. It's the best way to wake up—it makes it all worth it.

Advocacy is not a choice, it is a must

Judy Brewer

Grief was the first emotion I felt when I found out my son had a disability. This was followed by a painful cycle of grieving for the child that I imagined I would have, while making the huge adjustment that is involved in raising a child with extra needs. People around me reacted in various ways. Some were supportive, some ignored me for fear of not knowing what the right thing to say was, and others tried to comfort me with a variety of platitudes.

The most useful advice for me was to grieve; yes, because something had been lost, but to remember also that something had been found. As Emily Perl Kingsley (1987) attested in her beautiful piece called *Welcome to Holland*: after you've been there a while and you catch your breath, you look around and begin to notice that while it is not the place you dreamed of, it has its own special things as well.

Your response to this new challenge is your choice. You can continue to grieve and blame the world for its unfairness, wait for others to step in and do the work, or you can vow to move on so that you can put every ounce of your energy into finding the resources and supports that your child and your family are going to need to get through the years ahead. As a parent of a 16-year-old son with autism, as someone who lost far too much time in the grieving process, I recommend the latter.

I imagined a range of services kicking in, swooping my son up into various therapies and treatments that would give him the best start in life.

When my husband and I first heard those words, 'I think your son has autism', I tempered the shock with the thought that at least now we knew what the issue was; there would be an answer. I imagined a range of services kicking in, swooping my son up into various therapies and treatments that would give him the best start in life. Unfortunately, as all disability families know, this is never the case.

In frustration, I said to the psychologist who was our first professional of a very long line, 'Who is going to help us?' He answered '*You!* You are your son's best advocate.' Over the years since, this has proved to be true. In order to give our son the best chance at life, I have had to become something of an expert on autism. I have had to read, attend seminars, trawl the internet, and make connections with other families and professionals to learn the latest evidence-based treatments, and also to get the family support that we have needed to survive.

While there have been many ups and downs, and many stresses over this time, the one thing that has been constant has been our son's progress.

He has slowly achieved many milestones, and our goalposts continue to be moved as he now copes with mainstream secondary school and a vocational plan for the future. Perhaps this is being unrealistic, but I choose to keep the dream alive always, so that I have the motivation to continue to advocate for my son until maybe he can one day advocate for himself. This is not easy, but it is important.

The grief may never truly go, and life may never be as easy as I wished it would be, but the joy of seeing my child grow and find his own place in the world will make some of the sacrifice worthwhile.

But this is not how it should be in a country like Australia in 2011. My husband and I are among the lucky ones, in that we only have two children, and we have stable employment. Yet advocating for services for our child has many times taken us to the brink of despair. The enormous burden of caring can be too much for many families to cope with. To be not only a parent but a carer, teacher, therapist, and then an advocate as well: it is an enormous load for anyone to bear.

Before I entered the world of disability, I held this illusion of a caring society that provides adequate supports for families so that they can spend their time loving their children and not being exhausted through perpetual fighting for limited services. We need to make this illusion a reality. We need to make sure that a system of disability support is created. A system that provides for all children and adults, whether or not their family have the means and energy to seek out the care they need.

We need to work to see the phrase 'unmet need' obliterated from every disability report that the government tables.

We need to work together with other families, with service providers, professionals, bureaucrats, and parliamentarians to make equity and equality of opportunity for all a key priority of every policy initiative. That is the sort of Australia I dream of. That is the sort of future I want for my son, and for all the sons and daughters of families that have found themselves travelling down the road less travelled.

That is why all of us must find the time to advocate, not just for our own children but for all those who face life with additional challenges. Whether we are a family member or a professional, we have a role in building a different and easier path for those that follow us.

Please find the time to get involved.

Part 3

Interventions to promote skill development

14

Using a sensory diet to mediate behaviours of concern and to increase children's participation in daily activities

Lucinda Mora and Chris Chapparo

Introduction

The behaviour of children with a disability is complex. One possible contribution to the amelioration of problem behaviour that is not well understood is *sensory defensiveness*. This term refers to the way in which some children process non-noxious sensory input in everyday tasks as threatening. This qualitative study examined the impact of one type of intervention, *the sensory diet*, on reducing sensory defensiveness. Parents reported that positive changes to behaviour and increased participation in daily activity were easily achieved by purposefully scheduling a minimum of eight sensory-based activities into the day. This change was most likely to occur when using additional proprioceptive- (joint) and vestibular-(movement) based activities as part of the child's daily sensory experience.

The findings in this study describe the use of sensory diets from parent reports that were part of data collected for a pilot study. The study examined the impact of using a sensory intervention within a home context to improve behavioural responses and functional outcomes for children with a disability, behaviour problems, and sensory defensiveness. In this chapter, an overview of sensory-processing disorder and its impact on behaviour is presented, as well as a description of a sensory diet, and a rationale and current evidence to support its use. The qualities and components that were common across sensory diets used with 17 children will be described, and a case example will be used to demonstrate the clinical application in a home context.

Background to the study

Children with a disability and behaviour problems are a vulnerable group that is increasing in size within society. Prevalence studies report that 40 per cent of children and young people with intellectual disability experience severe behaviour and emotional problems (Emerson, 2003a). Behavioural intervention for this group of children predominantly focuses on home and school function. The relationship between problem behaviours (self-injury and stereotypy) and environmental situations that prompt those behaviours consists of a complex variety of contributing factors (O'Neill et al., 1990; Willis et al., 1993; Sameroff, 2000). One possible contribution to problem behaviour that is not well understood is the inability of some children to process sensory input that is inherent in a task (Ahn et al., 2004; Trott, 2002).

While many children with a disability have typical reactions to the sensory inputs of everyday life, some appear to interpret everyday sensations as threatening or noxious, showing signs of sensory-processing disorder (SPD) (Baranek et al., 2007; Dunn, 1999; Wilbarger & Wilbarger, 2002). The consequence is an extreme behavioural response to sensory dimensions of everyday tasks such as bathing, eating, and dressing, referred to as *sensory defensiveness*. Activities people think ought to come naturally to children, such as playing, making friends, doing schoolwork, and responding to a hug, are a struggle, and may contribute to social, emotional, personal, and learning problems. When sensory-processing styles are extreme, the ability of children to do their daily routines, tasks, and activities at home and school is compromised. This has been referred to as a *sensory-processing disorder (SPD)* (Miller et al., 2001), and the impact of this disorder on children and their families is substantial.

Parenting children who have an intellectual disability as well as sensory-processing disorder is difficult, and specific guidance to assist children and families to cope with everyday sensations is required (Cermak & Daunhauer, 1997; Mangeot et al., 2001; Murray-Slutsky & Paris, 2005; Reynolds & Lane, 2008; Schaaf et al., 2003; Schneider et al., 2008; Talay-Ongan & Wood, 2000). There is growing support for the use of a sensory-processing approach for such children and adults with intellectual disability (Baranek et al., 1997; Bright et al., 1981; Moore & Henry, 2002; Reisman & Hanschu, 1992; Soper & Thorley, 1996; Stagnitti et al., 1999; Wilbarger & Wilbarger, 2002).

Sensory-processing disorder (SPD)

The ability to process sensory information begins before birth, and continues to develop and adapt throughout life. The most rapid development occurs in early childhood. As a child's central nervous system matures, so do the sensory systems. Each of the senses develops at its own rate, but by the time a child enters preschool, children have learned to differentiate types of touch, visual, and auditory inputs, and regulate their responses to them. There is a wide range of what could be considered 'typical' responses to inputs. Genetics and environmental influences, as well as health and disability, play a huge role in how children respond to different types of sensory input (Williamson & Anzalone, 2001). While everyone experiences the occasional problem with processing sensory information, most people learn how to adjust and manage so that they can complete everyday tasks. Children with SPD are deficient in their ability to suppress (filter out) repeated or irrelevant sensory input, and fail to regulate selectively the sensitivity of cortical responses to additional incoming sensory stimuli (Davies & Gavin, 2007).

Children classified as having SPD by therapists are significantly different from their age-matched peers. Studies have shown that parents of children with SPD report aberrant behaviors that were prompted by specific everyday sensory events, whereas parents of children who appeared to be processing sensory inputs typically did not. Validity for these behavioural observations has been provided by electroencephalographic measures. These have shown differences between the two groups of children, with children with SPD displaying deficiencies in their ability to suppress repeated or irrelevant sensory input and their ability to selectively regulate the sensitivity of cortical responses to additional incoming sensory stimuli (Davies & Gavin, 2007). The decreased ability of children with SPD to suppress irrelevant stimuli is thought to contribute to behavioural manifestations such as distraction, impulsiveness, abnormal activity level, disorganisation, anxiety, and emotional lability (Cohn et al., 2000; Miller et al., 2001).

There is a significant relationship between sensory filtering and age, with researchers inferring that regulation of sensory inputs improves as children mature (Davies & Gavin, 2007; Freedman et al., 1987; Marshall et al., 2004). Alternatively, the sensitivity of children with SPD does not appear to change as a function of either biologically driven maturity (as during physical growth) or the accumulation of experiences across time (during learning), with children appearing to remain either *hyper*responsive or *hypo*responsive to sensory inputs occurring during everyday activity (Hanft et al., 2000; McIntosh et al., 1999).

Although occupational therapy using various sensory-based approaches has been trialled with children who have sensory-processing disorders, evidence supporting the effectiveness is controversial and inconclusive (Foss et al., 2003; Mulligan, 2003; Schaaf & Nightlinger, 2007). This has been partly a result of the heterogeneity of the populations studied, poor adherence to the principles of the particular sensory approach used, and use of research methodologies and outcome measures that do not assess functions that are most closely linked to regulation of sensation. Few studies have measured the impact of a sensory-based approach to behavioural management on aspects of home and family life that are important to individual children and parents. No studies reviewed before this pilot study measured outcomes of a sensory-based intervention that incorporated therapressure and sensory diet components and had been implemented by parents within the home context.

What is a sensory diet?

A sensory diet is one type of sensory-based intervention that has been widely used by occupational therapists to modify the effects of SPD in children. The term *sensory diet* was coined by Wilbarger (1984) to describe a strategy for developing individualised programs that provided planned and scheduled activities to address a person's sensory needs, so that behaviour remains purposeful. The term sensory diet uses a nutritional diet as a metaphor. That is, just as a nutritional diet involves three main meals a day with snacks in between and involves special knowledge about many complex factors, so does a sensory diet (Wilbarger, 1995). The purpose is to help children function better in a sensory world. All people require a unique amount and type of sensory input in order to maintain an optimal level of arousal, to regulate their mood and to perform their daily activities (Wilbarger & Wilbarger, 1991). Each person's diet will vary according to his or her goals, preferences, resources, and limitations. A sensory diet is considered an ecological approach to behavioural management, and requires collaboration between children, parents, therapists, and others. It is designed to be used in context, and in conjunction with other planned daily activities.

The way a person responds to sensory input is also unique. Some children crave sensory experiences, while others interpret sensory input as threatening (Dunn, 1999; Wilbarger & Wilbarger, 1991). The way children perceive sensory experiences can have an impact on their ability to engage in activities of daily living. Some may enjoy the sensory experience life offers, while others may be fearful about experiences that most people consider to be everyday, such as brushing one's hair. By understanding the sensory aspects of activities people seek out or avoid, clinicians can begin to understand people's behaviour from the perspective of their unconscious or conscious attempts to meet their sensory needs. Activities can either be reorganised or supplemented to ensure that a person is getting the right amount of sensory input during his or her day in order to be calm, concentrate, regulate mood, and participate in daily life. Central to the qualitative assessment of responses to sensory inputs and the need for a sensory diet are the answers to the following questions:

- Is there a *sensory contribution* to the child's presenting *anxiety, avoidance or hyperreactivity*?
- Is there a *sensory contribution* to the child's *intolerance to everyday objects* such as clothing and textured food?
- Is there a relationship between *responses to sensation* and *the family's struggle* to deal with the child within the daily routine (such as hypersensitivity)?

- Is there a *pattern of sensory preferences* across sensory modalities?

The Wilbargers (1995; 2007) have found that some sensory-based activities act like snacks to change a person's mood or arousal levels quickly and for a short duration, in a similar way to having a small snack between meals. Other activities are thought to have longer-lasting effects on mood and daily performance. The time of day when each person does sensory-based activities will also have an effect on how well he or she is able to stay calm and engage in everyday life. Thus the timing, duration, and intensity of activities throughout the day influences how easily people are able to stay calm, concentrate, and regulate their emotional state.

Components of a sensory diet

The Wilbargers (1991) recommended six components to be included in a sensory diet:

1 All activities in a sensory diet are prescribed after an indepth assessment of the child's context, sensory preferences, and needs.
2 All activities should occur naturally within the child's ecology, and should be sustainable.
3 Specific time-orientated activity routines—sensory-based activities—are prescribed: they can be done in a short time and repeated periodically throughout the day.
4 Changes in routines and interactions—consistent routines—are developed to increase predictability for the child, prepare for upcoming events, and help to seek out opportunities for sensory experiences that provide long-lasting effects. Clinicians also need to remain aware that interactions with people generate a lot of potentially disruptive sensory input for the child, in the form of voice, odours, eye contact, and touch.
5 Environmental adaptation—safe play—areas are created to provide spaces where the child can go if overstimulated and reduce disruptive stimulation.
6 Participation in play and leisure activities should meet the child's sensory needs; that is, clinicians need to determine what the sensory qualities of different activities are in terms of cost and benefit and assist the child to engage in these.

Senses utilised in sensory diet programs

Sensory diet programs employ the use of a child's senses—proprioceptive, vestibular, tactile, oral, auditory, and visual—based on his or her sensory preferences and needs. In order to have an understanding of the relevance of the different senses in a sensory diet, the function of each sense is outlined below:

- *Proprioception* is the sense that provides information about limb position, limb movement, and force (Kandel et al., 2000). This input relies on information from muscle, joint, and skin receptors.
- The *sense of movement and gravity* provides information about head movement through receptors in the vestibular labyrinth located in the inner ear. These receptors are activated by movement of the head and by gravity (Kandel et al., 2000).
- The *tactile sense* provides information about the environment via receptors located in the skin. It alerts a person to danger, and provides information about the qualities of objects in the environment (Kandel et al., 2000).
- *Oral structures* rely on several different senses working together to make sense of information in the mouth. It relies on the *gustatory, olfactory, proprioceptive and tactile systems* to provide information about texture, taste, pressure, vibration, movement, temperature, and pain. The nose receives olfactory information. and interprets whether the odour is a safe or noxious substance (School Therapy Services, 2001).
- *Vision* is the sense that detects visual images, and the eyes are the sensory receptors. The eyes take in information from the environment about the contrast between light and dark, colour and movement. Vision enables individuals to evaluate the environment, and recognise similarities and differences between object forms, sizes, and positions (Kandel et al., 2000; School Therapy Services, 2001).
- *Auditory information* is received through receptors located in the outer and inner ear, and is stimulated by noise and sound information. It receives information about volume, pitch, and rhythm. It enables individuals to distinguish between similar sounds, recall what is heard, and assists in the development of communication and literacy skills (Kandel et al., 2000; School Therapy Services, 2001).

Methodology

Study design

This study used two qualitative methods to address the following research questions:

1. How many and what *activities* were used in each sensory diet?
2. What were the *sensory qualities* of the activities?
3. *Who* implemented the intervention?
4. What *environments* was the intervention used in?
5. What were the therapeutic *goals* for the participants?

6 What *area of life* was the goal targeting?

First, a *directed qualitative content analysis* was used (Busch et al., 2005; Carley, 1993; Hsieh & Shannon, 2005; Minichiello et al., 1995) to examine themes in the documentation of sensory diets that were implemented by parents of children with intellectual disability and SPD. Content analysis is a way to understand qualitative data in the form of written text by counting the frequency with which words or concepts occur or are implied, and by the interpretive coding of data (Krippendorff, 2004). To conduct a directed content analysis, predefined concepts were developed for this study from research about sensory-processing disorder and use of sensory diets, and from terms that appear in italics in the research questions listed above (Hsieh & Shannon, 2005).

Second, a *qualitative critical case study* was used to further describe the use of sensory diets (Yin, 2003). Case study research designs have been acknowledged to contribute important information to the understanding of parenting issues and the behaviour of children with intellectual disability. In some instances they are the preferred method of determining intervention impact, because group methodologies do not yield the type of qualitative information sought from heterogeneous populations (such as children and families) and contexts (such as unique home environments) (Nott & Chapparo, 2008; Swan & Alderman, 2004). The case study is suited to situations where little is known about a new phenomenon (such as SPD and sensory diets), when studying problems in a real-life context (such as homes), and involving a number of complex human factors (such as intellectual disability and sensory defensiveness) (Salimen et al., 2006). Directed content analysis and case study methodology are being used in conjunction with randomised controlled trial methodology as part of a larger study that examines the impact of the sensory protocol in comparison to behavioural intervention in this group of children and parents (Chapparo & Mora, 2008).

The qualitative methods reported here have afforded the researchers a qualitative analysis of aspects of intervention outcomes and perceived changes in children's behaviour as a consequence of this particular sensory-based intervention that was not offered by quantitative approaches alone. Although the qualitative content analysis and case study approaches do not allow generalisation of findings, the findings further inform the results of quantitative analysis, the direction of research, and current clinical practice by describing both problems experienced by children with SPD and their parents, and what they perceived as useful solutions.

Participants

Seventeen children participated in the study. All were clients of Ageing, Disability and Home Care (ADHC), Department of Human Services NSW, and were receiving occupational therapy services. The age of the children ranged between 4½ to 11 years, with a mean age of 6½ years. Fifteen of the children were male and two were female. Three of the children had a mild intellectual disability, 10 of the children had a moderate intellectual disability, and four had a severe intellectual disability. Twelve out of the 17 children had a diagnosis of autism. Several of the children's experiences have been used to illustrate concepts relating to sensory diets. These children, Lachlan, Ted, Emilio, Jeremy, Ian, Milly, and Peter (pseudonyms used), lived at home with their families, and were assessed by therapists as experiencing sensory-processing disorder, characterised by severe sensory defensiveness.

Sensory diet intervention

The sensory diet intervention was designed to be used for a period of 6 to 12 weeks. It was refined in the first week, then monitored fortnightly. Interventions were activity based, and were scheduled into the children's daily routines to:

- provide additional sensory input, such as an arm wrestle at morning tea time
- prepare a child for a forthcoming event or interaction, such as wearing a weighted backpack to enter school
- provide a space where the child could go when overwhelmed, such as a rolling wheel
- provide participation in play activities, such as a climbing frame at the playground.

Table 14.1 outlines the interventions used in the sensory diets, categorised according to the primary sense used.

Data collection methods

Sensory diets

Data about individualised sensory diets were obtained for the 17 child participants. Each sensory diet had been generated by an occupational therapist trained in the sensory diet intervention, in collaboration with the parent or adult caregiver. The sensory diets were two pages long on average. The first page outlined the daily routine and the second page provided detailed descriptions of the sensory activities. As each sensory diet was developed within the context of a daily routine, sensory activities occurred at scheduled times and with key daily events; for example, at breakfast time a child would be given crunchy cereal.

Content analysis

Codes were generated for the content of the diets according to frequency of appearance of sensory activities, and according to the underpinning theoretical framework of sensory processing. Comparisons between the 17 sensory diets were made.

Table 14.1 Sensory diet interventions

Proprioception	
Being squashed by ball	Stomp feet
Squashing with pillow	Firm hugs
Wrap up and squeeze in blanket	Hand and foot massage
Pulling and pushing	Electric massager on hands and face
Swimming	Wipes table down with warm water
Arm wrestle	Spray from squeeze bottle
Climbing frame at playground	Sit on vibrating cushion to eat or travel
To bed with weighted blanket	Rough and tumble play
Sit to eat with weighted vest on	Popping bubble wrap
Carry weighted backpack to school	Firm rubdown with towel after wash
Sit with weighted lap bag	Sit among large, firm cushions
Animal walks to table	Running
Firm touch on head/shoulders	Jumping
Carries heavy objects	Walk the dog
Lift heavy objects	Crash on cushions
Action songs	
Vestibular	
Rolling on ball	Sit on moveable cushion to eat or do tasks
Bouncing on ball	Trolley ride at shops
Go in rolling wheel	Ride on scooter board
Going down slide	Dancing
Swinging	Riding scooter
Trampoline/mini-trampoline	Bike riding and tricycle
Rocking chair	
Tactile	
Messy play with shaving cream, dough	Play with hand fidget toys
Stand at back of line and get space	Push open newspaper door at school
Foot spa	Light touch on arm
Oral	
Eating chewy and crunchy food	Drink using straw
Use electric toothbrush	Blow toys
Chew toys	
Visual	
Increase light	Decrease light
Auditory	
Listen to music	

Behaviours of concern

The children's parents identified behaviours of concern and functional activities in which they hoped to see a change after implementation of the sensory intervention. Changes in the children's behaviour were obtained from documents that employed *goal attainment scaling (GAS)* (Kiresuk & Sherman, 1968) to measure the extent and direction of change. The descriptive content of behavioural change was reviewed in relation to this study, and is reported below. Quantitative results from GAS statistical analyses are reported elsewhere (Chapparo & Mora, 2008).

Findings

The findings of the study are presented below. It should be noted that the sensory diet was only one component of the intervention, therefore any change described can not be solely attributed to use of a sensory diet.

Behavioural changes

The types of behaviours of concern that parents identified included anxiety, agitation, crying in distress, tantrums, sleeplessness, hurting others, running away, protest vocalisations, not following rules, and stripping. These behaviours were mediated after the children received the sensory diet.

There were a few children who began to calm themselves down and were able to live their daily lives with a reduced 'heightened affect'. For example, Emilio lashed out at others less, Ian began to decrease the duration for which he made loud protest noises, Milly showed less distress, and Peter had fewer tantrums. Jeremy was able to stay asleep six out of seven nights, whereas previously he had woken almost every night during sleep time. Emilio, who previously ran away when out in the community, began to be able to walk beside his parents while out. Lachlan began to follow the house rules, such as having quiet time, which enabled his mother some time to get her daily chores completed.

These results demonstrated that family life became more manageable and community activities were able to occur without parents being concerned about their children's behaviour. These outcomes had a positive impact on the overall family functioning.

Frequency of sensory diet activities

Therapists programmed sensory-based activities into children's daily routines to enable children to be calm and participate in daily activities. On average there were 12 occasions of prescribed sensory-based activity during the day, however, most therapists prescribed eight per day. The number of sensory-based activities ranged from five to 28 per day. The duration of the activities varied from 30 seconds to 15 minutes; for example, a firm hug for 30 seconds, a bicycle ride for 15 minutes. These results suggest that clinicians may be able to make changes to children's behaviour with a minimum of eight sensory-based activities per day.

Frequency of the senses utilised

The proprioceptive, movement, tactile, oral, auditory, and visual senses were all used in the sensory diets with the 17 participants. During analysis of the

Table 14.2 Hierarchy of most utilised senses in the sensory diets

Sense	*Occasions of use*
Proprioception	31
Vestibular	13
Tactile	6
Oral	5
Visual	2
Auditory	1

data, a hierarchy of the most to least used senses emerged. Each activity used in the sensory diet was categorised by the primary sense utilised in the activity; for example, rolling on a ball primarily activates the vestibular receptors, whereas an arm wrestle relies more on the proprioceptors.

Proprioception was the most utilised sense in the sensory diets analysed. This was followed by activities that primarily targeted the vestibular system. The tactile system emerged as the third most used sense. The oral sensory system and the visual systems were the forth most utilised. The auditory system was used the least. See table 14.2 for the number of occasions of use of each sense.

In this study, sensory diets using primarily the proprioceptive and vestibular senses were more likely to assist in mediating behaviour and increasing participation in daily life. These interventions will be discussed further, as they were the most utilised senses in the sensory diets, and are the senses credited for having the most calming effect on exaggerated responses to perceived noxious sensory stimuli (Wilbarger & Wilbarger, 2007).

Sensory diet interventions relating to proprioception

Proprioception was the most highly utilised sense in the programs, and 31 proprioceptive interventions were generated for the participants. The qualities of the actions utilised in these interventions included squashing, pushing, pulling, providing pressure, lifting, vibration, and being contained in equipment that provided pressure. Some of the interventions were able to be implemented by the child independently, some required support from an adult, and others relied on a piece of equipment that the child could utilise independently or with adult assistance.

The outcomes of these interventions enabled extended participation in other daily life activities. Figure 14.1 shows a schematic representation of how proprioceptive interventions promoted participation. Self-care activities, such as eating and showering, were performed calmly and with comfort for the first time for Ted, Ian, and Milly. For example, Ted's mother provided firm touch to his head before he had a shower, and this enabled Ted to have a shower without distress.

Some of the interventions facilitated play between the child and the parent. Activities such as being squashed by a ball or wrestling with a parent produced

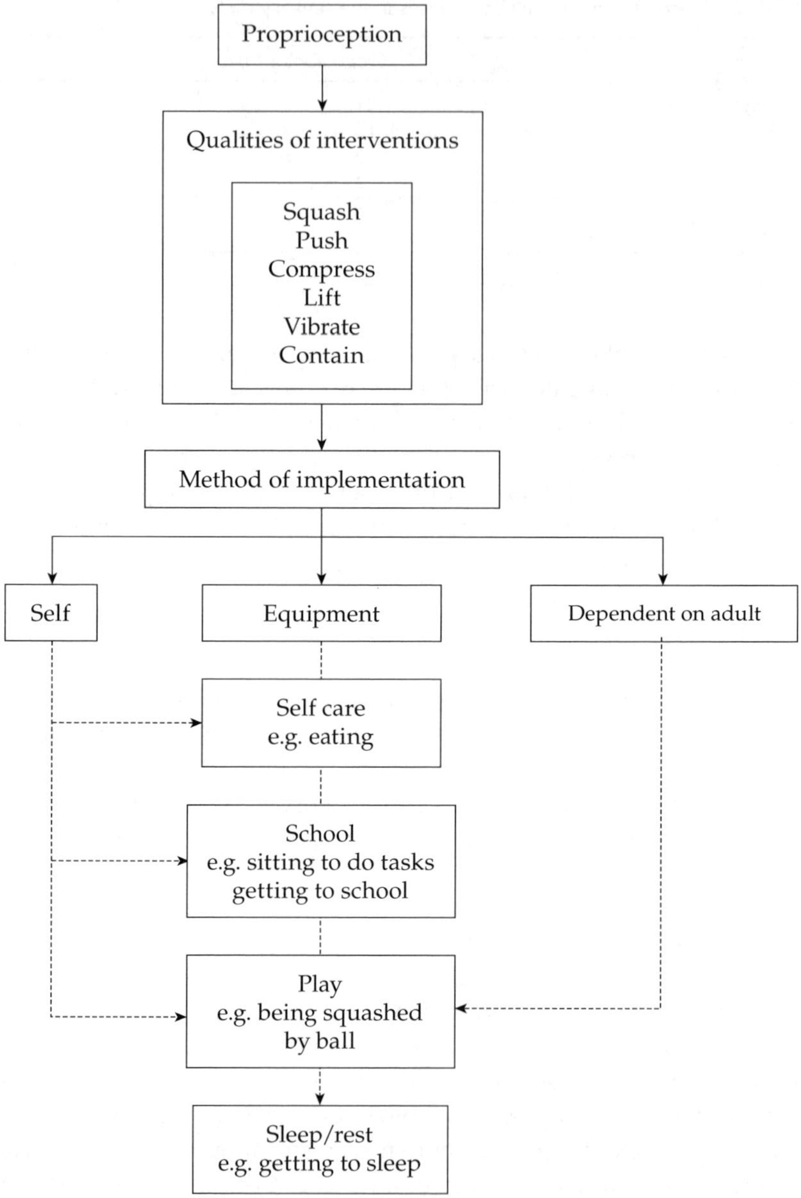

Figure 14.1 Proprioceptive interventions promoting participation in daily life

a playful social response. This was particularly relevant, as many of the parent's goals related to improving the child's opportunity for social experiences.

Proprioceptive interventions promoted the child's capacity to attend and participate in school-based activities, such as sitting down at a table to do lessons. In a classroom, some of these interventions were woven into the typical routine, and included activities such as handing out weighted activities to other students. Other interventions relied on the use of equipment, such as a weighted lap bag, to assist with regulating arousal and promoting concentration.

Finally Lachlan, Ted, and Emilio were assisted to get to sleep by parents giving them a back rub at the end of the day, as well as using weighted blankets on their beds to assist them to settle down for sleep time. Therefore, this study showed that the qualities of proprioceptive activities to consider in therapeutic programming include squashing, pushing, pulling, providing pressure, lifting, vibration, and being contained in equipment.

Sensory diet activities relating to movement and gravity

The vestibular system was the second most used sense used in the study to help the children to become calm and to enable participation in daily

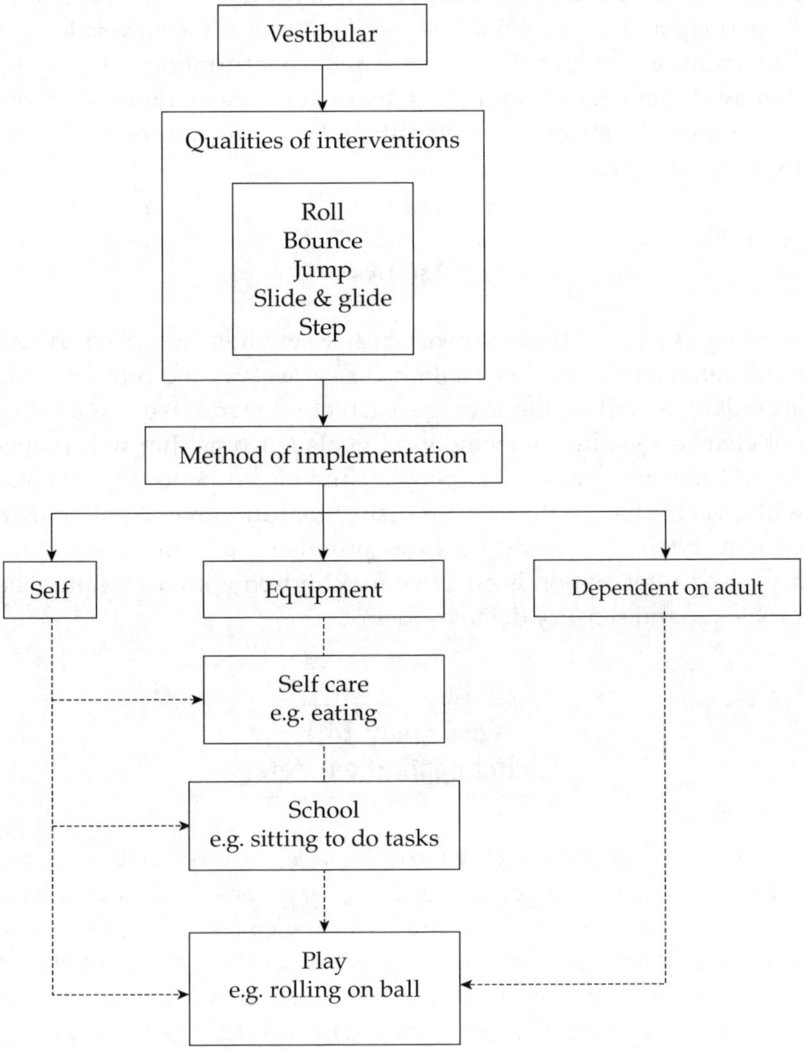

Figure 14.2 Vestibular interventions promoting participation in daily life

activities. Figure 14.2 provides a schematic representation of how vestibular interventions assist children to participate in daily life. The specific qualities of the vestibular interventions included rolling, bouncing, jumping, sliding and gliding, and stepping. Similar to the proprioceptive interventions, the vestibular activities were able to be implemented by the child, with assistance from an adult, or required a specific piece of equipment to facilitate the activity (see table 14.1 for details of the interventions).

Engaging in the vestibular activities enabled play, self-care, and school-related performance. However, play was the predominant performance area enabled by the vestibular activities. Eleven out of the 13 prescribed interventions related to play. Ian participated in one self-care activity while receiving a vestibular intervention. He was able to eat his meal while sitting on a moveable cushion. He usually found eating a noxious experience. Similarly, Emilio participated in a school task while sitting on a moveable cushion. This intervention facilitated calmness and concentration. Therefore, this study showed that when planning a sensory diet, the qualities of vestibular-based activities to consider include rolling, bouncing, jumping, sliding and gliding, and stepping.

Summary

The implementation of these sensory-based activities appeared to mediate children's behaviour problems, facilitated a calm state, and promoted participation in daily activities. On average, each child made two standard deviations of change relating to behavioural goals (such as 'Jim will reduce the amount of times he lashes out at people') and also functional goals (such as 'Jim will wash his hair in the shower') using goal attainment scaling (Kiresuk & Sherman, 1968). The study provides promising preliminary results that sensory-based intervention is effective for children with a disability, behaviour problems, and sensory defensiveness.

Case study 14.1
Clinical application: Peter

Peter was a 10-year-old boy with a moderate intellectual disability and autism. He lived with his parents and a younger sister and brother. Peter presented with tantrums every day, during which he screamed, cried, and occasionally pulled hair and pushed and kicked others. Peter was assessed to be sensitive to touch. He didn't like others being close to him, would get upset when lightly touched on his arm by family members, and removed his clothes 5 to 10 times per day because he disliked the feel of clothes on his body.

Table 14.3 Example of Peter's sensory diet

Time	*Key event in the day*	*Sensory activity*
6.30 a.m.	Breakfast	Drink using a straw
7 a.m.	Waiting for taxi	Jump on trampoline
7.45 a.m.	Getting in taxi	Tight hug goodbye
9.30 a.m.	School tasks	Making shapes with playdough
12.30 p.m.	Lunch	Run around yard
3.30 p.m.	Home from school	Jump on trampoline
7 p.m.	Bath time	Firm dry with towel after bath
9 p.m.	Bed time	Listen to quiet music

He was picky with the foods he ate, and would become distracted and upset with sounds in the background. He also required a lot of verbal prompting to play by himself for about two minutes. He interacted and played with his siblings once a month. His parents' goals during the sensory intervention were to decrease the frequency of his tantrums and how much he removed his clothes. His parents also wanted to increase how much time Peter spent playing by himself and with his siblings.

Peter's therapist prescribed eight occasions of scheduled sensory-based activities into his day (see table 14.3 for an example of his daily schedule). The majority of these activities were proprioceptive and vestibular based. The therapist suggested that Peter's parents show photos of these activities to let him know what was happening. In addition, his therapist recommended that a place be set up where Peter could go that was dark and quiet and also that Peter wear his most comfortable clothes.

After six weeks of intervention, Peter had a tantrum less than twice a week, he removed his clothes only once or twice a day, he played by himself for five minutes, and played with his siblings once a week. His parents were very happy with these changes, and reported that 'the tantrums are not happening this week at home, school, or respite'. They also noted that it was easy to implement the sensory activities at home, and that they were very helpful. These were very positive changes in the life of Peter and his family. This approach warrants careful consideration by practitioners working in this field.

Discussion

Findings of this study are consistent with others that have studied the effectiveness of sensory-processing interventions over the past few years. For example, single-subject research has shown some similar positive effects that resulted from efforts to decrease the child's hyper-responsiveness to sensory input (Case-Smith & Bryan, 1999; Linderman & Stewart, 1999) and deep pressure techniques (Edelson et al., 1999). The use of weighted vests (a technique to provide deep pressure sensation) has been evaluated, using single-subject designs, in children with pervasive developmental disorders, with results showing similar improvements in on-task behaviour and a decrease in self-stimulatory behaviours (Fertel-Daly et al., 2001; Smith et al., 2005; VandenBerg, 2001).

Descriptive articles (Olson & Moulton, 2004), research reviews (Mulligan, 2003; Schaaf & Miller, 2005), case reports (Kinnealey, 1998), and anecdotal parent reports support the views of parents in this study that behavioural changes can result from the use of sensory-processing interventions. Changes such as those found in this study, that included increased engagement, more goal-directed play, improved sleep patterns, reduced anxiety, and increased tolerance for change, have also been reported by others (e.g., Candler, 2003; Cohn, 2001; Paul et al., 2003; Stonefelt & Stein, 1998). The finding in this study that parents found the use of the sensory diet easy to manage is novel, and should be followed up with further research.

On one hand, these cumulative research findings offer hope to parents of children with behavioural problems that may be linked to sensory-processing disorder. On the other hand, the findings are of concern to those therapists and parents who believe that they see positive changes in the children treated using a sensory diet approach, and want to base their practices on strong evidence. There are clear limitations in the research, with sample sizes of this and most other studies being quite small. As stated previously, individual gains may be masked by lack of distinction between the use of the sensory diet and other sensory-processing approaches in this study. Nonetheless, the findings of this study suggest that the decision to provide parents with a sensory diet to assist with management of behavioural problems that are linked to sensory defensiveness should be considered as part of an overall behavioural strategy to enhance children's occupational performance. Further research is required to produce solid evidence that use of a sensory diet is effective.

Conclusion

Sensory diets are used by occupational therapists to influence behavioural change and improve participation in daily life activities (Candler, 2003; Cohn, 2001; Paul et al., 2003; Stonefelt & Stein, 1998). This study found that behaviour problems (such as anxiety and agitation) relating to sensory defensiveness were mediated after children received a sensory diet, which improved the overall quality of family and community life. Therapists using this treatment will need to program a minimum of eight sensory-based activities throughout the day in order to create behavioural change and to increase participation in school, play, self-care, and sleep/rest. The therapeutic program will need to include primarily proprioceptive- (joint) and vestibular- (movement) based activities.

These findings are consistent with other research (Edelson et al., 1999; Fertel-Daly et al., 2001; Smith et al., 2005). Of note is the parental perception that sensory diets are easy to implement. Further research is required to explore intervention utility and implementation. The sensory diet is an effective and easy-to-use treatment for children experiencing behaviour problems related to sensory defensiveness.

15

Communication for life: Promoting communicative competence for mental health and well-being

Donna White

Introduction

Children and adolescents with intellectual disability have *complex communication needs (CCN)*, experiencing difficulties acquiring competency in communication. These young people are also at risk of emotional and behavioural disturbances, and psychopathology. It is the emergence of *challenging behaviours* used by young people with intellectual disability that signals that they may be experiencing significant communicative, emotional, behavioural, or mental health difficulties. Providing support is about 'seeing beyond the behaviour … and dealing with the reasons why' (Cross, 2004, p. 10) in order to a make a difference for young people with intellectual disability in the long term.

This chapter will consider briefly those behaviours of young people with intellectual disability that cause concern for families, carers, and clinicians, and may indicate a specific communication impairment or disturbance of their emotional, behavioural, and mental health status. The challenges that young people with intellectual disability have in achieving communicative competence will be described, and how difficulties across communication domains have an impact on their mental health status discussed. The use of *augmentative and alternative communication (AAC)* will also be explored as a strategy for promoting communication competence from an early age to prevent emotional, behavioural, and mental health disturbances.

Challenging behaviours

When children or adolescents with intellectual disability exhibit behaviours that challenge family, carers, and others within their environments and community, there may be many reasons (Cross, 2004). As part of a functional behavioural assessment, clinicians will investigate underlying factors that may be contributing to the *challenging behaviours* displayed by young people. These may include physiological causes (such as behavioural phenotypes, medications, and sensory impairments) or environmental influences (such as physical surroundings, relationships or interactions with others, restricted opportunities, or undesired activities) (White, 2001). Once these factors have been examined, it is important that the form and function of observed behaviours are examined in order to interpret the intent of the behaviour.

Behaviours of concern, or challenging behaviours, may involve young people with intellectual disability causing harm to themselves (self-injury), property (such as throwing objects and breaking windows), or others (such as hitting, punching, or scratching). Severe behavioural difficulties may result in exclusion from their home (through family stress and breakdown), school, or community, and require alternative care and schooling arrangements, or detention. These socially inappropriate or maladaptive behaviours can be interpreted as a form of communication that occurs because of an inadequate communication system, or they can be seen as behavioural determinants of emotional and behavioural disturbances, or diagnosed psychopathology (Baumgart et al., 1990; Di Marco & Iacono, 2007; Donnellan et al., 1984). Ascertaining the meaning and underlying cause of such behaviours is complicated by *'diagnostic overshadowing'* (Bernard & Turk, 2009) and *'behavioural overshadowing'* (Di Marco & Iacono, 2007). This is where possible symptoms of mental health problems in young people with intellectual disability are overlooked because they are seen as being part of their intellectual disability.

It has long been established within the literature that there is a link between communication difficulties and challenging behaviours in young people with intellectual disability (Baumgart et al., 1990; Donnellan et al., 1984). There has also been an association found between communication difficulties and mental health in typically developing children and adolescents that can be applied to young people with intellectual disability (Cross, 1999; 2004). This association is complex and multifaceted, although longitudinal studies have indicated that complex language disorders in childhood that persist into adolescence and young adulthood increase the risk of poor psychosocial outcomes and psychiatric disturbances in later life (Clegg et al., 2005; Snowling et al., 2006; Whitehouse et al., 2009). Snow (2008) noted that achievement of communicative competence in childhood was a predictor for positive mental health outcomes in adolescence and adulthood. The next section will consider the development of communicative competence and its effect on mental health outcomes.

What is communicative competence?

Communication is the use of verbal and nonverbal methods to exchange information with others. Partners in this dynamic exchange make sense of the communicative behaviours used by others to determine the intent and meaning of interactions. From birth, these exchanges between children and caregivers facilitate the development of children's linguistic, social, cognitive, and emotional knowledge and skills. Integration of these skills assist children to develop a level of competence to enable them to be active and effective communication partners within their communities and throughout their lifespan (Prizant & Wetherby, 1990; Light, 2003). Such integration is known as *communicative competence*, and is influenced by environmental factors, relationships with caregivers, and interactions with others (Cross, 2004). Children gain competence through development of knowledge and skills in:

- *language content (semantics):* understanding and conveying meaning through words
- *language form (syntax):* the structure of language, including the sound system, grammar, sentence structure, and narratives
- *language use (pragmatics):* being able to use language appropriately in a variety of contexts.

Typical development of communicative competence

In the prelinguistic stage of communication development (birth to approximately 18 months), typically developing children use behaviours (such as vocalisations, facial expressions, and body movements) in response to their internal states and the environmental context. Caregivers interpret these responses as being communicative, and make inferences about the meaning of children's behaviours (McCathren et al., 1996). Caregivers then respond to children in a way that is sensitive to children's communication needs, scaffolds their learning, and encourages acquisition of communication skills (White, 2001). As children grow and learn through these interactions, their communicative behaviours become more intentional (8–10 months). Children learn to use informal or idiosyncratic means of communication (such as eye gaze, vocalisations, and gestures) to request, establish joint attention, and engage in social interaction (Prizant & Wetherby, 1990). As children develop further (12–18 months), their understanding of language and interactions increases, and their communicative intentions become more symbolic (single words), then linguistic (use of two or more word combinations). They use words to request objects and actions, comment and share information, and engage in communicative games and routines (Hill & Coufal, 2005; McCathren et al., 1996).

The early childhood (18 months to 2 years) and preschool (3–5 years) stages of communication development are characterised by a rapid increase in children's knowledge and use of words and word combinations (semantic relations to simple sentence construction) to fulfil a range of communicative functions (such as request, comment, negate, or respond). As development continues, there is a rapid increase in children's receptive and expressive vocabulary, ability to convey meaning, understanding and use of structural language, and the ability to use language in a variety of situations (Cross, 2004).

By the end of the preschool stage, children have acquired fundamental communication skills and a have a basic level of communicative competence. At this stage, children have started to interpret their own and others' emotional states, and use language to express their experiences (Giddan et al., 1995). Furthermore, the level of competence achieved in this stage predicts acquisition of communication skills in the school years and adolescence required for 'transition to literacy [leading to positive] self-esteem, school attachment [and] mastery of an increasingly complex range of written and spoken discourse genres' (Snow, 2008; p. 7). These skills in turn promote positive mental health and well-being in children and adolescents.

In the school years (5–11 years), children continue to develop their level of competence through extension of their word knowledge, sentence length and complexity, use of narratives and conversation, as well as acquisition of literacy skills (Reed, 2005). In this stage, there is a change in language requirements and the need both to understand and use more specific and technical vocabulary (such as words with extended meanings, semantic categories, and definitions), and abstract or figurative language (including humour and idioms) as they progress through the education system (Smith, 2005; Starling, 2003; van Mourik & Roberts, 2003). The development of *self-talk* or *inner voice* is important during this period for verbal organisation and flexibility, and learning self-control and regulation of behaviours associated with internal emotional states (Cross, 2004; Giddan & Milling, 1999). All of these skills assist children in acquisition of the pragmatic skills necessary for understanding and expressing complex emotions, personal problem solving, peer mediation, conflict resolution, and establishment of relationships with family and peers that will provide emotional support for positive mental health in the long term (Giddan et al., 1995; Hill & Coufal, 2005; Snow, 2008).

Adolescence (11–20 years) is a time of psychological change and development, with increased emotional, cognitive, and linguistic growth occurring during this period. Adolescents learn to become independent, consolidating a sense of personal identity and establishing roles within their communities (Smith, 2005). This independence is achieved through the development of sophisticated communication skills across a range of contexts that enables them to be flexible and adaptable to the increased rate and complexity of interactions (Smith, 2005). Examples include the extension of skills in information and communication technologies (ICT, including internet, email, SMS, and texting), use of 'teen talk' specific to peer groups (Starling, 2003), appropriate interpersonal skills, and being able to 'code switch' between language requirements for different forms of oral and written discourse (such as joking with peers compared to the demands of oral presentations, debating, written reports, and essays in the classroom) (Starling, 2003). A high level of communicative competence in these skills ensures that adolescents achieve academic success, thus promoting positive self-esteem and personal identity (Snow, 2008). Snow (2008) noted that the level of communicative competence (particularly oral language) achieved in adolescence reflects 'a range of early protective factors, such as secure attachment; child-focused parenting; adequate exposure to and experience with a variety of linguistic forms and opportunities; exposure to prosocial role models; consistent and developmentally appropriate educational input; and access to specialist services along the way if needed' (p. 8). Indeed, these factors need to be kept in mind when considering communicative competence in young people with intellectual disability and the mental health impact of developmental difficulties through childhood and adolescence.

Communicative competence development in young people with intellectual disability

Acquisition of communication skills for children and adolescents with intellectual disability follows a developmental pattern similar to that described above, and can be seen as a continuum from non-symbolic to symbolic skill acquisition (Beukelman & Mirenda, 2005). However, the rate of skill acquisition, level of communicative competence, and functional ability achieved will depend on:

- intrinsic variables, such as individuals' cognitive and/or neurological status (Sevcik, 2006) and psychosocial attributes, such as patterns of attention, social responsiveness, motivation for learning and communication, and resilience (Light, 2003)
- extrinsic variables, such as the demands of an individual's environment, including responsiveness of communication partners (Light, 2003; Prizant & Wetherby, 1990).

According to studies conducted in the UK and Australia, 45 per cent of individuals with an intellectual disability had significant communication impairments or complex communication needs (Department of Health, 2007; Perry et al., 2004), and up to 80 per cent have some communication impairments (Scottish Executive, 2000). The patterns of development along the continuum of intellectual disability (from severe to milder levels) often result in different communication profiles. These are briefly described below.

Communication profiles of young people across the levels of intellectual disability

Some young people with intellectual disability do not progress beyond the preintentional level of communication development, are non-symbolic, and have difficulties understanding and interacting with the world around them. Often young people at this stage of communication do not learn that they need to attend to or interact with objects, people, and events in their environment, and thus do not know how to engage in appropriate communicative exchanges (White, 2001). They may use communicative behaviours that are idiosyncratic and unconventional (facial expressions, physical movements, gestures, and vocalisations) or challenging (screaming, grabbing, hitting, or throwing) in their 'best attempt to transmit a message or meet a need' (Bopp et al., 2004; p. 5). These behaviours may result in fewer opportunities for the young person to have a positive impact on his or her environment (Beukelman & Mirenda, 2005). Thus, the road to communicative competence may become an isolating experience, with the young person having limited skills to enable connection with the world, establish relationships, and express thoughts, ideas, and feelings (Light, 2003; White, 2001).

Young people with more moderate levels of intellectual disability develop symbolic skills and use verbal communication. These young people may have been identified from an early age as having communication difficulties because of their intellectual disability and need for specialist services (such as early intervention and special education support). They may also have been introduced to a range of multimodal AAC systems (discussed shortly) through childhood and adolescence to assist development of receptive (including activity schedules, behaviour scripts, and visual timetables) and expressive skills (including choice boards, request cards, chat books, and communication books) (Beukelman & Mirenda, 2005; ScopeVIC, n.d.). Even with these supports, achievement of functional communication skills and competence across communication domains may not be guaranteed in the long term.

At the other end of the intellectual disability continuum, young people with milder levels of intellectual disability have unique communication needs. These young people often appear to be competent communicators because of their fluent verbal skills, but may have significant undiagnosed communication difficulties in receptive, expressive, pragmatic, and literacy skills that persist into adolescence and adulthood (White, 2011). They may attend mainstream schools with additional unidentified learning needs or attend schools for children with 'emotional or behavioural disturbance', and have limited access to specialist services (Hall, 2000). Communication partners overestimate the communication skills of these young people, use language at a higher level than they can understand, and expect a level of competence in interactions beyond their skill level (Kevan, 2003; Smidt et al., 2007). These difficulties place young people at a disadvantage in interactions in school and community settings. They may appear to be uncooperative or oppositional when asked questions (White, 2011), uninterested, not motivated, or detached, and revert to 'safe' interpersonal communicative behaviours (such as nodding, shrugging, 'dunno', 'maybe') when in social settings, leading to further disadvantage (Snow, 2008).

Young people with milder levels of intellectual disability may feel the stigma of difference, more so than those with greater levels of disability, in the struggle to compare themselves with and seek acceptance by others. They may feel alienated and disconnected (Starling, 2003), and in the struggle for identity may easily be drawn to groups with antisocial and delinquent behaviour patterns. They may not acknowledge (or be aware of) their disability, thereby placing themselves at a disadvantage, and engage in 'at risk' or offending behaviours as a consequence of exploitation, deficits in knowledge, skills, and experience, or an inability to 'function responsibly in a complex world' (Cockram, 2005; p. 75). They also have complicated clinical profiles, which may include comorbid mental health diagnoses, limited social networks or social isolation, complex family systems, poor academic outcomes, drug and alcohol abuse, and acquired brain injury (White, 2011).

As discussed, children and adolescents with varying levels of intellectual disability are confronted by a range of difficulties that have an impact on their ability to acquire competent communication skills and achieve the positive outcomes of their typically developing peers. A literature review of the specific difficulties in the communication domains of 'content, form, and use' experienced by young people with mild to moderate intellectual disabilities is summarised in table 15.1.

Augmentative and alternative communication (AAC) and environmental challenges

The significant communication impairments (as outlined in table 15.1) experienced by young people with intellectual disability have an effect on their ability to function within the community, and to establish and maintain social interactions. AAC systems are used to support and extend development of functional communication skills. An *augmentative and alternative communication (AAC) system* refers to a 'compilation of methods and technology designed to supplement spoken communication for people with limited speech or language skills' (Wilkinson & Hennig, 2007; p. 58).

AAC technologies use multimodal approaches to enhance communication development and include symbols that may be unaided (such as body movements, facial expressions, touch cues, gesture, or sign language) or aided

Table 15.1 Communication difficulties experienced by young people with mild-to-moderate intellectual disability

Communication domain	*Difficulties*
Content and semantics	• Delayed development in both receptive and expressive skills • Limited vocabulary: use of 'survival' vocabulary, non-specific language, word-finding problems • Verbal language lacks information and meaning • Requires longer to process information • Difficulties understanding questions (e.g., yes/no, either/or, 'who, what, where, why' questions): suggestibility, acquiescence or 'yea-saying' • Difficulties understanding instructions longer than three key elements: context-dependent; watches others • Difficulties understanding abstract or complex language that includes higher-level language: takes literally: – concepts e.g., time, emotions – word meanings and definitions – analogies and lexical ambiguities – figurative language (e.g., humour, slang, idioms, irony, metaphors, similes, proverbs) – problem solving. • Difficulties learning to read: sight words, re-read to obtain meaning
Form and syntax	• Delayed vocal development, articulation difficulties, and decreased fluency • Delayed development of first words and word combinations • Difficulties understanding and using grammatical markers, e.g. tenses, negatives, conjunctions (and, because) • Difficulties understanding complex sentence structures • Reduced sentence length, fragmented, and word order confused • Difficulties with recounting experiences, stories, narratives: leaves out detail, poor sequencing, confabulation • Difficulties generating written language
Use and pragmatics	• Difficulties in unfamiliar situations: requires contextual information • Difficulties using appropriate linguistic forms in different contexts (e.g. politeness, 'code switching') • Reduced use of communicative functions and initiations • Difficulties in conversation: topics inappropriate, repetitive, and tangential; poor turn-taking • Difficulties understanding or using appropriate nonverbal behaviours (e.g. personal space, body language, intonation, volume control, speech rate) • Difficulties signalling and responding to communication breakdown • Poor social responsiveness and difficulties understanding requirements of social contexts, social rules, nuances of establishing friendships with peers

Source: adapted from Abbeduto & Hesketh, 1997; Abbeduto et al., 2007; Landa, 2007; White, 2011

(such as objects, photos, symbols, or written text) (Beukelman & Mirenda, 2005; Wilkinson & Hennig, 2007). *Aided AAC systems* may incorporate low-technology aids (such as communication boards, visual schedules, paper, and pen) or high-technology aids (such as voice output communication aids and computer-based technologies or devices) (Wilkinson & Hennig, 2007). Yet, regardless of the communicative modes or aids used in interventions with children and adolescents with intellectual disability, it is important that they are used to assist the development of language comprehension, production, and use in interactions (Sevcik, 2006). In this way, young people may be able to achieve a level of communicative competence that promotes positive interactions, mental health, and well-being. However, there may be environmental factors in young people's lives that interfere with the successful use of AAC and impede their ability to develop functional communication.

Cress and Marvin (2003) indicated that, for a child with multiple developmental needs, the burden of care, and focus on medical and physical interventions in early childhood, often takes precedence over the introduction of a communication system for the child. In situations such as these, 'children may move on to the preschool years with under-developed, limited communication repertoires, and restricted access to formal AAC modes' (Cress & Marvin, 2003; p. 254). Light and Drager (2007) also noted that preschoolers with CCN were often introduced to limited modes of communication (such as gestures, communication books, and simple technologies with digitised speech output) and a restricted number of communicative functions (such as requesting wants and needs), which limited their opportunities and interactions with communication partners.

Additionally, Downing (2005) indicated that there were many challenges for adolescents with severe disabilities who were included in general classrooms. She found that, in this environment, additional effort was required to ensure that adolescents who used AAC were given opportunities for sharing information, expanding their communicative functions (through greetings and farewells, rejecting, making requests, and commenting), using multimodal communication, and being given age-appropriate vocabulary and messages for social language. Smith (2005) also reviewed literature that indicated that some communication aids did not allow for the rapid rate of communication and flexibility of topics and vocabulary required for adolescent interactions.

Furthermore, it has been noted in the literature and clinical practice that there is a growing number of young people with intellectual disability who no longer use their AAC systems because of operational, self-image, and identity issues (Clarke et al., 2001; Smith, 2005). Light and Drager (2007) proposed that it was the interaction between communication partners, social context, and purpose of interaction that determined the effectiveness of AAC systems and whether individuals continued to use them in the long term. The following case examples illustrate some of the barriers to using AAC that young people with intellectual disability may have when they experience changes and unfamiliar environments.

Case study 15.1

A child with a moderate level of intellectual disability started at a new school. She understood and used speech, key word signing, and photos for communication. Her new teachers and peers had difficulties understanding her speech, did not know any signs, and used line drawings only in the classroom. The child had difficulties participating in class activities and interacting in the playground. She began hitting out at others, throwing things, and screaming, which resulted in suspensions from school.

Case study 15.2

An adolescent with a mild level of intellectual disability would not use his symbol diary and schedule systems because it made him look different and 'uncool' among peers in his mainstream school. He became anxious and confused when he forgot the routine or when changes occurred. The increased anxiety and comprehension difficulties resulted in aggressive outbursts at home, leading to family stress.

Case study 15.3

A young adult with a moderate intellectual disability and autism spectrum disorder (ASD) had used multimodal AAC systems (such as activity schedules and a conversational topic book) at his special school, but when he started in a supported work place, these were outdated. His AAC systems did not have the necessary vocabulary for following work tasks, engage in conversations, or establish new friendships. This resulted in reduced participation in work activities and withdrawal from others in the workplace.

These clinical examples reflect the difficulties that young people with intellectual disability and complex communication needs experience because of inadequate communication systems, communication partners who don't understand their unique needs, and the impact of changes in environmental and social contexts. Lack of competence in dealing with these demands increases a young person's vulnerability to mental health issues (Smith, 2005), and can exacerbate existing behavioural challenges. It is important therefore, for clinicians to be aware of these environmental challenges and assist young people's communication partners to overcome barriers that may exist.

The *participation model* (Beukelman & Mirenda, 2005) provides a useful framework for AAC assessment and intervention for young people with intellectual disability. This model takes into consideration young people's current and future AAC needs, and barriers to participation by 'planning for today and tomorrow'. This framework may assist in planning AAC strategies across the lifespan to reduce the risk of mental heath disturbances.

The impact of communicative competence on mental health

Epidemiological studies have shown that 31 to 50 per cent of young people (4–19 years) with intellectual disability have significant emotional, behavioural, or psychiatric disorders (Cormack et al., 2000; Einfeld & Tonge, 1996b; Einfeld et al., 2006; Hastings & Mount, 2001). There are many factors that increase the risk of individuals with intellectual disability experiencing emotional and behavioural disturbances, and psychopathology. These include developmental (such as cognitive impairment), biological (physical health, epilepsy, or sensory impairments), psychological (adverse life events and poor attachments), and social (deprivation, family dysfunction, parental stress, or mental health) risk factors (Dosen, 2005b; Dykens, 2000; Emerson et al., 2005; Hatton & Emerson, 2004; Koskentausta et al., 2007; Kwok & Cheung, 2007; IASSID, 2001). However, it is the cumulative effect of these factors that increases the risk of mental health disorders.

Curran and Kyrkou (2008) noted that the key elements for emotional development included expression and recognition of emotions in self and others, self-regulation, establishment of relationships, and recognition of a sense of self. Acquisition of these skills requires a high level of communicative competence that many young people with intellectual disabilities do not achieve, especially those who have more severe levels of intellectual disability, such that their communication skills are pre-symbolic or even pre-intentional. Emotional and interpersonal skills will be affected by difficulties with semantic competence (such as limited vocabulary to describe emotions, poor comprehension of ambiguities and subtleties of language), narrative competence (such as being able to understand one's own experiences and share these with others), and pragmatic competence (such as knowing rules of conversation and using a flexible repertoire of social skills). In fact, reduced competence in these areas has been identified as part of the communication profile of young people with emotional and behavioural disturbances and mental health disorders who access services (Anger, 1999; Koskentausta et al., 2007; Russo, 2004). Having communication impairments and mental health disturbances can be 'a frustrating and lonely experience for both the child and the family' (Russo, 2004; p. 113). This affects their quality of life and has an impact on young people's relationships with family members and peers, coping in social situations, academic success, employment opportunities, self-esteem, and personal identity, thus affecting mental health outcomes (Hill & Coufal, 2005; Russo, 2004; Snow, 2008, Starling 2003).

A review of the literature on young people with mild to moderate intellectual disabilities revealed that the clinical presentation of emotional and behavioural disturbances or mental health disorders is through:

a *internalised behaviours,* such as withdrawal, thought problems, cyclical mood and behaviour changes, emotional reactivity, depression, and anxiety (Bernard & Turk, 2009; Dekker et al., 2002; Hartley et al., 2008)
b *externalised behaviours,* such as hyperactivity, disruptiveness, antisocial behaviours, aggression, self-injurious behaviours, non-compliance, and inattentiveness (Bernard & Turk, 2009; Brereton et al., 2006; Hartley et al., 2008).

An *inner voice* (also referred to as *internal language, inner speech* or *private speech*) is dependent on a young person's level of communicative competence, including acquisition of a symbolic system in order to develop an internal representation of experiences, and also narrative skills (Cross, 2004; Prizant & Wetherby, 1990). The internalised and externalised behaviours associated with emotional and behavioural disturbances may reflect young people's ineffective communication skills, including difficulties in developing an inner voice that allows them to regulate and modulate their inner (emotions and arousal levels) and external environments (Audet & Hummel, 1990; Anger, 1999). An inner voice is related to self-control, and helps 'mediate between intention and action' (Cross et al., 2001, p. 229).

An inner voice also helps with reflecting, organising information, formulating ideas, and being able to interact effectively with others (such as repairing communication breakdown, negotiating, and problem solving) (Audet & Hummel, 1990; Anger, 1999; Prizant & Wetherby, 1990). Young people with intellectual disability who have not developed an inner voice may have behavioural outbursts or violent reactions in response to emotional upsets or threatening situations, as they are unable to consider the consequences of their actions or an alternative response (Cross, 2004). Therefore, if young people with intellectual disability have significant difficulties acquiring basic functional communication skills, then using an 'inner voice' for internalising thoughts and regulating behaviours is going to be particularly difficult. Such difficulties may have implications for emotional and interpersonal skill development, and mental health outcomes.

Communication for life: promoting communicative competence for mental health and well-being

As noted, acquiring a level of communicative competence required for positive mental health is difficult for children and adolescents with intellectual disability. Difficulties with communication development, in conjunction with increased developmental, biological, psychological, and social risk factors, limit young people's capacity to achieve the positive mental health outcomes of their typically developing peers. Therefore it is necessary to attempt to bridge the gap and promote communicative competence across the lifespan through AAC interventions.

AAC interventions have been utilised with children and adolescents with intellectual disability since the mid 1980s (Beukelman & Mirenda, 2005), with an extensive research base supporting its use with this population. AAC has been demonstrated to:

- support development of expressive and receptive communication skills
- promote the use of a range of communicative functions across contexts and interactive partners
- reduce problem or challenging behaviours
- provide a foundation for later linguistic development
- support academic learning, participation in the educational curriculum, and literacy development
- support the establishment of peer relationships
- promote acquisition of skills required for post-school employment and community living (McNaughton & Bryen, 2007; Ratcliffe & Cress, 1998; Sevcik, 2006; Sturm & Clendon, 2004; Wilkinson & Hennig, 2007).

Communicative competence can be developed by using multimodal AAC strategies within naturally occurring routines, play situations, and social contexts, such as home, school, and the community (Nurcombe et al., 2001). Involvement of communication partners (family members, peers, and other professionals) is essential in any AAC intervention. Parent training programs, such as the Hanen Center's *It Takes Two to Talk* (for parents of children with language delay) and *More Than Words* (for parents of children with ASD), teach parents how to facilitate communication development in everyday situations (see <www.hanen.org>).

Light (1989, cited in Light, 2003) proposed that the attainment of a level of communicative competence using AAC requires the integration of knowledge, judgment, and skills across four domains:

- *linguistic competence:* receptive and expressive skills in the form, content, and use of spoken language and the 'linguistic code' used in AAC systems, and the ability to switch between codes
- *operational competence:* the ability to produce and sequence unaided symbols (such as gestures and signs), and access to low- or high-technology aided AAC systems
- *social competence:* pragmatic skills (discourse and communicative functions) and interpersonal skills (being active and responsive in interactions)
- *strategic competence:* compensatory strategies to manage limitations in the other domains.

Review of the AAC and language intervention literature has revealed numerous strategies that can be used to promote communicative competence in young people with intellectual disability. Some of these strategies have a strong evidence base, and other strategies have been included because they have been found to work in clinical practice. The selection of specific communication goals and intervention strategies should always be based on a thorough communication assessment, consideration of factors associated with the presence of challenging behaviours, and with multidisciplinary consultation. The strategies described below focus on promotion of communicative competence in young people with mild-to-moderate levels of intellectual disability in order to prevent mental health disturbances. The main aim of the strategies is to integrate AAC modes with young people's natural speech in order to achieve effective communication (Hustard & Shapley, 2003).

Development of linguistic competence

The aim of augmenting spoken language with AAC is to extend young people's understanding of different linguistic codes (such as speech, symbols, and signs), assist with learning the meanings of symbols or signs (content or semantics), and provide models for combining and ordering words, symbols, and signs for generative language (form or syntax) (Mirenda, 2008; Romski & Sevcik, 2003). AAC can facilitate the expansion of vocabulary (semantics) that is essential for a range of communicative functions (pragmatics) (Anger, 1999; Burkhart, 2008; Downing, 2005), such as:

- *directing attention*
- *requesting:* for example, objects and actions, social routine, permission, information and clarification; asking questions
- *rejecting and protesting*
- *self-expression and assertion:* for example, showing off, expressing feelings, asserting independence, negotiating and bargaining
- *naming and commenting:* for example, commenting on an action or object; describing
- *giving and sharing information and stating opinions*
- *social interaction:* for example, greeting, acknowledging, turn taking, relating events, talking about past and future, teasing, making up stories to share information, initiation, maintenance and termination of conversations.

Acquisition of a vocabulary and a repertoire of communicative functions can be achieved by immersing children in language-rich environments where communication partners use opportunities within daily routines to provide language models and prompt appropriate use. Examples of early intervention approaches for promotion of communicative competence in children with intellectual disability are described below.

Aided language stimulation (ALS)

Aided language stimulation (ALS) (Goossens et al., 1992) is an approach developed for children requiring AAC systems that uses a total-immersion approach (Beukelman & Mirenda, 2005). The communication partner simultaneously uses spoken language and points to symbols on a communication display, thus modelling how symbols can be used naturally and interactively in activities. This technique requires the use of topic boards for activities, and provides an opportunity for language mapping aimed at increasing receptive language skills (Dada & Alant, 2009). Romski and Sevcik (2003) noted that the essential elements of this approach were 'engineering the environment, including overlays and selecting vocabulary specific to daily activities' (p. 149).

Although studies on the use of ALS have been limited to small samples, this technique has been shown to increase symbol comprehension and production in three children with moderate intellectual disability (Harris & Reichle, 2004), increase the syntactic performance on manual communication boards for four out of nine participants after a week's intensive intervention (Bruno & Trembath, 2006), and facilitate the acquisition of target vocabulary items across three activities for four children following a three-week intervention period.

BLADES therapy

BLADES therapy (based on the Bristol Language Development Scales) (Gutfreund et al., 1989, cited in Sherwood, 2004) focuses on semantic and pragmatic development. There is limited research on this approach, however, Sherwood (2004) reported positive results using BLADES therapy that incorporated parent training (two sessions) and parent–child group intervention (six sessions) over an eight-week period. Evaluation of the intervention revealed that the majority of parents indicated that their children's communication skills had improved, and they felt that they had changed the way they interacted with their child.

The main feature of BLADES therapy (Sherwood, 2004) is the acquisition of verbs to promote two-word phrases across five categories: *possession* (ownership, such as 'got'), *location* (movement, such as 'sit down', 'go'), *experience* (inner thoughts and feelings, such as 'want', 'like', 'listen' and 'hear'), *attribution* (physical properties, such as 'that's a …' or 'open'), and *function* (ideas peculiar to people or objects, such as 'what do?', 'eat', 'drink', or 'play') (Sherwood, 2004). Teaching strategies involve (a) *mapping*: making the meaning obvious to the child while modelling the word at the critical time; (b) *having the child say the word* by prompting, such as the use of object and gestural aids and 'waiting'; and (c) *generalisation* of the new verb phrases into daily routines, interactions, and book-sharing activities using pragmatic functions for 'controlling the environment … giving or receiving information … expressing a feeling' (Sherwood, 2004; p. 11).

This technique has been used in clinical practice with children with mild-to-moderate intellectual disability by augmenting the strategies with additional AAC (signs, photos, symbols, symbol workbooks). BLADES therapy provides a structured developmental framework for extending beyond the one word, sign, or symbol level, and teaching functional vocabulary that incorporates parent training and generalisation, which is particularly important for children with intellectual disability.

Development of operational competence

The use of multimodal AAC systems, including both unaided (such as gestures and signs) and aided (with photos or symbols) modes, will promote development of operational competence. Burkhart (2008) noted that teaching young people with intellectual disability to use 'multiple systems is far more powerful than the use of any one system' (p. 4). Such teaching assists young people to be flexible and adaptive to meet the requirements of a variety of communication partners and situations, thereby enabling them to be more efficient and effective communicators. The ability to use AAC systems depends on a young person's level of communication, including his or her symbolic representational skills, memory skills, scanning abilities, and discrimination skills (Burkhart, 2008; Rowland & Schweigert, 2003). A young person will also use an AAC system that is meaningful, motivating, and organised (such as *pragmatic organisation dynamic displays*, engineered displays; Burkhart, 2008) so it is accessible.

In more recent times, researchers and clinicians have been exploring ICT or 'funky gadgets' (Gillett & DePompei, 2004; Ireland, 2007), such as smart phones and personal data assistants (PDAs), as AAC aids. Adolescents with intellectual disability may be more likely to use these aids than other forms as they are more acceptable to peers; however, they require literacy skills (Gillett & DePompei, 2004). Westby (2010) noted that accessing these types of technology required more than the ability to decode the written word; it required *visual literacy* for images and video, *computer literacy* for computer use (and devices) and software, and *media or technology literacy* in order to understand digital and multimedia formats on the internet. The *Multiliteracies Map*, developed in South Australia, provides a four-dimensional approach to teaching multiliteracy skills in schools, and can assist with observing, assessing, and planning typically developing children's literacy learning. For more information on *Multiliteracies Map* see <http://www.earlyyearsliteracy.sa.edu.au/> and Westby, 2010. For ideas for general literacy instruction for those with complex communication needs see Clendon & Erickson, 2009).

Development of social competence

Social competence relies on the acquisition of pragmatic skills and interpersonal skills, which includes effective use of communicative functions and discourse, and being an active and responsive communication partner (including showing interest in interactions, responding to questions and comments, and showing consideration for others) (Burkhart, 2008). Young people with intellectual disability need to be given a range of social experiences to have the opportunity to learn these skills. Such opportunities include, for example, setting up child-directed activities, with opportunities to make choices, experience control over their environment, and interact with peers (Burkhart, 2008; Light & Drager, 2007). Some specific AAC strategies that can assist with development of these skills are outlined below.

Talking Mats™

Talking Mats is a low-technology augmentative communication framework that assists young people with intellectual disability to understand and express their views and feelings about choices in their lives (Cameron & Murphy, 2002; Murphy & Cameron, 2008). Picture symbols are used to represent topics being explored, options, and emotions, or feelings about each option. Murphy and Cameron (2008) found that *Talking Mats* enabled individuals with intellectual disability with receptive language skills at three or more *information carrying words (ICWs)* (understanding of three or more key ideas in sentence) to express their views effectively and reliably.

Social Stories™

Social Stories was initially developed for children with ASD. *Social Stories* 'describes social situations in which an individual might have difficulty identifying salient social cues, expected behaviours, and consequences of behaving in various ways' (Reynhout & Carter, 2007; p. 173). *Social Stories* was developed by Carol Gray, who provided specific guidelines for writing a social story using six sentence types: *descriptive* (describe what to do), *perspective* (thoughts and feelings of others), *affirmative* (reassures child), *directive* (appropriate behavioural response), *control* (analogies), and *cooperative* (who can assist child) (Crozier & Tincani, 2007). The stories are written from the child's perspective, and are implemented by reading them to the child or recording them onto audio or video (Reynhout & Carter, 2006).

Social Stories is not an AAC intervention, however, the stories have been used with children and adolescents with intellectual disability, augmented with photos, drawings, and symbols. Research has yet to provide adequate evidence of the effectiveness of this technique. Nonetheless, some small-scale studies have indicated behaviour change following the use of *Social Stories* (Crozier & Tincani, 2007; Reynhout & Carter, 2007). An individual's levels of cognitive and communicative functioning appear to be important considerations when implementing *Social Stories* (Reynhout & Carter, 2006).

Comic Strip Conversations

Comic Strip Conversations were also developed by Carol Gray for young people with ASD. They form a visual communication strategy that involves simple drawings (using stick figures, colour, speech, and thought bubbles) to represent concretely a conversation between two or more people (Barnhill, 2002).

They can assist a young person to process and understand interactions, and support social and emotional understanding. There is very little research evidence on the use of this strategy. However, in clinical practice comic strip conversations have been used to explain major life changes, support retelling of events, match emotional expression with thought and language processes, develop theory of mind, structure social interactions, support activity choices, and facilitate transition (Quinn, 2006).

Development of strategic competence
Beukelman and Mirenda (2005) noted that interventions for strategic competence focused on teaching compensatory and repairs strategies for when young people with intellectual disability experience communication breakdown or interaction difficulties. Strategies may include teaching young people to repeat what has been communicated, rephrase, or use another communication mode. It is also important to teach communication partners how to manage breakdowns in communication and ways to prompt young people to use their repair strategies.

Conclusion

The majority of young people with intellectual disability will have some communication difficulty that affects the way in which they understand the world around them, express their basic needs, wants, thoughts, and feelings, and relate to their families, peers, and others in the community. The complex interrelationship between cognitive, communication, emotional, and social development means that a difficulty in one area will have an impact on development in other areas. Thus, ineffective communication systems will affect the way young people with intellectual disability interpret their internal states and regulate their responses, and how they negotiate personal and social encounters by engaging with others in an active and responsive manner.

The presence of severe behaviours in young people may mask an underlying communication difficulty or mental health disturbance. The challenge for families and professionals is to be proactive and support communication development from childhood and across the lifespan, to reduce the risk of emotional and behavioural disturbances and poor mental health outcomes later in life. Black and Devine (n.d.) stated, 'Good mental health is about the ability and opportunity to enjoy life, to deal with disappointment and sadness, and to have a positive sense of well-being and self-worth' (p. 2). Promoting communicative competence through the use of AAC strategies facilitates multimodal communication in order for young people with intellectual disability to connect with others, exert control over their environments, and develop relationships with their families, peers, and others in the community, thus promoting positive mental health.

Acknowledgments

The author gratefully acknowledges Teena Caithness and Martine Fourie (ADHC Statewide Behaviour Intervention Service) and Professor Teresa Iacono (LaTrobe University) for their review and helpful contributions to this chapter.

16

Building life skills in children with intellectual disabilities

Victoria Grahame

Introduction

Children with an intellectual disability are particularly vulnerable to additional emotional and behavioural problems. Social and emotional cognitive skill-building programs that teach children with intellectual disabilities problem-solving skills and coping strategies can reduce the risk of psychopathology. However, children and adolescents with an intellectual disability often have difficulty developing problem-solving skills and coping strategies, and will therefore need developmentally appropriate interventions that build on their existing abilities. This chapter will discuss appropriate and effective interventions that help individuals with an intellectual disability develop these skills.

Intellectual disability is a common developmental problem of childhood, occurring in approximately 1.38 per cent of the school-aged population in Australia (McCleod & McKinnon, 2007). Furthermore, research has suggested that children with an intellectual disability are particularly vulnerable to additional emotional and behavioural problems such as attention deficit hyperactivity disorder (ADHD), conduct disorders, and anxiety (Emerson, 2003a). In an Australian epidemiological study, Einfeld and Tonge (1996a) found that 41 per cent of children with an intellectual disability aged between four and 18 years had a clinically significant emotional or behavioural disorder. However, what was of concern was that the authors reported that fewer than 10 per cent of the children and young people identified had received any specialist mental health services. It has also been suggested that as many as one-third of children and adolescents referred to mental health services for behaviour problems in school have undiagnosed learning disabilities (Kauffman, 1997).

It therefore appears that the experience of having an intellectual disability has a substantial effect on the psychological development of children and adolescents. This may not always lead to a comorbid psychiatric diagnosis, however, additional problems, such as low self-esteem, negative attributions for success, and poor social competence, should still receive attention from clinicians. If left untreated, they will further complicate learning, schoolwork, and relationships, and may lead to future mental health problems.

This suggests that the psychological and social difficulties that are characteristic of children and young people with intellectual disabilities can often be more problematic than the disability itself, as it will set them apart from peers both intellectually and socially. This, therefore, highlights the need for developmentally appropriate treatment services for this at-risk group of children. There are a number of programs that focus on generic social and emotional cognitive skill building as a means of reducing psychopathology. However, this chapter will focus on programs that build resilience through the use of effective coping strategies, and the development of problem-solving skills.

What types of interventions are available?

Children and young people with intellectual disabilities need interventions that will build age-appropriate life skills and improve their ability to cope with the social demands of everyday life. Skill-based approaches, such as social skills training and anger management, are familiar interventions that usually teach children specific skills in a group setting. However, research and clinical opinion highlight the inadequacy of social skills training as the sole intervention for emotional and behaviour difficulties (Bullis et al., 2001). That is not to say that the development of social competence is not important, as research clearly indicates that it is an essential life skill for children to master, because of the strong association between poor social skills and psychopathology (Matson et al., 2000). However, in terms of building psychological resilience and reducing behavioural risk factors, social skills programs should only ever be one component of a multifaceted treatment package. Similarly, anger management programs often fail to target the underlying deficits, such as poor emotional regulation and a lack of age-appropriate coping strategies.

In contrast, the skill deficit model is a more developmentally appropriate approach that focuses on (a) assessing what the child is capable of; (b) using this assessment to identify the life skills that the child needs to develop; and (c) teaching these skills in a developmentally appropriate manner by building on the child's existing skill level. This is a more practical approach, which is often used in one-to-one work with an individual where sessions can be tailored accordingly.

Problem solving

Problem solving is an essential life skill that teaches children how to deal with day-to-day challenges. To be good at problem solving, children need to acquire critical and creative thinking skills that will help them think about options and evaluate their possible consequences. When do children acquire these skills? Theories of cognitive development suggest that by the age of eight years children enter the concrete operational stage, which means they are able to think more logically, but still have difficulty with abstract reasoning and considering a range of alternatives (Vernon, 2002). They are also able to recognise and communicate feelings more effectively, suggesting that this stage has a positive impact on their problem-solving abilities.

Is this similar for children with an intellectual disability?

Research suggests that adolescents with intellectual disability have difficulty reaching early instrumental thinking milestones (such as word recognition, spelling, and computation), which results in poorer problem-solving strategies in general (Fidler et al., 2005). Research also indicates that individuals with intellectual disabilities are often slower at retrieving information from long-term memory, and thus acting on that information, suggesting poor verbal reasoning skills (Bjorklund, 2005).

It therefore appears that the language demands of cognitive techniques such as problem solving can be problematic for young people with intellectual disabilities, especially as verbal instruction is often the predominant approach to teaching these skills. However, problem solving can be enhanced for these children by providing a choice of possible solutions using visual cues such as pictures and animations (Bernard-Opitz et al., 2001), and through effective instruction (Swanson, 2001).

It is also important that the specific components and methods used to teach problem-solving techniques are appropriate to the developmental level of the child or young person. For example, adolescents with intellectual disabilities are often given social skills programs designed for younger children in an attempt to match their level of cognitive functioning, but this ignores the real-life social dilemmas that they face (Baker, 2003).

The use of group treatment programs to teach problem-solving skills rather than individual approaches are more commonly reported in the literature. Two examples of group interventions that could be appropriate and effective for this population are (a) the *Stop, Think, Do social skills training program*, which includes three separate manuals covering the age range from four to 15 years: early years (Petersen, 2002), primary school (Petersen & Adderley, 2002), and middle school (Petersen, 2004); and (b) the use of *augmentative and alternative communication (AAC) strategies* for developing emotional intelligence and problem-solving skills.

Stop, Think, Do social skills training program

Stop, Think, Do is an Australian social skills program (Petersen, 2002, 2004; Petersen & Adderley, 2002) developed for use in schools with children who

Table 16.1 Problem-solving steps from Stop, Think, Do social skills training

STOP (red light)	'You *feel … because* (problem)'. The aim is to develop perceptual, self-control, and communications skills.
THINK (yellow light)	*'What could we do?' 'What might happen then?'* This aims to develop cognitive, consequential thinking skills
DO (green light)	*'Do it!'* This aims to develop verbal and nonverbal behavioural skills

Sources: adapted from Petersen, 2002, 2004; Petersen & Adderley, 2002

have social emotional difficulties. The program aims to develop emotional social intelligence and social problem-solving skills. The program has been shown to be effective in a special school for secondary school children with mild to moderate intellectual disability and emotional and social problems (Beck & Horne, 1992). Beck and Horne (1992) reported that students developed a broad range of social skills, such as the ability to cope with teasing in a non-aggressive manner, resolving conflict with peers and siblings at home, and thinking before they acted.

The key problem-solving steps are taught using traffic light symbols to cue the skills (see table 16.1). The program has an accompanying book, *Stop and Think Learning: A Teacher's Guide for Motivating Children to Learn Including those with Special Needs* (Petersen, 1995), which contains ideas on how to modify the program for students with special learning needs or disabilities.

Augmentative and alternative communication (AAC)

Bloom and Bhargava are Australian speech pathologists (see <www.innovativeprogramming.net.au>) who have developed *augmentative and alternative communication (AAC)* strategies for developing emotional intelligence and problem-solving skills. Their manual, *Using AAC to Develop Emotions and Problem Solving Skills* (Bloom & Bhargava, 2004) utilises a social-cognitive approach to help individuals with communication difficulties and/or additional disabilities (such as individuals with autism, Asperger's syndrome, and Down syndrome) to gain better self-control over their emotions and improve their problem-solving skills. Bloom and Bhargava (2004) break the problem-solving process down into sequential steps, using AAC strategies such as social stories and multimodal teaching methods, to help the individual understand what concept is being illustrated at each step. This is outlined in table 16.2.

Struggling children

Some children will have difficulty with problem solving, as it entails a deeper level of cognitive processing, requiring the individual to make a best judgment, given the particular situation. Social problem solving also requires a child to think about how different people see or understand problems

Table 16.2 Steps in developing emotions and problem-solving skills

Step 1	Define the problem by identifying the relevant information; for example: 'What is the problem?'
Step 2	Identify the goal of the problem; for example: 'What will happen if the problem disappears?' 'What will happen if the problem is fixed?'
Step 3	Analyse the problem: break it down into smaller parts
Step 4	Explore possible solutions to achieve the goal
Step 5	Determine a solution that results in a win–win situation for everybody involved by considering their feelings
Step 6	Implement the best solution and evaluate the results

Adapted from Bloom & Bhargava, 2004

differently (perspective taking), which requires good abstract reasoning abilities (Bloomquist, 2006). If children have difficulty acquiring these skills, a more traditional behavioural approach can be used as an alternative, where the individual is taught specific strategies to be applied in a given situation. The cognitive approach is clearly preferable for teaching problem solving, as this encourages children to develop flexible thinking.

There are also a number of social skills programs that teach social problem solving as a small component of the program. These include the *Talkabout* series by Kelly (1996), a social communication skills package specifically designed for children and young people with learning disabilities. There is also *Space Travellers: An Interactive Program for Developing Social Understanding, Social Competence, and Social Skills* (Carter & Santomauro, 2004), which is an interactive social skills program. It was developed for students with autism spectrum disorder (ASD) and other social cognitive challenges, and takes students on a journey into space, where they learn major social skills. The skills taught include understanding emotions, feelings, and thinking patterns, reflective problem solving, stress release, dealing with bullying, goal setting, and self-regulation. There is also a version of the program designed for preschool children titled *Pirates: An Early-Years Group Program for Developing Social Understanding and Social Competence for Children with Autism Spectrum Disorders and Related Challenges* (Carter & Santomauro, 2007), which covers similar topics.

Coping strategies

As part of the problem-solving process, children need to be able to think of possible answers to their identified problem (for example, 'What can I do about it?'). As discussed earlier, this is quite a complex cognitive process. It requires children to (a) generate alternative solutions; and (b) evaluate the potential appropriateness or consequences of each solution, given the initial problem. However, more practically, children also need to have real experience of what is a possible helpful or unhelpful solution (*coping strategy*). Children will often learn different coping strategies (what works when) through their experiences. This is supported by research that has suggested that the pathway to healthy coping behaviour requires children to have opportunities to overcome manageable levels of distress (opportunities to learn) (Cole et al., 1994; Stifter et al., 1999).

It has been suggested that challenging behaviour in children with intellectual disabilities is associated not so much with the effectiveness of the child-coping skills as with his or her high levels of frustration (Jahromi et al., 2008). For example, research has suggested that children with Down syndrome may have insufficient experience of practising coping strategies that help overcome negative arousal, for instance, learning how to manage emotions such as frustration. It is hypothesised that the reasons for this are that some mothers compensate for their infants' lower levels of arousal by intervening earlier in response to low-intensity signals, thereby resulting in children not learning how to cope with the situation by themselves (Sorce & Emde, 1982). Furthermore, it has been suggested that children with high levels of frustration would have better social and behavioural outcomes if they were able to develop emotion regulation skills (Eisenberg et al., 1995).

In conclusion, in promoting psychological well-being, it is important to help children learn how to deal realistically with what they can and cannot change in their lives. These skills can be developed through the use of *cognitive behaviour therapy (CBT)*, which helps them understand the connection between thoughts, feelings, and behaviours. A review of the literature on CBT for children and young people indicates that task-orientated problem solving and social problem solving are often core components of many CBT programs (Christie & Wilson, 2005).

There is also the *PATHS program (Promoting Alternative Thinking Strategies)* (Greenberg & Kusche, 1998), which is an American intervention that targets children's development of effective coping strategies. It has been shown to be appropriate and effective for children with developmental disabilities. The PATHS curriculum is a comprehensive program for promoting emotional and social competencies, and reducing aggression and behaviour problems in primary school-aged children.

The curriculum consists of developmentally based lessons designed to be used by teachers and school counsellors, but also includes information and activities for parents to use at home to improve generalisation of skills taught. The program has been evaluated with a variety of special needs students, for instance, children who are deaf or hearing-impaired, or who have mild intellectual disability, language delay, and learning disabilities, and has shown promising results (Greenberg et al., 1995; Greenberg & Kusche, 1998). These studies indicated that, following intervention, the special needs group of children had significantly improved their social problem-solving skills and emotional understanding, and that they were significantly less likely to provide aggressive solutions and more likely to provide positive social solutions to interpersonal conflicts. These results were maintained at the one year and two year follow-up assessments.

In reviewing these programs, it appears that there is a trend towards early intervention and prevention through the school system. Many of the programs are being run in classrooms by teachers, and delivered to all children, in an attempt to build resilience and prevent the development of emotional and behavioural problems.

Attention

Attention deficit hyperactivity disorder (ADHD) is the psychiatric disorder most frequently diagnosed in association with learning and intellectual disabilities (Emerson, 2003a). The presence of ADHD has been found to further impair education and school adjustment, as well as compromise social interaction and family life for these children (Loveland & Tunali-Kotoski, 1997). This raises the question of whether these children need a different type of intervention program.

Research indicates that children and young people with ADHD, especially those with problems of self- control, often have deficits in cognitive processes that have an impact upon their ability to engage in planning or problem solving (Kendall 1993; Spence & Donovan, 1998). For example, aggressive children have been found to possess limited problem-solving skills and generate fewer verbal solutions to difficulties (Lochman et al., 1991). It therefore appears that children with intellectual disabilities and ADHD would benefit from being taught problem-solving skills. The question is whether they need to be taught in a different way.

Soo and Bailey (2006) reviewed attentional functioning in children with ADHD and learning and intellectual disabilities. They found that few studies had qualitatively investigated the similarities and differences in the attentional profiles of children with learning and intellectual disabilities, children with the inattentive form of ADHD, and children with the combined symptoms of inattention and hyperactivity-impulsivity. However, they argued that what was known so far about the attentional profiles of these children suggested that interventions need to consider the possible differences in attentional profile, and that this would allow for greater specificity in interventions. Researchers further argued that improving attentional functioning would have positive knock-on effects for many other abilities and skills that are reliant on age-appropriate attentional skills. This would lead to secondary gains in the children's school-based learning, behavioural problems, and organisational and social skills.

There are currently very few specific programs for children with an intellectual disability and ADHD. The closest is the *Alert Program for Self-regulation: How Does Your Engine Run?* (Williams & Shellenberger, 1994), which was originally designed to support children with attention and learning difficulties (ages 8 to 12 years), but has been adapted for preschool children through to adults. The program does not target social and emotional cognitive skill building, but may be an essential prerequisite for children with severe attention problems who have difficulty maintaining concentration within a group setting.

The *Alert Program* aims to help teachers, parents, and therapists work with the child to choose appropriate strategies to change or maintain states of alertness, to develop self-control skills. The development of self-control skills will help a child to participate more effectively within a group situation, as such children will be able to listen and follow directions, as well as control internal feelings.

Involving parents

Research has indicated that caring for a child with a learning or intellectual disability with additional emotional and behavioural problems was often associated with an increased risk of mental health problems and stress for parents (Baker et al., 2003). This suggests that effective management of emotional and behavioural disorders in children with intellectual disability should include parent education, as well as support and management of any parental mental health problems. Therefore it is not surprising that the above studies showed a trend towards involving parents in the intervention. The inclusion of parents in these programs has a number of additional benefits, such as increasing how techniques are generalised, and providing parents and children with a common language to discuss problems.

Conclusion

It appears that there are a number of programs available that focus on social and emotional cognitive skill building, problem-solving techniques, and coping strategies, as a means to reduce psychopathology. There is also a trend towards early intervention and prevention by involving parents and teachers in the intervention.

However, not all programs are appropriate and effective for children and young people with intellectual disabilities. Therefore, in selecting a program, it is essential to examine whether there is any research literature supporting the program for the intended client group. It is also important to remember that group treatment programs should only ever be one component of a multifaceted treatment package, especially when working with children who display high levels of emotional and behavioural problems.

17

Developing emotion-based social skills in children with autism spectrum disorder and intellectual disability

Belinda J. Ratcliffe

Introduction

Autism spectrum disorder (ASD) is a pervasive developmental disorder characterised by core difficulties in social and communication skills, as well as restricted and repetitive behaviour. ASD is commonly associated with intellectual disability. Children with intellectual disability have delayed social and emotional skills, generally commensurate with their overall skills. However, children with intellectual disability and comorbid ASD have deficits in social and emotional skills that are more than expected given their overall abilities. These social and emotional skill deficits in children with ASD may be one of several contributing risk factors to the very high prevalence of mental health issues in this population. Thus, interventions to promote social and emotional skills may provide an avenue to promote the mental health and well-being of children with ASD and intellectual disability. This chapter outlines current research and resources in the area of social and emotional skills.

Emotion-based social skills training (EBBST) (Wong et al., 2004) was developed to enhance the mental health and well-being of children with ASD (without intellectual disability) by developing social and emotional skills. EBSST was modified to meet the additional learning needs of children with ASD and comorbid intellectual disability. The implementation of *EBSST for children with ASD and mild intellectual disability* (Ratcliffe et al., 2010) is presented through a case study of Luke. This case highlights that existing clinical resources can be modified to meet the learning needs of children with intellectual disability. Moreover, the case suggests that child mental health and well-being can be promoted by means of clinical development of social and emotional skills.

Autism spectrum disorders and intellectual disability

Autism spectrum disorders (ASDs) fall under the broad umbrella of *pervasive developmental disorders*. The three autism spectrum disorders include *autistic disorder, Asperger's disorder,* and *pervasive developmental disorder, not otherwise specified (PDDNOS/atypical autism)*. Children with ASDs have difficulties with the quality of their social and communication skills, as well as difficulties with restricted, repetitive, and stereotyped patterns of behaviour, interests, and activities (American Psychiatric Association, 2000). Each of the three core features in the 'triad of impairment' can be represented on a continuum of severity. For example, an individual with a severe level of impairment in social skills will not necessarily have the same level of impairment in communication and/or behavioural skills. This implies that there is considerable variability in the presentation of children with ASD.

Current estimates are that ASD occurs in one of 150 children (Matson & Shoemaker, 2009). Approximately 50 to 70 per cent of all children with ASD have an intellectual disability.[1] Of those children with an intellectual disability, approximately 30 per cent have mild to moderate intellectual disability, and 40 per cent have severe to profound intellectual disability (Fombonne, 2003). In general, research suggests that childhood IQ level is negatively correlated with overall negative adult outcome (Billstedt et al., 2005). This suggests that children with ASD and intellectual disability represent a particularly vulnerable and important population to consider in clinical treatment.

Typically developing children tend to make progress in their social and emotional skills in an ordered sequence, with simple skills that develop in early life, becoming more elaborated, sophisticated, and established over time. Although there is no universal timetable for the acquisition of social or emotional skills, tables 17.1 and 17.2 respectively provide a guideline for the sequence of social and emotional skills in typically developing children.

Children with intellectual disability, without autism, have delays in social and emotional skills, commensurate with other areas of their development and behaviour (Kraijer, 2000). For example, a ten-year-old child with an intellectual disability who is functioning cognitively at the level of about a six-year-old child would be likely to have social and emotional skills also at the

1 Intellectual disability refers to significantly sub-average intellectual functioning, as measured by an IQ score less than 70 on individually administered tests of intelligence as well as concurrent deficits in adaptive behaviour (American Psychiatric Association, 2000).

Table 17.1 Guideline for the development of social skills in typically developing children

Age (years)	*Social skills*
2	• Social awareness is limited • Play tends to be solitary • Toddlers will closely observe and copy adults and other children
3	• Parallel play develops: children play alongside one another, with some interaction • Beginning to learn to share and take turns • Beginning to learn to manage physical aggression
4–5	• Can approach others and ask to join in • Cooperative play develops • Beginning to learn to play fairly and abide by rules • Start to play group games, which are more complex and organised • 'Special' friendships begin to form • Beginning to learn to be assertive and to ask others to stop if they are being annoying
6–8	• Beginning to learn to be a 'good winner' and a 'good loser' • Can empathise with others in distress and offer appropriate support • Conversation skills develop: listening and turn taking • Negotiation skills develop: including others in decision-making, learning to decide together and make suggestions rather than boss others around • Asks an adult for support when needed • Able to say 'no' to peers when appropriate
9–12	• Beginning to learn to speak confidently in front of a group • Beginning to learn to respect the opinions of others

Source: adapted from McGrath & Francey, 1991

level of about a six-year-old. In contrast, children with ASD have delays in social and emotional skills more than expected, given their development in other areas (Bolte & Poustka, 2002; Kraijer, 2000). Thus, for example, a ten-year-old child with ASD and intellectual disability who is functioning cognitively at the level of about a six-year-old would be likely to have social and emotional skills at the level of about a two- to three-year-old.

The pronounced difficulties in social and emotional skills in children with ASD can manifest in a variety of ways, depending on the individual presentation of the child. Social skill excesses and deficits in ASD have been studied much more extensively in the empirical literature (see for example, Matson & Wilkins, 2007) than emotional skills. However, in general, empirical research and clinical experience suggests that children with ASD have social and emotional skills that are delayed and disordered, and can often be thought of as being more consistent with the skills of a young child or toddler. For example, in the social domain, children with ASD may tend to:

- show less awareness of others
- engage in solitary or limited play
- prefer their own company
- appear awkward and unsure
- lack motivation to interact socially with others

Table 17.2 Guideline for the development of emotional skills in typically developing children

Developmental sequence	*Progression*
1 Children's emotions emerge	The four key emotions are: • SAD (sad, blue, gloomy) • MAD (angry, irritable, furious) • BAD (guilty, anxious, fearful) • GLAD (happy, joyous, peaceful, content)
2 Children develop emotional self-awareness	• Simple declarations of emotions (e.g., 'I'm sad') • Develop more complex reasoning and greater understanding • By 5-6 years: can hold more than one feeling at a time but in same 'emotional cluster' (e.g., happy and excited; not happy and nervous). At this point children believe opposing feelings are directed towards different things. • By 8-11 years: children understand that multiple and contrasting feelings towards the same event are feasible, but not at the same time (e.g., they can be happy and sad about the same event, but not at the same time) • By 10–12 years: children can hold two or more very different feelings towards the same object or situation simultaneously
3 Children recognise others' emotions	• By 2–5 years: identify others' positive and negative emotions based on obvious physical and body cues (e.g., facial expressions), focusing on only one emotion at a time • By middle childhood: identify others' emotions based on more subtle contextual cues (e.g., take into account situational cues) • Older childhood: identify shades of meaning and combinations of feelings, and ability to assess another person's probable mental state • Develop awareness that the same events do not always lead to the same outcomes
4 Children learn to regulate what they are feeling	• Children gradually learn to manage their emotions so that they are not totally overwhelmed by them, so they can interact with others more effectively • Rather than a 'progression', children tend to develop strategies to regulate emotions, which expand along with the development of verbal, physical, and intellectual abilities (e.g., suppressing the expression of certain emotions; soothing one's self; seeking comfort; avoiding or ignoring certain emotionally arousing events; changing goals that have been thwarted; interpreting emotionally arousing events in alternative ways)

Source: adapted from Kostelnik et al., 2006

- show interest in younger or older children, but not same-aged peers
- experience difficulty understanding social norms
- have poor social problem-solving abilities.

Similarly, in the emotional domain, children with ASD may have difficulties with:

- understanding their own emotions
- showing facial expressions congruent to the situation
- attending to others' emotional communication

- imitating others' emotions
- inferring how another person feels
- displaying emotional extremes or flat affect
- managing their emotions.

There is a high prevalence of mental health issues in children with intellectual disability. For example, Einfeld and Tonge (1996b) found that 40.7 per cent of Australian 4–18-year-olds with intellectual disability have 'emotional or behavioural disorders'. However, children with ASD experience significantly higher levels of psychopathology than young people with intellectual disability without comorbid ASD (Brereton et al., 2006; Gillberg & Billstedt, 2000). Studies involving community samples (unselected for psychiatric disorders) of children with ASD have found approximately 72–73 per cent of children have at least one other mental health issue in addition to ASD (see for example, Brereton et al., 2006; Leyfer et al., 2006).

One challenge in this area of research is that assessment and diagnosis of these comorbid mental health issues in intellectual disability are complex. Despite this, there is evidence that children with ASD experience significantly higher than expected levels of both internalising and externalising disorders than the general population of children with intellectual disability. For example, children with ASD are at risk of internalising disorders, including comorbid anxiety or fears (Bellini, 2003; Brereton et al., 2006; Leyfer et al., 2006), obsessive compulsive disorder (Leyfer et al., 2006; McDougle et al., 1995), and mood disorders (Brereton et al., 2006; Leyfer et al., 2006; Ghaziuddin et al., 2002). Children with ASD are also at risk of externalising disorders, including attention deficit hyperactivity disorder (ADHD) (Brereton et al., 2006; Goldstein & Schwebach, 2004) and challenging behaviour (Murphy et al., 2009).

Research examining possible reasons for the high levels of comorbid mental health issues in children with ASD is sparse. However, research from typically developing children suggests poor social skills and poor social supports may be a contributing risk factor to the development of mental health issues (Spence, 2003). Thus, it is plausible that social and emotional skills deficits may be one of several risk factors for the development and maintenance of emotional and behavioural disorders in children with ASD. Interventions to provide social and emotional skills may provide one of several points of intervention to promote mental health and well-being.

Interventions to promote social and emotional skills

Research and published resources

Existing empirical research in the area of interventions to promote social and emotional skills in ASD has focused almost exclusively on social skills (for reviews, see Scattone, 2007; Matson et al., 2007; McConnell, 2002). In general, these reviews suggest that social skills interventions have been successful in producing positive changes in the social behaviour of children with ASD. However, similar to the developmental disability research, there are significant methodological limitations inherent in the ASD literature. Participant samples are often small and heterogeneous in regard to age, gender, comorbid issues, and level of disability. There is a clear bias to conduct social skills interventions with verbal children without intellectual disability. Studies often fail to demonstrate generalisability of skills to the 'real world'. Moreover, where interventions have been found to be successful, research often isn't published in sufficient detail to replicate key components of the intervention, and treatment manuals are rarely published for dissemination to clinicians in the field (McConnell, 2002). To date, no empirical study has explicitly examined the impact of social skills intervention on mental health and well-being in children with ASD and intellectual disability.

There are several published clinical resources available for clinicians to help promote social and emotional skills in children with ASD. However, in general these resources lack the empirical literature to support their use. There are several other problematic issues with the published curricula at this time. Current resources tend to be aimed at children with ASD without intellectual disability (high functioning autism and Asperger's disorder). They tend to incorporate a bits-and-pieces approach to teaching social and/or emotional skills, rather than being presented in a coherent developmentally orientated framework. Parent and/or teacher training is often not included in resource packages, and if it is included, is often done as a handout only, which suggests a lack of attention to supporting children to further develop and generalise skills in 'untrained' settings.

Despite these limitations, current published resources can be clinically helpful and provide a basis for developing social and/or emotional skills interventions. Table 17.3 provides a sample of published resources to promote the development of social and emotional skills and suggestions for possible clinical applications in children with ASD and intellectual disability. Clinicians must utilise these and other resources critically, considering their appropriateness for individual children. Programs may need to be modified to meet individual learning needs, particularly if children have a comorbid disability, behavioural, or mental health issues.

Emotion-based social skills

Emotion-based social skills training (EBSST) (Wong et al., 2004) is one program that aims to bridge the gap between empirical literature and published resources. EBSST was originally designed to meet the needs of upper primary school-aged children with *high functioning autism* and *Asperger's disorder* (Wong et al., 2004). In particular, this intervention was designed to enhance the mental health and well-being of children with ASD and their parents by developing social and emotional skills.

Table 17.3 Sample of published resources for development of social and emotional skills and possible clinical applications

Name of program	*Brief description*	*Clinical applications*
PALS Social Skills Program: Playing and Learning to Socialise (3rd edn) (Cooper et al., 2007)	A social skills program for children aged 3–6 years, consisting of ten 20–30 minute lessons on the following topics: greetings; turn-taking; talking and listening; play; sharing; asking for help; identifying feelings; empathy; overcoming fear and anxiety; managing frustration; calming down and speaking up	• This program has been used in childcare settings for children with internalising and externalising problems (many of whom did have associated developmental delay in one or more areas) rather than specifically for children with intellectual disability. However, use of concrete, visual teaching materials such as role-play with puppets, videotape vignettes and songs with actions suggest this resource could be easily adapted for children with intellectual disability • Teacher and parent handouts are included to promote generalisation of the 'skill of the week'
Social Skills Activities For Special Children (Mannix, 1993)	A program to develop social skills in primary school-aged children. It provides ready-to-use lessons with 142 reproducible activity sheets, which are split into the following areas: 1 Accepting rules and authority at school 2 Relating to peers 3 Developing positive social skills	• This program is designed to be used by teachers in the classroom. However, it could be easily adapted for individual and/or group intervention • This program is probably most appropriate for children with intellectual disability who have skills in basic reading and writing (prerequisite to complete worksheets) • Letters to parents outlining key teaching points are provided to promote generalisation of skills at home
Promoting Social Success: A Curriculum for Children with Special Needs (Siperstein & Rickards, 2004)	A curriculum designed to improve social skills of students with mild intellectual disability (and other learning difficulties). Arranged into five units (between 5 and 22 lessons; 30–45-minute lessons per unit) each of which builds on the last: • Unit 1: Introductory lessons • Unit 2: Understanding feelings and actions: emotional and behavioural regulation • Unit 3: Using social information: noticing and interpreting cues • Unit 4: Planning what to do: problem solving • Unit 5: Making and keeping friends: social knowledge	• Designed for 'self-contained and inclusive classrooms'. However, the authors note that it could be adapted for use in small groups outside the classroom • Provides suggestions for activities to promote generalisation • Uses a range of visual strategies to reduce verbal load and make lessons concrete (e.g., using footprints on ground as visual aid for commencing role-play)

Name of program	*Brief description*	*Clinical applications*
Social Skills Training for Adolescents with General Moderate Learning Difficulties (Cornish & Ross, 2003)	A 10-session social skills program aimed at 13–17-year-old students with moderate intellectual disability. Aims to develop the following skills: listening and paying attention; monitoring spoken language; monitoring body language; recognising strengths; assertiveness; recognising feelings; confidence; conflict resolution; and empathy	• Concrete with reduced literacy demands • Letters to parents and weekly homework tasks for the adolescents to promote generalisation • Provides guides on multisource and modal assessment of social skills
The Transporters (Golan et al., 2006)	An interactive DVD format involving 15 five-minute episodes about 15 different emotions involving imaginary toy vehicle characters who have emotional experiences and adventures. 'Easy' and 'hard' quizzes follow each episode. This program aims to help children enhance their understanding of the causes of emotions and of emotional expressions	The series was created especially for children with autism spectrum disorder (ASD) who find it hard to recognise causes of emotion and facial expressions of emotion. However, would also be appropriate for young children with intellectual disability. It could be adapted for individual or small groups
My Book Full of Feelings: How to Control and React to the Size of your Emotions (Jaffe & Gardner, 2006)	An interactive workbook that aims to teach primary school-aged children to identify and assess the intensity of and respond appropriately to their emotions	• Originally designed to be used individually for children with ASD • This program could be adapted for children with intellectual disability who have skills in basic reading and writing (prerequisite to complete workbook) • Could be adapted for small groups • This book has laminated pages for use with a non-permanent marker allowing for the pages to be wiped and reused
The Way to A: Empowering Children with Autism Spectrum and Other Neurological Disorders to Monitor and Replace Aggression and Tantrum Behaviour (Manasco, 2006)	An interactive workbook aimed at understanding and managing a particular emotion: anger	• Originally designed to be used individually for children with ASD • This program could be adapted for children with intellectual disability who have skills in basic reading and writing (prerequisite to complete workbook) • Could be adapted for small groups • This book has laminated pages for use with a non-permanent marker allowing for the pages to be wiped and reused

EBSST assumes that emotional skills are embedded in social interactions, thus emotions in the context of social situations are targeted, rather than pragmatic social skills. For example, a typically developing eight-year-old child would have the ability to perceive emotions, be developing insight into the feelings and thoughts of others, and have some cognitive strategies to regulate his or her own emotions. The child would use these abilities to regulate social interactions. However, an eight-year-old child with ASD may be taught the skills of conversation initiations but lack basic insight into his or her own emotions, emotions of others, and emotional regulation, and thus lack the ability to engage in appropriate social interactions. Thus, EBSST draws on theories of emotional development, as well as emotional intelligence (Mayer et al., 2000), to offer a specific social skills intervention that also considers the level of emotional development of the child with ASD. EBSST has been evaluated in a pilot study, and is currently in a randomised control trial (Wong & Heriot, 2009). To date, findings are suggestive that EBSST is clinically effective.

Given the high level of comorbid intellectual disability in children with ASD, and the high risk of mental health issues in this population, EBBST was adapted to meet the learning needs of children with ASD and mild intellectual disability. *EBBST for children with ASD and mild intellectual disability* (Ratcliffe et al., 2010) also aimed to enhance mental health and well-being in children (and their parents) by developing social and emotional skills. An overview of the EBBST for children with ASD and mild intellectual disability (Ratcliffe et al., 2010) curriculum is outlined in table 17.4. A pilot of the program was conducted in 2008, when groups of up to six children were seen for three modules (each consisting of five sessions), with breaks in between modules. Parent sessions were held concurrently to child sessions.

To modify EBSST (Wong et al., 2004), the individual learning needs of upper primary school-aged children with ASD and comorbid mild intellectual disability were considered. In terms of teaching content, developmentally appropriate emotional skills were targeted, with greater emphasis placed on targeting and consolidating early to middle childhood emotional skills. Teaching methods were also tailored to support children's cognitive and language abilities. Thus, modelling and visual supports or *augmentative and alternative communication systems* (such as pictures or line drawings, video social stories, and video story movies) were used to supplement verbal language wherever possible.

The pace of information delivery was slowed to allow for children's processing capacity. Information was also kept concrete, and repetition of key learning points was provided through presentation of the same information using a variety of teaching methods (rather than the same information presented repetitively in the same way). Further detail regarding the teaching methods employed in this program is outlined in the case study below. Also in keeping with a developmentally oriented intervention, structured breaks and games were utilised to increase children's motivation and concentration.

Table 17.4 Curriculum for EBBST for children with ASD and mild intellectual disability

Modules	*Child curriculum*	*Parent curriculum*
		Promote generalisation and maintenance of child skills via:
One 5 × 90-minute weekly sessions	Identifying emotions	Psychoeducation
Break: 2 weeks		
Two 5 × 90-minute weekly sessions	A Emotional problem solving B Understanding others' emotions	Parent cognitive behaviour therapy (CBT)
Break: 2 weeks		
Three 5 × 90-minute weekly sessions	Managing emotions	Training parents as 'emotion coaches'
Break: 2 weeks		
Booster session 1 × 90-minute session	Skills consolidation	Training in self-monitoring and evaluation
		Source: Ratcliffe, 2010

Case study 17.1
Luke

Luke was a 10-year-old boy with a confirmed diagnosis of autistic disorder using the *Autism Diagnostic Observation Schedule (ADOS)* (Lord et al., 1999) and *Autism Diagnostic Interview–Revised (ADI-R)* (Rutter et al., 2003). Luke also had a mild intellectual disability, confirmed using the *Wechsler Intelligence Scale for Children–Fourth Edition (WISC-IV)* (Wechsler, 2003) and the *Adaptive Behaviour Assessment System–Second Edition (ABAS-II)* (Harrison & Oakland, 2003). Luke was currently enrolled in an 'IM' class (for students for mild intellectual disability) in a NSW Department of Education primary school. Luke lived at home with both of his parents and his seven-year-old brother. His mother was concerned that Luke was a 'worrier' and didn't cope well with change. Luke also had difficulty 'reading' social situations, and his mother felt that he was often socially inappropriate. Luke's teacher reported that he was a loner at school, preferring his own company.

Luke was enrolled in a pilot study in 2008 for *EBSST for children with ASD and mild intellectual disability* (Ratcliffe et al., 2010) in an outpatient setting, along with five other children with similar presenting issues. His mother attended concurrent parent sessions. Pre-intervention assessment of social skills using the *Social Responsiveness Scale* (*SRS*, formerly known as the *Social Reciprocity Scale*) (Constantino, 2002) indicated an overall moderate impairment in social skills, as indicated in parent and teacher reports. The parent and teacher reports also noted that Luke presented with significantly elevated emotional and behavioural issues, as measured by the *Developmental Behaviour Checklist (DBC)* (Einfeld & Tonge, 1992).

EBSST for children with ASD and mild intellectual disability (Ratcliffe et al., 2010) employs a uniform teaching framework for each session, within modules that include four key teaching elements. The key teaching elements and some samples of Luke's work in a session on feeling 'worried' from module 1 ('Understanding own emotions') are outlined below.

Key teaching element 1: Provide a visual worksheet to support skills development

Module 1 of the training focused on teaching children to understand the four primary emotions: happy, sad, worried, and angry. Children were taught to link social situations with the different feelings that they might have in these situations. They were also taught to rate the intensity of their feelings. Each feeling was the focus of one session within the module. A *feelings strength bar visual worksheet* was developed for each of the four feelings. Note that the feeling worried strength bar worksheet in figure 17.1 was clear and concrete, incorporating pictures as well as words, and colour coding to support the learning needs of a child with intellectual disability.

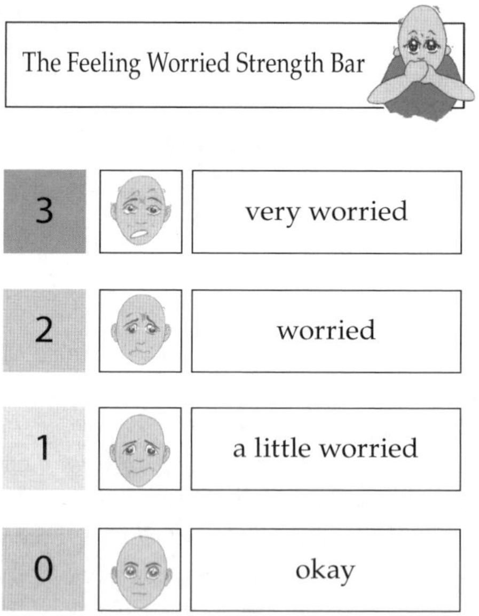

Figure 17.1 'Feeling worried strength bar' from module 1

Source: Ratcliffe et al., 2010

Key teaching element 2: Teach the skill using visual supports

The 'feeling worried strength bar' was introduced using a DVD social story with the following script:

> There are lots of different things that make me feel worried. Sometimes I feel okay. Other times I feel a little worried. Sometimes I feel worried. Other times I feel very worried. We can use a strength bar to describe how strong our feelings are in different situations. Let's practise using the feeling worried strength bar in different situations (Ratcliffe et al., 2010; Youth work, module 1, p. 18).

Children then watched a video story movie showing an actor, Adam, in different situations that made him feel different intensities of worried. For example:

- Adam feels OK when his friend is running late
- Adam feels a little worried when he got stuck on his homework
- Adam feels worried when he spilt something on his shirt
- Adam feels very worried when he thinks about meeting new people.

Following each scene, the children watched Adam while he modelled labelling his feeling, and the intensity of his feeling, on the feeling worried strength bar. DVD video social stories, story movies, and modelling were use extensively throughout the intervention to introduce and teach emotion-based social skills. Luke frequently reported that the 'best thing' about the group was watching the Adam DVDs.

Key teaching element 3: Practise the skill and use the visual worksheet in the clinic setting

Following each of the video clips showing 'Adam' in situations that made him feel different intensities of worried, children were invited to show how worried they would feel in that situation by standing next to the number on a floor sized 'feeling worried strength bar'. Later in the session, children were asked to 'draw, write or stick a picture of something that made them feel worried', and then 'draw an arrow to how worried it makes you on the feeling worried strength bar'. In this activity, Luke felt worried, a number two on the 'feeling worried strength bar', when he was 'all alone at school'.

Key teaching element 4: Practice the skill and use the visual worksheet in the 'real world' via a takeaway task

Children were asked to complete a takeaway task, which involved completing a visual worksheet for a 'real life' situation during the week when they felt worried, and rate the intensity of the worried feelings on the strength bar. As shown in figure 17.2, Luke felt very worried, a number three on the feeling worried strength bar, when 'mum left her keys in the car and I was very late to school'.

Each of these four key teaching elements was incorporated into the sessions in module 1 (identifying emotions). Each teaching element was also incorporated into module 2 (emotional problem solving and understanding others' emotions) and module 3 (managing emotions).

Outcomes

Following completion of the 15 sessions, and at the six-month followup, Luke was found to have made and maintained clinically significant improvements in his social and emo-

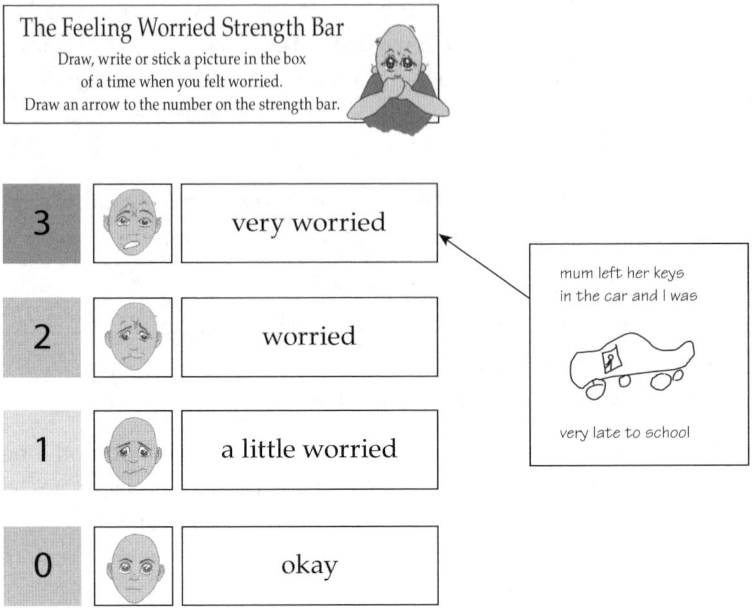

Figure 17.2 Luke's feeling worried strength bar takeaway task
Source: Ratcliffe et al., 2008

tional skills. Post-intervention, Luke's social skills (as rated on the social reciprocity scale through parent and teacher report) were found to fall just within the normal range expected for his age. Luke's emotional and behaviour issues had also improved, with particular clinically significant improvement reported in the anxiety domain (as measured using the developmental behaviour checklist).

Qualitatively, Luke's mother reported that 'Luke has always had difficulties with language; however, for the first time he now has a language to talk to others about his feelings—because the skills were taught in a visual way.' At home, Luke's mother felt she was 'a lot better off, as I know what to do to help Luke understand and manage his feelings'. She further reported that the intervention had 'rubbed off' on the family: 'Everyone can use the skills—we will use these skills throughout Luke's life.' At school, Luke's teacher reported that Luke 'is better able to deal with other children's behaviour [and] comfort other children when they are upset'. Taken together, these findings suggest that Luke made clinically significant improvements in his emotion-based social skills that appeared to have generalised from the clinic into the home and school settings. In addition, Luke's mental health and well-being appeared to have been enhanced.

Conclusion

Difficulties in social and emotional skills may be an important risk factor for the development of mental health issues in children with ASD and intellectual disability. Interventions to promote social and emotional skills may be an important avenue to promote the mental health and well-being of this population. However, there is limited empirical literature available to guide clinicians on intervention approaches and how to promote the social and emotional skills of children with ASD and intellectual disability. Published resources are available; however, they often lack an evidence base and therefore need to be used critically. *EBSST for Children with ASD and Mild Intellectual Disability* (Ratcliffe et al., 2010) is a program designed to enhance mental health and well-being by developing social and emotional skills. The case of Luke was presented to highlight the key teaching elements of this program, and the adaptations that are needed to meet the needs of children with intellectual disability. Clinicians are encouraged to utilise evidence-based resources where possible, and adapt existing resources to meet the individual learning needs of children with ASD and intellectual disability to develop social and emotional skills.

18

Promoting healthy sexual lives for young people with learning difficulties

Cheryl Jones and Jane Chivers

Introduction: sexuality: it's not just about sex

A useful definition of sexuality takes us beyond the narrow confines of biology, that it is just about sexual intercourse between a man and a woman, and reproduction. Sexuality is a normal part of human development that is expressed through every life stage. Gender, sexual identity, reproduction, and sexual orientation are all aspects of sexuality. Beliefs about sexuality are influenced by biology, and also the social, cultural, religious, legal, and political worlds in which people live. Sexuality is expressed in many ways, not just through sexual activity, and may be demonstrated through the varied roles and relationships that people have.

In this chapter, the term *person with a learning difficulty* is used to encompass any young person whose disability or mental health diagnosis has an impact on his or her learning capacity. There is an emphasis on young people with an intellectual disability. *Sexuality education* is used as a broad term that includes a range of actions from providing information to delivering formal structured education.

Regardless of their ability, all young people have the right to education, information, and support to enable them to experience their sexuality in a positive way and to have safe, healthy relationships. This support can influence their sexual health, and their ability to make informed decisions, develop relationships, and stay safe. Lack of support in this vital area of a young person's development may lead to less positive outcomes, including exploitation, vulnerability to abuse (Blanchett & Wolfe, 2002; Servais, 2006), and contact with the criminal justice system. It may also lead to poor health, including risk of sexually transmissible infections including HIV.

What do young people with learning difficulties need and want?

In the authors' experience of providing sexuality education, young people with learning difficulties want the same experiences and opportunities as their peers. To enable this, it has been identified that young people with a learning difficulty need:

- information about their changing bodies and the integrity of their body
- rules about social sexual behaviour
- to be in safe environments free from abuse
- people who will support them towards developing positive sexuality and not see it as a problem
- skills in developing and maintaining friendships
- opportunities to develop intimate relationships
- opportunities to take risks that will enable them to become more independent
- access to health services
- people to advocate with them for their rights.

Why don't people talk about sexuality more often?

Professionals, parents, and carers will often say that sexuality education is the domain of experts and therefore it is someone else's responsibility (Chivers & Mathieson, 2000). However, if sexuality is seen as a normal part of human development, young people need to be supported in the same ways as for their intellectual, physical, social, and emotional development. Anyone supporting a young person needs to consider his or her role in sexuality education. There are a number of issues that impede carers and professionals from taking on this task. These issues include: lacking the confidence to teach young people with learning difficulties; fear that talking about sexuality may create problems; a belief that this education is not necessary; confusion about duty of care and other legal issues; anxiety about conflict with parents and other staff; and personal cultural, and religious beliefs (McConkey & Ryan 2001; Chivers & Mathieson, 2000; Löfgren-Mårtenson, 2004).

Often young people with learning difficulties are stereotyped as asexual, or there are concerns they will be sexually inappropriate and unable to control themselves. One of the consequences of this is that education may be withheld purposely or not seen as important. Parents and carers may not want to provide education for fear of awakening sexual interest and creating problems. Even if people can get past these barriers, and do provide some sexuality education, it may be more focused on dangers and avoidance of risk rather than on aspects of positive sexuality, such as love, intimacy, pleasure, and fun.

Good practice in providing sexuality information and education

Planning and preparation

A supportive environment, where the young person feels he or she has permission to ask questions, seek information, and receive accurate positive responses from approachable people, is important. While the provision of sexuality education and information should be a planned process, that should not take away from the day-to-day opportunities that arise as teachable moments. An assessment of the person's existing level of knowledge and skills will ensure that education and information is accurately focused. It cannot be assumed that the person will have even basic knowledge, such as names for private body parts.

It is important to address misinformation and myths that may be believed by young people, for example, that masturbation leads to blindness or that they will not get pregnant having sex for the first time (Blanchett & Wolfe 2002). Garwood and McCabe (2000), in a comparative study of pre-knowledge of men who participated in a sex education program, report that misinformation included that HIV is transmitted by coughing, sneezing, and kissing; also, some believed that sexual intercourse is 'bad'.

Two tools that can assist in assessing a young person's knowledge about sexuality issues have been developed in Victoria. The first of these tools is *Human Relations and Sexuality: Knowledge Awareness Assessment for People with an Intellectual Disability* (Family Planning Victoria, 1997). This tool is designed to identify knowledge about the body, concepts of private and public places and behaviours, sexual activity, and other topics. The second assessment tool is *Assessment of Sexual Knowledge (ASK)* (Butler et al., 2003), which includes a *problematic sociosexual behaviour checklist* that can be administered by trained clinicians. Other information to consider includes sexual health history, such as impact of medications, medical conditions and syndromes, contraceptive use, lifestyle and environment, sexual activity, and sexual orientation.

Collaboration among the key people in the person's network, including parents and support workers, will enhance the effectiveness of sexuality education (Blanchett & Wolfe, 2002). People who have close personal or professional relationships with the person will be in a position to create opportunities to reinforce skills, answer questions, and use teachable moments. Young people are strongly influenced by the values and agenda of family and staff. There may be some resistance to young people's rights to sexual expression. Carers and staff can benefit from information about sexuality to assist them to develop a more positive perspective.

Many people with a disability are victims of sexual assault. Goodfellow and Camilleri (2003) reviewed research over the previous decade and reported that incidence could be as high as ten times that of people without a disability. Any person providing sexuality education should be prepared to respond to a disclosure of past or current abuse. Knowledge of mandatory reporting, support services, and organisational procedures is essential.

What to include in sexuality information and education

Sexuality is a private area of people's lives, and education brings it out into a more public arena. Education can be as readily used to control people's behaviour as it can be used to open up opportunities for them. While sensitivity to culture and personal values is appropriate, this needs to be balanced with the provision of accurate and contextually useful information. The trainer needs to reflect on his or her own personal values, concerns, and beliefs, and how these may influence what information is provided and how it is delivered.

When information or education about sexuality is provided, trainers tend to focus on danger, risk management, and protection (Blanchett & Wolfe, 2002). There is a need to balance this by focusing on the emotional aspects of sexuality, such as skills in forming, developing, and ending relationships (Garwood & McCabe, 2000). Comparative studies of sexuality education curricula reported that two areas that are absent in much sexuality education are pleasure and sexual diversity, including homosexuality. Löfgren-Mårtenson (2004), in her study of young people attending dances, reported that homosexuality in young people with an intellectual disability was often misinterpreted by carers and parents as friendships or as misdirected sexual expression. Sexual orientation is often ignored, or attempts are made to adjust it. Also, when sexuality education discusses positive sexuality (such as pleasure, intimacy, caring, and sexual diversity), the young person may be better equipped to make informed choices about his or her sexual life.

Research and clinical practice have found that education is most effective when received from a young age, and that it should reflect a comprehensive developmental framework. Such frameworks have been developed by McDonagh and colleagues (2000), who identified four main domains of sexuality education, and suggested possible sequences for teaching topics. These frameworks are outlined in table 18.1.

How to teach sexuality information and education

Most professionals working in the disability area have experience in supporting the development of skills and knowledge in many areas of a young person's life. It is often personal discomfort or lack of role clarity that can inhibit them in the area of sexuality. Yet the principles and methods are similar. Programs and resources can be tailored to suit the person's current level of knowledge, learning style, and capacity. They are delivered in ways that use the person's individual communication methods. Using visual resources and drama or role-play assists learning for many people.

It is important to provide key messages and give examples that emphasise social norms, acceptable behaviour, and how the law reinforces rules about

Table 18.1 Frameworks for sexuality education and possible sequences for teaching topics

Framework	*1*	*2*	*3*	*4*
Domain	*Sexuality*	*STIs/AIDS*	*Relationships*	*Health and hygeine*
Possible sequence of topics	• Self-awareness and self-esteem • Body parts and functions • Puberty • Feelings • Sexual feelings • Being sexual – what does it mean? – legal rights – decision-making and assertiveness – protective behaviour • STIs and HIV/AIDS • Pregnancy and contraception	• Self-awareness and self-esteem • Sexuality • Sexual relationships, rights, and responsibilities • Decision-making • Sexual health and diseases • HIV/AIDS • Signs of STIs • Transmission • Preventing diseases • Condoms: how to use and where to buy • Safe sex: practices and communication skills • Protective behaviours • Testing (STIs): rights and procedures • Testing (HIV): rights and procedures • Treatment	• Self-awareness and self-esteem • Feelings about others and choosing friends • Circle concept: different types of relationships – communicating – making friends – maintaining relationships – different things we do with friends – appropriate behaviour • Sexual relationships • Consequences of being sexual • Caring for ourselves and our partner • Rights and responsibilities • Preventing STIs, including HIV • Problem solving	• Body parts and functions • Feelings: body awareness • Self-awareness and self-esteem • Nutrition and exercise • Feeling healthy and feeling ill • Health care • Contagious and communicable diseases • STIs and HIV/AIDS • Using medical practitioners and health services

Source: adapted from McDonagh et al., 2000

sex and relationships. Using terms for body parts and sexual activity that are accurate and generally socially acceptable is good practice. The use of slang should be avoided, because it can be offensive or have negative connotations. Peer interaction can be an effective learning process, so consider presenting information in a group setting. Progress of learning should be monitored frequently to check that key messages are being understood.

There are many educational resources that use accurate explicit images. If using explicit material, explain to the person what will be shown and seek their consent. It may be necessary also to seek agreement of parents or guardians. Always let the person know that he or she can stop the learning or say no at any point. The use of pornography as an educational tool is not appropriate and is likely to be illegal.

Using opportunities in everyday situations will reinforce learning. For example, contemporary TV drama can be used to illustrate relationships, both healthy and unhealthy. Although at times it may be necessary to provide support and education to deal with specific issues—for example, masturbation in public—this could also be considered an opportunity to open the discussion about what other education might be needed and how best to provide it.

The following case study demonstrates a simple process for developing and supporting a collaborative approach to learning by assessing knowledge and learning styles, identifying learning needs, working in partnership, using appropriate resources, and creating opportunities for practice.

Case study 18.1: Ricky

Ricky was 11 years old, and had autism and a moderate intellectual disability. He lived at home with his parents and siblings, and attended a special class in a mainstream school. His parents contacted the local disability caseworker, anxious to get help regarding how to provide sex education to Ricky. They were keen to take on this role but did not know where to begin. Ricky's school was to commence sex education classes, but his parents were concerned that the information would be too complex.

Through parent interview, a simple assessment was done of their understanding of Ricky's current level of knowledge. Ricky participated in the interview and was able to demonstrate a basic knowledge of male and female private body parts. Effective ways to help Ricky to learn were identified.

Ricky enjoyed computer-based and visual learning. The caseworker liaised with the school to review the mainstream sexuality education program, and was able to modify the information to suit Ricky's learning style. The content was simplified and condensed into key messages. The focus was on puberty, friendships, and protective behaviours, as these were relevant to his learning needs. Ricky's parents were further supported with the provision of information and resources.

Through the program, Ricky continued to gain knowledge relevant to his developmental needs, and his parents felt more confident in their role as educators. They were equipped with knowledge and resources, and had access to professional support as required. A collaborative approach was developed between the family, the school, and the disability service to support ongoing learning, and a plan was developed to extend Ricky's sexuality education as he developed. Ricky was provided with opportunities to practise and develop appropriate social interactions through participation in a local dance class and a sporting group.

Being proactive rather than reactive

Often clinicians only receive referrals around sexuality when there is a problem or issue for a young person. This approach can reinforce people's anxieties and beliefs about sexuality being a problem. A more proactive approach is underpinned by education and supporting a positive approach to sexuality. Clinicians can work in partnership with schools, parents, and carers to support young people proactively to develop healthy sexual lives.

This can commence from early childhood, when parents can set the basis for future sexuality education. Clinicians can play a role in this early work by having discussions with families about the importance of planning for this part of their children's education in the same way that they do for other aspects of their development. Concepts of private and public places, learning names for body parts, setting boundaries around behaviours, and preparation for puberty are all important at this time. Learning in these areas can be incorporated in a range of other skill development areas; for example, opportunities arise when teaching toileting skills to name private body parts and reinforce concepts of private places and behaviours.

It is sometimes assumed that there are few resources to assist in talking about these issues with young people, staff, and families. However, there has been considerable work done, both internationally and in Australia, to develop a wide range of resources, including easy English health booklets, plain English teaching materials, interactive computer games, DVDs, websites, anatomically correct dolls, as well as some culturally specific resources. One resource that is readily available is *Sex Safe and Fun* (FPA Health (now Family Planning NSW), 2006). This is a free, easy English teaching resource that has been widely distributed throughout NSW, Australia, and internationally. It supports people to talk about sexuality by delivering positive messages about safety, consent, privacy, fun, and caring. It was originally developed for adults with a learning disability, but it has been used extensively with young people over the age of 16 years.

Sex Safe and Fun was created in close discussion with young people with learning difficulties, who provided input on the written and visual content. Young people with a learning disability wanted a book that was explicit, so they could really understand the messages, but had pictures that were not so realistic that they would cause embarrassment. This resource is easy to use, and has the acceptance of a wide range of people, including professional staff, teachers, parents, disability workers, sexual health workers, youth workers, and people with learning difficulties themselves.

The resource has two parts: (a) a colourful booklet using comic-style pictures with key messages about good and bad touching, safe sex practices, sexual diversity, and consent; and (b) a *Reader's Guide* that gives clear brief directions about how to talk with the person about the pictures in the booklet. The guide provides practical general information about providing sexuality education. It explains the importance of gaining consent from the person before delivering information, how to prepare, implement and provide feedback, and reinforcement.

The guide can be used as a whole program, as groups of topics, or individual units can be used to address particular issues. A major strength of the resource is that it promotes positive and healthy sexual behaviour, both in individual and group learning situations. It also assists in creating environments that are supportive of people's learning by giving permission to talk about sexuality and providing clinicians, carers, and staff with the tools they need to make them confident in carrying out this task. A selection of resources designed for young people with learning difficulties are outlined in table 18.2.

Opportunities

For education to be integrated, it needs practice, and practice requires opportunity. Young people are more likely to be restricted and organised by others in regards to their social interactions. They accept that parents and staff will make such decisions for them (Löfgren-Mårtenson, 2004). Opportunities for practising romantic relationships skills, dating, and expressing their sexuality in less public and scrutinised ways need to be constructed by staff and carers, as they are less likely to happen without this support. This requires creativity and advocacy. Lumley and Scotti (2001) noted that efforts to address sexuality education must move beyond knowledge to behaviour. They recommended that person-centred planning and a team approach are necessary to enable application of knowledge and skills acquired in an education program.

Education alone is not enough

In an ideal world, an educative approach would equip all young people with the knowledge and skills they need to have healthy sexual lives. However, some young people will require more support, because their behaviour

Table 18.2 Selected educational resources

Resource	*Description*
Feel Safe: CD-ROM (Family Planning Queensland, 2002)	This interactive CD-ROM supports the development of protective behaviours and assertiveness skills
Friendships and Dating: Information about Relationships for Parents, Carers and Young People (Shine SA, 2009)	This booklet uses cartoon-style pictures and straightforward information to guide appropriate choices about relationships
Jason's Private World (Life Support Productions, 2002a) *Kylie's Private World* (Life Support Productions, 2002b)	These animated DVDs cover a range of topics from puberty to relationships to sexual interactions in an engaging and accessible manner
Love and Kisses (Family Planning NSW, 2007)	A DVD that presents people with intellectual disabilities, describing their thoughts and experiences of relationships and sexuality, and asserting their right to be treated as adults
Special Boys Business (Anderson et al., 2007) *Special Girls Business* (Angelo et al., 2005)	These two books teach about puberty through the use of colourful cartoons with simple factual information that young people readily respond to
Responding Positively to Sexual Behaviours: The Traffic Lights Model (Family Planning Queensland)	This DVD provides a guide for professionals to identify, assess, and respond to sexual behaviours that may cause concern in school settings

continues to cause problems for themselves and others, and perhaps brings them into contact with the criminal justice system. In these situations, it is important to ensure that people are assessed comprehensively so that their needs are identified and appropriate therapeutic services provided.

It is a commonly held belief that inappropriate sexual behaviour occurs because of lack of sexual knowledge. A review of the research conducted by Lindsay (2005) on sexual offending and intellectual disability reported on several motivations for offending, with poor sexual knowledge being only one aspect. However, it is still acknowledged that intervention should include the provision of education. Furthermore, there should also be a focus on the provision of opportunities that promote positive relationship building, appropriate sexual behaviour, and encouragement to engage with the wider community.

Conclusion

Sexuality is a normal part of the development of all young people. They need to learn how to experience their sexuality in positive, safe, and healthy ways. Education is the responsibility of parents, carers, and professionals working together. There are many resources that will assist in assessing knowledge and providing ways to talk about sexuality.

While it is acknowledged that some young people will need support to manage particular difficulties with their sexual behaviour, the provision of sexuality education provides an appropriate framework for any intervention. There is a need to focus on the provision of clear basic knowledge, but it is of equal importance that young people are provided with opportunities to develop and maintain relationships. Enlightened future approaches to promoting positive sexual lives for young people with learning difficulties will see an emphasis on early, stage-appropriate education, positive risk taking, and the encouragement of opportunities for healthy sexual expression.

19

Transition: More than an event

Debra Corfield and Kate Brearley

The only constant in life is change (Heraclitus, c. 535–475 BCE)

Introduction

All people experience transitions in the course of their lifetimes. Transitions are important and often complicated periods of change and adjustment in the lives of any child, young person, or adult. However, when the child or young person at the centre of the process also has an intellectual disability, the transition may become more complex and challenging as a range of factors and systems interact (Jacobson & Wilhite, 1999; Janus et al., 2008; Teeters Myers, 2006). While it is debated whether people with intellectual disability experience more transitions than their typically developing peers (Coe et al., 1999; Emerson & Hatton, 2007; Hatton & Emerson, 2004), exposure to this process of change is a certainty. As such, practitioners have an opportunity, if not a responsibility, to support the children and young people with intellectual disability with whom they work to negotiate these periods of transition successfully.

What is transition?

The concept of transition is not new. However, much of the existing transition literature adopts a narrow scope by focusing on specific life events and contexts (Kralik et al., 2006). Life-change events commonly studied in the lives of people with intellectual disability include starting school (Janus et al., 2008; McIntyre et al., 2006), moving from primary to high school (Repetto & Correa, 1996), leaving school and commencing work or post-school programs

(Boardman, 2003; Heslop et al., 2002; Kohler, 1996; Nuehring & Sitlington, 2003; Rapanaro et al., 2008), moving out of home (Bigby, 2000), and moving from paediatric to adult health care services (Blum et al., 1993; While et al., 2004). Although periods of transition are associated with these and many other events across the lifespan, it can be limiting to conceptualise transition as an event alone.

Transition is more than an event. It is not the day a child with intellectual disability starts school or begins to access respite services. It is a dynamic and interactive process of change and adjustment that occurs as the child or young person moves from one phase, condition, place, or set of circumstances to another. While transition is always embedded in a particular context, it is not a discrete event in itself (Department for Children, Schools and Families/ Department of Health, 2008; Department of Health/Department for Education and Skills, 2006; King et al., 2005; Kralik et al., 2006). As shown in figure 19.1, transition involves three phases over time: (1) planning and preparation; (2) the provision of individualised supports and systemic linkages; and (3) integration and follow-up in the receiving context.

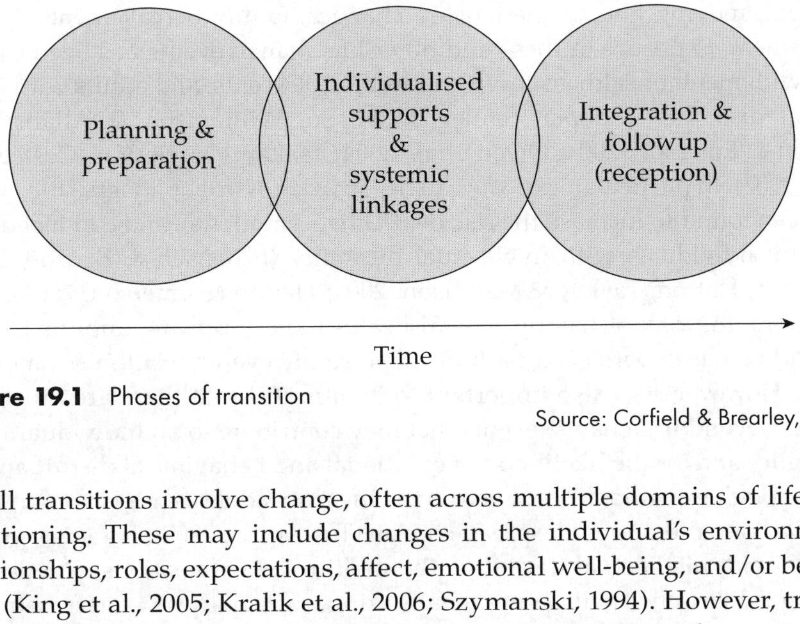

Figure 19.1 Phases of transition

Source: Corfield & Brearley, 2009

All transitions involve change, often across multiple domains of life and functioning. These may include changes in the individual's environment, relationships, roles, expectations, affect, emotional well-being, and/or behaviour (King et al., 2005; Kralik et al., 2006; Szymanski, 1994). However, transition is not simply another word for change. Instead, it is the process of adapting to these life changes that is central to the conceptualisation and understanding of transition (Kralik et al., 2006). Transitions both influence and are influenced by the individual and others in their support network. Therefore, transitions may necessitate a period of significant change and adjustment not only for the individual but also for a range of stakeholders (King et al., 2005).

Transition and mental health and well-being

In terms of the clinical significance of transition, it has long been established that stressful life-change events, such as moving house or the death of a loved one, can place an individual at increased risk of physical and mental health issues (Hulbert-Williams & Hastings, 2008; Paykel, 2001; Tiet et al., 2001). Life-change events have been identified as a risk factor for mental health issues across the lifespan for people with and without an intellectual disability. Emerson and Hatton (2007) found that exposure to two or more negative life events significantly increased the likelihood of conduct disorder, emotional disorder, and hyperkinesis in children with and without an intellectual disability. Further, they found that exposure to these events was significantly higher for children with intellectual disability. This supports Hatton and Emerson's (2004) earlier finding that children with intellectual disability were more likely to experience a greater range of adverse life events than their typically developing peers.

Owen and colleagues (2004) found that the life-change events most commonly reported by individuals with intellectual disability included staff changes, moving house, relationship changes, family bereavements, injury, and illness. Exposure to these and other life-change events has been associated with mental health issues in children, adolescents, and adults with intellectual disability (Cooper, Smiley, Morrison, Williamson & Allan, 2007; Hatton & Emerson, 2004; Owen et al., 2004; Tsakanikos, Bouras, Costello, & Holt, 2007). In particular, exposure to negative, stressful or adverse life events has been found to increase the risk of affective, emotional, and conduct disorders in individuals with intellectual disability (Esbensen & Benson, 2006; Hastings, Hatton, Taylor, & Maddison, 2004; Hatton & Emerson, 2004). Furthermore, the risk of having mental health issues appears amplified if the individual has experienced multiple adverse life events (Hatton & Emerson, 2004). However, it is also important to be mindful that there are other risk factors beyond life-change events that may contribute to an individual's vulnerability and/or the likelihood of emotional and behavioural disturbance.

Although transitions occur across the lifespan, adolescence is known to be a period of rapid and widespread change (Tur-Kaspa, 2002). For some young people with intellectual disability, the multitude of transitions experienced during adolescence will prove challenging, perhaps even overwhelming. Moreover, as the risk of mental health issues increases with exposure to an increasing number of life-change events, adolescence may present a period of particular vulnerability. However, it is apparent that the way an individual experiences transition and adjusts to life changes, irrespective of his or her age, can have significant implications for mental health and well-being. Therefore, the provision of supports through these times of change is one way of enhancing an individual's coping mechanisms, moderating the risk of mental health issues, and promoting quality of life for children and adolescents with an intellectual disability.

The child or young person experiencing transition

It is widely acknowledged in the literature that a person-centred approach to transition is needed when supporting children and young people with intellectual disability (Attfield, 2009; Department for Children, Schools and Families/Department of Health, 2008; Department of Health/Department for Education and Skills, 2006; King et al., 2005; Kohler, 1996; Michaels & Ferrara, 2005). A *person-centred approach* is an individualised and flexible approach that draws on the strengths, needs, and desires of the individual with intellectual disability. However, in practice, transition planning continues to be done *for* children and adolescents with intellectual disability rather than *with* or *by* them. For example, Heslop and colleagues (2002) explored the transition experiences of young people aged 13 to 25 years. They found that, despite the existence of legislation and guidance on transition, more than 40 per cent of children and young people surveyed had little or no involvement in their transition planning. Moreover, they found that one-fifth of young people had left school without a transition plan. This highlights the need for practitioners and educators to listen to the views of individuals with intellectual disability, facilitate their active participation, and foster their self-determination skills in this process (King et al., 2005; LaCava, 2005).

One way of assisting the child or young person to participate in transitions is through the use of *augmentative and alternative communication (AAC) systems* (Beukelman & Mirenda, 2005; Brewster, 2004; LaCava, 2005), such as *Talking Mats* (Cameron & Murphy, 2002). AAC systems provide the young person with a helpful scaffold for expressing their needs and making decisions and choices at points of change. In turn, these resources can be used to identify key actions and communicate information to the child or young person throughout the process.

Other people involved in transition

The impacts of transition are not limited to the child or young person with intellectual disability. Rather, a broader view is needed to consider the influence that transition has on the child's or young person's support system (Hudson, 2003). This system may include family, friends, peers, professionals, and members of the community (Kim & Turnbull, 2004; Szymanski, 1994). These stakeholders both contribute to, and are affected by, the transition process in varying ways and to varying degrees (Jacobson & Wilhite, 1999; King et al., 2005). For example, significant points of change (such as starting or finishing school) can be a source of stress and even sorrow for parents, as they are reminded of the discrepancies between normative expectations and their child's circumstances (Hanline, 1991). King and colleagues (2005) suggested that factors such as caregiver isolation, burnout, and stress can also complicate transitions, contributing to and/or being an outcome of the transition process. Attfield (2009) offered a personal account of her experience of supporting her son through a period of transition. She described her son's move to a residential special school as 'probably the most stressful time of all … [that was] a huge 18-month battle … finally achieved … when he was 14, but only at considerable detriment to our own mental health' (Attfield, 2009, p. 36).

Attfield (2009) suggested that, although an individualised and person-centred approach to transition is vital, it is also important to consider the views of the individual's family and friends to promote the well-being of all. Transitions present a significant period of change and adjustment for children and young people with intellectual disability, their families, and other stakeholders. Therefore, ensuring good communication, coordination, and collaboration is essential in good transition practice (Attfield, 2009; Heslop et al., 2002; Hudson, 2006; Kim & Turnbull, 2004; Nuehring & Sitlington, 2003; Stoner et al., 2007).

The impact of transition across life domains

In the same way that transition not only affects individuals but also their support network, the impacts of transition are not limited to one area or aspect of an individual's functioning. Transition can affect multiple domains of life and functioning, including the individual's environment, relationships, roles, expectations, affect, and behaviour (Department of Education, 2008; King et al., 2005; Stewart et al., 2007; Szymanski, 1994). These domains need to be considered in the planning, development, and provision of comprehensive transition supports for children and young people, irrespective of the actual life-change event.

Although the impact of transition across life domains will be explored below with reference to the individual with intellectual disability, it is important to highlight that these domains apply equally to others within the support network. For example, when a child or young person begins to access centre-based respite for the first time, his or her family also experiences a significant period of transition. Parents and siblings may find that their home environment, relationships, interactions, and behaviour change as a consequence of the role of caregiver being transferred to a service provider, albeit for a brief period of time. Families may also experience a wide range of contrasting emotions, such as guilt and relief, as the expectations of the family as individuals, and as a unit, shift and evolve.

Transition and the environment

People do not exist in a vacuum; they grow, develop, and live in constant interaction with the world around them. The environment provides both a physical space and a link with personal histories, culture, experiences, relationships, memories, and a sense of self (Jacobson & Wilhite, 1999). People and their environments have reciprocal effects on each other, and therefore must be considered as interdependent (Brofenbrenner, 1979).

The degree to which the environment adequately meets the needs, desires, and preferences of the individual has important implications for adjustment (King et al., 2005). When a good 'fit' exists between children with intellectual disability and their environments, then positive outcomes can be expected (such as participation in meaningful activities). Conversely, a poor 'person–environment fit' is likely to result in negative outcomes, such as dissatisfaction or the presence of challenging behaviour (Swanson & Fouad, 1999). The person–environment fit can become compromised during periods of transition because of direct changes in the physical environment (such as home renovations or moving house) or changes in other domains, which then have an impact on that environment (for example, addition of a new sibling at home or a new child in the classroom).

When supporting children and adolescents with intellectual disability, it is important to inform them about and prepare them for changes in their environment and/or routine. This could be achieved through the use of AAC systems such as *Social Stories* (Gray, 1995), *Comic Strip Conversations* (Gray, 1994), and routine schedules. *Lifestyle and environment reviews*, which identify discrepancies between the individual's needs and their supporting environments, may also provide a mechanism for the development of strategies to achieve an optimal person–environment fit.

Transition and relationships

Relationships are critical in the lives of all people. They can provide safety, support, stimulation, confidence, self-esteem, a sense of self, and historical affiliation (Forrester-Jones et al., 2006; Jacobson & Wilhite, 1999). At times of transition they can also offer a significant source of support, which aids in coping and well-being, and provides a buffer against stress (Hanline, 1991). For this reason, it is paramount that individuals with intellectual disability and their families are supported to maintain relationships and utilise both their informal and formal networks through periods of transition. It is also important to be sensitive to the implications of transition for the broader system of support (as discussed earlier).

In some situations, transition can signal the end of relationships (Bridges, 2004; Jacobson & Wilhite, 1999). For example, when a young person changes or leaves school, his or her relationships with teachers typically end, and friendships with peers may also be lost or weakened. The significance of such losses is often overlooked, and individuals may report feeling lonely or missing particular people (Jacobson & Wilhite, 1999; Runnion & Wolfer, 2004). This may be further complicated if the child has a history of loss, bereavement, or unresolved grief. To help a child or young person with intellectual disability to adjust to these changes it is important to provide opportunities to say goodbye. Acknowledging and recording significant and changing relationships in a child or young person's life using life-story books, scrapbooks, photo albums, or memory boxes can also be of help (Runnion & Wolfer, 2004).

Transition may also signal the beginning of new relationships (Bridges, 2004; Jacobson & Wilhite, 1999). For some children with intellectual disability, the process of forming new friendships can be particularly difficult (Runnion & Wolfer, 2004). Again, AAC systems, such as a *Chat Book* or *A Book About Me* (Bloomberg et al., 2004) can be helpful ways of supporting a child or young person in interactions to share information about themselves.

Transition and roles

Like all people, individuals with intellectual disability fulfil a range of roles in different contexts of their lives. These may include child, sibling, friend, student, worker, housemate, and partner. These roles bring both privileges and responsibilities, and are critical in the construction of a positive sense of self, self-esteem, and hopefulness (King et al., 2005). For this reason, continuity of roles throughout transition is beneficial. The alignment of roles with the strengths, skills, needs, and goals of the individual and their circle of support is also considered vital.

As roles influence the way in which events are perceived and responded to, they have significant implications for an individual's adjustment to transition (King et al., 2005; Stewart et al., 2007). Transition often leads to the adoption of new roles and responsibilities, as well as changes to existing ones (King et al., 2005; Stewart et al., 2007). Therefore the provision of information and skill development opportunities can assist an individual to prepare for and adjust to these changes in roles. This may also assist to resolve discrepancies between new role demands and existing skills, knowledge, and resources (King et al., 2005).

Transition and expectations

All people hold expectations for themselves, others, their routine, and the world around them. These are based on existing schemas, and influence the way individuals anticipate, interpret, and participate in daily life (Parkes, 1993). Change is interpreted in relation to these existing expectations and schemas. Therefore knowledge of an individual's history can offer helpful clues about how he or she might respond to future points of change. This may also offer intervention and support ideas to promote the individual's adjustment and well-being, drawing on what has worked well in the past.

During periods of change, information is often acquired that is at odds with an individual's existing schemas or expectations (Parkes, 1993). This can prove challenging for any individual, but particularly for individuals who rely on the predictability and consistency provided by familiarity and a structured routine. As such, it is essential that children and young people with intellectual disability are prepared for transition to reduce discrepancies between their expectations and experienced reality. This preparation includes communicating to children and young people about what changes they should expect, what others will do, and any specific requirements or things that they may be asked to do. AAC systems, such as calendars, checklists, and illustrated transition books, can be helpful means of communicating and clarifying expectations. Providing opportunities for questions, acknowledging concerns, and highlighting aspects that will remain constant during the transition can also be a source of reassurance for individuals.

Transition, affect, and emotional well-being

During periods of transition, individuals with intellectual disability can experience a wide range of emotions, including excitement, apprehension, anxiety, and loss (Jacobson & Wilhite, 1999). Parkes (1993) noted that in transition the familiar becomes unfamiliar, and this can affect an individual's sense of security and emotional well-being. Even positive life changes, such as making a new friend, can result in stress (King & Anderson, 2002).

Researchers have found a strong association between life-change events and an increased risk of mental health issues, including the presence of mood disorders in both children and adults with and without intellectual disability (Emerson, 2003a; Esbensen & Benson, 2006; Hastings et al., 2004; Hatton & Emerson, 2004; Owen et al., 2004; Tiet et al., 2001; Tsakanikos et al., 2007). Emerson (2003a), for example, found that exposure to potentially stressful life events increased the likelihood of emotional and anxiety disorders in children and adolescents with intellectual disability. Interestingly, Esbensen and Benson (2006) found an association between life-change events and depressive symptoms was present regardless of whether the individual perceived the event as negative or positive. They also found that as more negative or positive events were experienced, more depressive symptoms were reported.

To support children or young people to adjust to the emotional impacts of transition it may be useful to develop a toolkit of strategies that promote wellness. Strategies might include:

- ensuring opportunities to talk with others about how they are feeling, and offering validation and empathy
- providing a structured routine, encouraging exercise and participating in enjoyable activities

- teaching problem-solving skills and relaxation strategies
- promoting a healthy diet and good sleep hygiene
- seeking professional help and advice about medication and other therapeutic options.

Transition and behaviour

Given the observable nature of behaviour, changes in this area of life are often the first to be noticed when individuals experience difficulty coping with transition. For children with intellectual disability and autism spectrum disorder (ASD), these behaviours may reflect their resistance to and/or difficulties adjusting to the change (Sterling-Turner & Jordan, 2007). Life-change events have been found to be positively correlated with challenging behaviours, including irritability, lethargy, stereotypical behaviour, hyperactivity, non-compliance, inappropriate speech, and aggressive/destructive behaviours (Esbensen & Benson, 2006; MacHale & Carey, 2002; McIntyre et al., 2006; Owen et al., 2004). Changes in everyday patterns of behaviour, such as sleeping and eating, have also been observed during periods of transition (Jacobson & Wilhite, 1999). Interestingly, while stressful life events are associated with an increased risk of behavioural difficulties, positive life events are not (Esbensen & Benson, 2006). This suggests that the way in which an individual perceives a change (as positive or negative) has implications for the likelihood of behaviour problems.

Behavioural difficulties can interfere with a child's functioning and participation in daily life, and can be a source of significant stress for his or her family and wider support system. With this in mind, the presence of challenging behaviour may increase the likelihood of life-change events occurring. For example, Alborz (2003) found that challenging behaviour was one of several factors reported by families as contributing to their decision to seek alternative accommodation for their child with intellectual disability.

When challenging behaviour is present, it is important that an assessment is conducted in order to understand the underlying function and make meaningful recommendations for intervention and support. For those who already have existing behaviour support strategies, these should be reviewed in preparation for the transition, then monitored and updated throughout the process. Additional strategies or supports that focus specifically on the transition process may also be needed to reduce the likelihood of problem behaviours. For example, visual learners (such as those with ASD) and young people with limited verbal skills often benefit from videos about the transition, *Social Stories* (Gray, 1995), and activity schedules. These tools and strategies act as useful primers that increase the predictability of the change event (Sterling-Turner & Jordan, 2007). These AAC systems can provide an introduction and give information about new settings (such as how to get there, how to find your way around, the key new people, and the activities that will occur). The option of viewing videos and reading *Social Stories* repeatedly can provide valuable learning and reassurance.

The following case study illustrates some of the issues and challenges faced during transition by children and young people with intellectual disability. It also highlights many opportunities to provide creative and proactive supports that promote emotional and behavioural well-being.

Case study 19.1: Billy

Billy is a 16-year-old young person with a moderate intellectual disability and a history of severe and persistent interpersonal and emotional difficulties. He has lived with his maternal grandparents since he was an infant; however, because of their declining health and increasing difficulty managing his behaviour, they recently reached the difficult decision to relinquish care. Billy was placed in emergency respite care while a more appropriate and longer term option was identified.

This accommodation change occurred at a point of crisis, with little preparation and support for Billy. It was a change that provided Billy's grandparents with a much-needed break; however, it also caused them tremendous guilt and sorrow. Billy also struggled to adjust to the change. For him the move was much more than a change in residence. He was being cared for in an unfamiliar place, by unfamiliar people, and he did not know what to expect or who he could trust. With the exception of Billy's schooling, his life and routine had been turned upside down. The respite staff reported that Billy appeared highly anxious and withdrawn. He cried and regularly asked when he would be going home. He self-injured and attempted to assault other clients several times a day. Respite care staff did their best to support Billy with the little information they had available. However, on several occasions they needed to call for police assistance.

This transition was anything but seamless and anything but smooth. The people in Billy's support system agreed that things needed to be done differently if future transitions were to be more successful. When a more suitable accommodation placement was identified, a transition team was established to work with Billy in preparing him for the upcoming change and to assist him with the adjustment required. This team included his grandparents, school teacher, respite staff, speech pathologist, behaviour support practitioner, and the manager of the new accommodation service. A number of goals were identified, including that Billy maintain regular contact with his grandparents, as requested by his grandmother.

Using visual supports, the speech pathologist and behaviour support practitioner asked Billy about what he wanted to know about his new home. He said that he wanted to know what his bedroom looked like, whether the other people who lived in the group home liked Harry Potter, and whether the house was near his school. This formed the beginnings of Billy's transition plan.

A Social Story (Gray, 1995) was developed to explain to Billy what was happening, when and why. A short video was also made to introduce Billy to his future home, its staff and co-residents. Billy watched this video repeatedly, and took great pleasure in reciting people's names. Staff were provided with training, support protocols, and scripts to guide their interactions with Billy to ensure consistency in the information being conveyed. The move was framed as a positive and exciting part of growing up that many people experience as they become young adults. However, Billy's anxiety and concerns were also acknowledged and validated.

Billy's grandparents continued to have regular contact with him throughout the transition, and helped him make a memory box containing small mementos and reminders of the fun times they had shared. They also included a phone card in the box so Billy could call them whenever he wanted. As Billy met and got to know the staff and residents at his new home, this memory box was often a good icebreaker in establishing new relationships. Billy appeared to enjoy showing other people photos and trinkets from his life.

Having been prepared for the move, Billy's anxiety was much lower than was anticipated. Although he continued to display self-injurious behaviour in his new group home, the number of incidents was relatively low. Staff reported that he was engaging more with them and his co-residents each day. He continued to have daily phone calls with his grandparents, and continued to attend school. Billy's adjustment continued to be monitored, and support from the speech pathologist and behaviour support practitioner continued. It was recognised by his transition team that their coordinated, collaborative, and comprehensive approach to transition greatly contributed to the positive outcomes achieved by both Billy and his support network.

Conclusion: implications for practice

As shown in the case study above, transition goes beyond the particular point in time at which change occurs. It is a complex and interactive process of change and adjustment that involves many people, and has implications across multiple domains of life. Therefore, the scope of transition should be broad, and consider the perspectives, goals, strengths, skills, and needs of individuals with an intellectual disability and their wider support systems. This requires clinicians, practitioners, educators, families, and others to identify the individuals in the support system, and determine how each may contribute to and be affected by the transition process.

Participation, information sharing, and collaborative decision-making are essential during transition. These processes may be enhanced by the structuring of a safe and supportive environment, the forging of respectful relationships, and the use of communication strategies tailored to the individual's needs. While a range of communication tools and AAC systems have been discussed, only those that are matched to the individual's communication skills should be used. For example, visual systems such as *Talking Mats* and picture-based timetables or routine schedules would not be meaningful or helpful for a person with a more severe intellectual disability who does not have symbolic language skills.

Careful consideration of the potential impact of transition across life domains, particularly for the individual with an intellectual disability, is also warranted. This will allow for the identification of actions that promote continuity and well-being, and reduce or remove adverse outcomes (such as relationship or role losses, emotional distress, or challenging behaviour).

Throughout the transition process, individuals with intellectual disability and their support systems require different kinds and degrees of support. Consequently, it is neither possible nor appropriate to suggest a one-size-fits-all solution. For example, although some children with intellectual disability respond best when provided with considerable notice for upcoming transitions, for others this could be extremely anxiety-provoking, and thus a shorter lead time is preferable, albeit with other components of planning in place.

When supporting children and adolescents with intellectual disability through periods of transition, clinicians, practitioners, and educators are encouraged to focus on the unique qualities of each individual, each family and support network, and each set of circumstances. Flexibility is also important, given that needs change over time, even across periods of transition.

Although researchers are yet to establish best practice standards in relation to transition, some features of good transitions have been described. Drawing on the current literature (e.g., Heslop et al., 2002; Kohler, 1996; Stewart et al., 2006), eight guiding principles are presented for consideration when supporting a child or young person with intellectual disability through transition. These principles, listed in table 19.1, provide a checklist for good transition practice.

Putting these guiding principles into action and developing the associated transition strategies may involve a significant amount of time and commitment from a number of people from the individual's support network. Therefore it is important that transition planning commences early to allow sufficient time to undertake this work. It is acknowledged, however, that in some circumstances the timeframes for transition can be limited. Therefore,

Table 19.1 Guiding transition principles

1	Be goal orientated
2	Be individualised
3	Incorporate choice
4	Provide skill development opportunities
5	Offer good information flow, communication, and resources
6	Be collaborative and well coordinated
7	Promote continuity
8	Be comprehensive: consider implications across time, life domains and the service system.

the challenge to clinicians, practitioners, educators, families, and support staff is to think creatively and with flexibility to find ways to best implement these principles of good transition practice within the available time and resource constraints.

This chapter has sought to identify and explore the linkages between key elements of transition. Briefly, it is suggested that an understanding of the individual with intellectual disability and his or her specific circumstances should be central to any transition planning or support process. A broad view that encompasses the wider support system and considers the impacts of transition across life domains is also needed. This is fundamental in promoting a holistic and comprehensive approach to any transition.

Acknowledgments

The authors gratefully acknowledge Martine Fourie (senior clinical consultant, Statewide Behaviour Intervention Service, Office of the Senior Practitioner, Ageing, Disability and Home Care, Department of Human Services, NSW), and Vivienne Riches (senior research fellow, clinical senior lecturer, and psychologist, Centre for Disability Studies) for their contributions to this chapter.

Part 4

Interventions to promote mental health

20

Mental illness and intellectual disability: The concepts, the evidence, and the clinical skills

David Dossetor

Introduction

This chapter describes the development of the scientific concepts of intellectual disability and mental illness, including challenging behaviours. The empirical practice and limitations of adult psychiatry in intellectual disability are described, and in particular the problem of recognising depression. There is a growing understanding of the multifactorial nature of mental illnesses and challenging behaviours in the context of a holistic model.

Although family care can best provide for children with intellectual disability, and parent training has the best evidence of efficacy, the biological drivers of disturbance have a major impact on quality of life, and require a skilled multidisciplinary team and a range of services. The mental health problems of young people with severe intellectual disability particularly lead to an emphasis on a developmental perspective to the bio-developmental-psycho-social-cultural model of understanding. The chapter also looks at the need for different theoretical models, for example, for attention deficit hyperactive disorder (ADHD) in intellectual disability. It may be more useful, because of greater clinical face validity, to conceptualise some mental health disorders, such as autism and ADHD, as developmental disorders. The special needs and problems of young people with intellectual disability are driving the development of a range of subspecialty clinician skills in different disciplines.

This chapter emphasises the critical role psychiatry has made in enabling deinstitutionalisation and community care for many. All psychiatrists should have a holistic understanding of the needs of young people with intellectual disability and contribute a neuropsychiatric framework.

The chapter is divided into two sections: section 1 is on adult psychiatry of intellectual disability; section 2 is on child and adolescent psychiatry of intellectual disability, and looks at the mix of workforce skills required to provide for this population of special need.

1 Adult psychiatry of intellectual disability

Distinguishing intellectual disability and mental illness

Although intellectual disability and mental illness were mentioned in ancient times, it was in the thirteenth century that the English King Henry II demonstrated a humane view, passing legislation to make these people wards of the king. Prerogativia Regis provided for care of their lands, but distinguished 'natural fools' from 'lunacy', as 'lunatics' were expected to recover and resume such responsibilities (Harris, 2006). However, accounts of such 'community care' suggested that, although some people were treated humanely by family and parish, others were chained or locked up and mistreated 'for the devil in them'. Even today, because of significant poverty in Africa, in order to go to work a single mother may have to lock up her child with intellectual disability (Adnams, 2008).

Treatment versus rehabilitation

The modern notions of intellectual disability and mental illness arose subsequent to the development of asylums in the eighteenth and nineteenth centuries for the 'insane' and 'feebleminded'. Admission to these institutions was on the judgment of a magistrate, and was intended to protect vulnerable groups who could not cope in society. The better institutions provided a 'moral' culture, with fresh air and fresh water, and were frequently identified by their fine rural real estate and the landmark water tower. Harris (2006) noted that Seguin's text of 1866 described how people too disabled to learn from classroom instruction still benefited from training, similar to the rehabilitation movement for those with mental illness. Seguin (as cited in Harris, 2006) also identified different levels of intellectual disability: idiocy, imbecility, and feeblemindedness (severe, moderate, and mild), but the intelligence test as an empirical measure of intellectual disability was not developed until 1905 by Alfred Binet and Theodore Simon (Harris 2006).

The Industrial Revolution led to the development of science in medicine, and accordingly medical superintendents were appointed to manage and study their charges. For example, Langdon Down in 1866 identified several types of intellectual disability, including his Down syndrome, well before genes had been discovered. With the recent epidemiology on the association of intellectual disability and social and economic adversity (Emerson, 2004), it can be speculated that the social and economic adversity of the Industrial Revolution also contributed to the proliferation of individuals with intellectual disability and mental illness in institutions.

Access to and protection from mental health institutions

The legal framework of the *Mental Health Act* 2007 remains an important part of the gatekeeping process of the mental health system in New South Wales (NSW). It provides access to treatment for serious mental illness in the absence of insight and protects the individual from the abuse of psychiatrists and their institutions, particularly with independent monitoring by the Mental Health Review Tribunal. Accordingly, access to psychiatric services is dependent on the notion of (a) an illness of the functioning of the brain that warrants psychiatric treatment; or (b) disordered behaviour that needs an assessment for the presence of a psychiatric illness.

Psychiatry and phenomenology

The term *psychiatry* means 'healing of the soul or mind' (Stevenson, 2007). It is taken as an assumption that subjectivity and conscious mindfulness are fundamental to the human condition. The models of mental illness come from studying people who were too disabled (and often bizarre) to participate in the community, and who neglected themselves or put themselves at risk. Psychiatry is based on the examination of the individual's subjectivity. Psychiatry was described by eminent philosopher psychiatrists, such as Bleuler and Kraeplin in the nineteenth century, whose works classified these deviant moods and thoughts into mental illnesses. This process is termed *phenomenology*: the practice of describing the patterns of phenomena of the mind (Alexander & Selesnick, 1966).

From these origins, the diagnostic classifications of the American Psychiatric Association's (APA) *Diagnostic and Statistical Manual of Mental Disorders* (DSM) and the World Health Organization's (WHO) *International Classification of Diseases* (ICD) developed. The classification processes of the DSM and ICD are still based on a committee of experts who debate and research the best way to classify these abnormalities of subjectivity, associated with social impairment and dysfunction.

Medical advances and deinstitutionalisation

The rise of medicine and the science of healing brought notable progress in treating mental illness. These medical advances led to significant *deinstitutionalisation* of people with a progressive increase in community care. The start of the decline of psychiatric institutionalisation arose with the development of penicillin (1940s) for treating general paresis of the insane (neurosyphilis), and chlorpromazine (1950), which was the first major tranquilliser for psychoses, especially schizophrenia. Lithium (first reported in 1949) as a treatment of manic depression has saved more lives of the mentally ill than any other medication.

Deinstitutionalisation led to rehabilitative approaches to treatment of people with mental illness, with integration of services into mainstream hospitals and community support. Mental illness remains real and harmful. This has been illustrated by a recent report stating that the main cause of maternal death is not directly a result of the process of childbirth but to suicide from postnatal depression (Cliffe et al., 2008). Although better treatment and community integration of services is associated with more accepting views of mental illness, it is still treated with stigma and denied the concern shown to other illnesses. Yet people with mental illnesses have an increased risk of death by suicide, and suicide is second only to accidents as the main cause of death in youth.

In the last 10 years, the introduction of *selective serotonin reuptake inhibitor antidepressants (SSRIs)* has been associated with a reduction in suicide rates in the Western world. Indeed, temporary reversal of access to SSRIs in Japan, because of fears that they increased suicide attempts, led to an increase in deaths because of loss of availability. Both lithium and the SSRIs have been shown to prevent cell death of neurones, particularly in the hippocampus (crucial for memory) in the presence of depression and bipolar disorder.

Epidemiology and the economic costs

It is the public health and epidemiological approach to health that has raised the political importance of psychiatry, highlighting the cost to the community of psychiatric morbidity and mortality. The World Bank and WHO now put the economic cost of mental health, particularly depression, ahead of other diseases in developed and developing countries. The success of the contribution of psychiatry to humanity is a result of what has been described as a combination of 'evidence-based medicine' with 'values-based practice' (Fulford, as cited in Fannon, 2008).

Psychiatry in intellectual disability: part of mainstream skills, subspecialty, or neither?

Mental illness or disorder is defined as 'psychological or behavioural pattern or syndrome that occurs in an individual and causes distress or disability that is not expected as part of normal development or culture' (DSM-IV) (APA, 1994). For several decades it has generally been recognised that those with intellectual disability suffer from the full spectrum of mental disorders experienced by the general population, but that these may present in different ways. Commonly used diagnostic criteria, such as those used in the fourth edition of the *Diagnostic and Statistical Manual of Mental Disorders* (DSM-IV) (APA, 1994), or in the tenth version of the *International Statistical Classification of Diseases and Related Health Problems* (ICD-10) (WHO, 2007), can be difficult to apply in this group.

Methodical approaches to recognising mental illness in intellectual disability is a recent phenomenon. *The Diagnostic Manual–Intellectual Disability* (DM-ID) (Fletcher et al., 2007) is a textbook of diagnosis of mental disorders in persons with an intellectual disability. It was developed by the National Association for the Dually Diagnosed (NADD) and the American Psychological Association (APA), and authored by an international (mainly American) expert group. The group reviewed the strength of the evidence supporting each diagnosis and the adaptations of diagnostic criteria required for persons with an intellectual disability. The quality of scientific evidence was evaluated in keeping with the criteria of the Cochrane Collaboration, where the best evidence is from multiple randomised control trials and the least good is the opinion of experts or from case series. The level of scientific evidence is generally poor, mainly based on cohort studies and expert opinion. The Royal College of Psychiatrists published a similar guide in 2001, titled *Diagnostic Criteria for Psychiatric Disorders,* for use with adults with learning disabilities or mental retardation. This guide provided a consensus of current practice for adults with moderate to profound intellectual disability leading to ICD-10 diagnostic categories. Sometimes it is not the criteria that need alteration but the method of eliciting the necessary information.

It has been noted that children and adults with intellectual disability are one of the most underserved populations in the USA. The situation in Australia is also poor (AMWAC, 1999), as these individuals fall through the cracks of both disability and mental health service systems. Although 40 per cent of young people with intellectual disability have significant mental health problems, only 9 per cent of these received services skilled in mental health and intellectual disability (Einfeld & Tonge, 1996b). A further 31 per cent received help from disability or mental health services. This finding is not dissimilar to that made about other child mental health disorders, as found in the *National Mental Health and Wellbeing Survey* (Sawyer et al., 2001).

This difficulty accessing services partly reflects the history of funding for individuals with intellectual disability. For example, in New South Wales, funding moved from health to social services (Family and Community Services) in 1987, and to disability services in 1999 (now known as Ageing Disability and Home Care, Department of Human Services NSW). There is therefore no historical ownership or funding for mental health of this special needs population. The lack of a recognised subspecialty of psychiatry in Australia means that there is a lack of advocacy for services for individuals with these mental health needs.

Special problems of phenomenology and reliability in intellectual disability

Diagnostic criteria and reliable interviews for the psychiatry of adults with intellectual disability have been developed in the last 10 years. They are yet to be established for children and adolescents. People with intellectual disability may have additional difficulties (such as cognitive and verbal), which in turn lead to difficulties in articulating abstract or global concepts, such as depressed mood. Part of the problem is that subjective mental phenomena cannot be elicited reliably below an age of seven years or an IQ of 45 (Brugha, 1988). Reliance on observable behaviours meant that it was not until the 1980s that psychiatry recognised depression in children, and down to the level of seven years. Yet it is a strongly held assumption that criteria symptoms are identifiable, and the recognition of psychiatric diagnoses is possible regardless of level of intellectual disability or age.

Failure to identify comorbid psychiatric disorder in people with intellectual disability has been attributed to the problem of these people giving answers to please interviewers in assessments and, of course, the problems of diagnostic overshadowing, where the presenting problem is attributed to the intellectual disability. The majority of those who have intellectual disability have a disability in the mild range. There is a growing literature validating psychiatric disorders in this population. However, the greatest problems occur in reliably recognising and validating major psychiatric disorders in those with moderate or severe intellectual disability or with major developmental disorders such as autism.

Approaches to classification: phenomenology or factor analysis?

The DM-ID (Fletcher et al., 2007) provides a multidimensional framework, and is based on diagnostic criteria that are 'generic'; that is, they can be applied to all individuals independent of age, ethnicity, culture, gender, or comorbid medical or mental conditions. For many diagnostic categories, the expert committees determined that the diagnostic criteria 'didn't need' modification, and that they could also be applied to individuals with moderate, severe, and profound intellectual disability. For other diagnostic categories there were modifications of the criteria. Obsessive compulsive disorder (OCD) and post-traumatic stress disorder (PTSD) were not classified under anxiety disorders, but given separate chapters because of their underdiagnosis and importance to the intellectually disabled population. Further, behavioural diagnostic criteria were added for those with severe or profound intellectual disability.

The expert group used for the development of the DM-ID (Fletcher et al., 2007) acknowledged that a number of different approaches to diagnosis had been proposed over the last 20 years. Such approaches included the dimensional approach used by Sovner and Hurley (1986) and a factor analysis approach used by Einfeld and Tonge (1996b) with six factors. However, Aman's review (1991b) of a range of factor analyses of symptom checklists, suggested seven factors for types of behaviour. Given the lack of consensus or an evidence base for many decisions, the expert group concluded that peer discussion and committee agreement was the best way forward in the diagnosis of psychiatric disorder in individuals with intellectual disability. They resolved that at least DSM methods were a means of giving people with an intellectual disability the same entitlement to mental health services as non-disabled people. Clinical usefulness of the DM-ID was tested in 2006 with a field trial of clinical data on 900 individuals, using 80 clinicians from 11 countries. The evaluation concluded that the DM-ID was user friendly and enabled clinicians to be more specific about the diagnosis than using the DSM-IV text revision (DSM-IV-TR) (APA, 2000).

Problems in eliciting symptoms in intellectual disability

The special problems and considerations in diagnosis in intellectual disability (DM-ID) (Fletcher et al., 2007) are described below.

1 Baseline exaggeration or the increase in frequency and intensity of existing maladaptive behaviours during the course of a mental illness, such as increase in self-injurious behaviour at a time of stress.
2 Intellectual distortion or the effects of intellectual limitations, such as saying 'Yes' to 'Hearing voices' from not understanding the question.
3 Psychosocial masking of symptoms that are recognised within a developmental framework; for example, an individual with moderate intellectual disability believing that he can drive a car might indicate grandiosity and therefore exhibit a symptom of mania.
4 Cognitive disintegration, disorganisation, or psychotic behaviour through lack of cognitive reserve and stress or problems coping.
5 Existence of symptoms that are seen as appropriate for a child (such as talking to oneself out loud, fantasy play, pretend friends) but would be abnormal in an adult of normal intellect.
6 Families and professionals alike are at risk of attributing behaviour to serious psychiatric disorder where none exists, especially when individuals with intellectual disability present with behaviours and interaction skills of chronological younger children. These developmentally understandable behaviours can be maintained throughout their life.
7 The inability of individuals to articulate their losses or stresses, or changes in physical health, or problems of health treatment.
8 Changes in behaviour due to stress can be misconstrued as a serious mental illness. Such stress may be related to environmental change (a change of teacher, staff member, classroom, accommodation arrangement, or frequency of family visits) or to the anniversary of a loss. Such changes may be precipitants of stress that carers do not identify.
9 Specific considerations in mental health assessments include:
   - anxiety symptoms, which frequently go unnoticed by family or carers, and need careful eliciting
   - vegetative symptoms, which are important, and may be sourced from sleep charts, mood charts, dietary records
   - changes in activity or cognitive capacity, and in particular any decline in functional capacity, is important, and may be identified from school or work records.
   - mood changes, which may be expressed typically or in terms that are implausible or delusional, such as referring to important figures as dead, or no longer caring

- both mania and depression, which can present as irritability, sometimes with explosive anger
- normal ebullience and elation, which may not be recognised as part of hypomania
- delusions and hallucinations, which are frequently very difficult to distinguish from a range of normal developmental phenomena such as concrete thinking, pretend friends, stereotypic thinking, and imagination, particularly in the context of autistic spectrum disorder (ASD). Evidence of a psychotic process is best indicated by a pervasive change in the trajectory of social engagement and independence skills (Dossetor, 2007; Hollis, 2008)
- substance abuse and suicidal or homicidal ideation, which need to be considered
- vigilance for physical or sexual abuse, which need to be kept in mind as communication difficulties, greater dependency, and the large numbers of carers make people (especially girls) vulnerable to such exploitation.

Despite these cautionary observations, there is no guidance on dealing with these errors, for example, when one rule or another might apply. In practice, trusted expertise is the only standard; that is, significant experience or mentoring as a psychiatrist with people with an intellectual disability.

What psychiatric disorders are found in intellectual disability?

Studies from USA

The New York State Institute for Basic Research in Developmental Disabilities did a study that found one (and frequently more) psychiatric disorder in 60 per cent of 4468 clients, three-quarters of whom were in out of home residential settings (Tsiouris et al., 2008). The main DSM-IV psychiatric diagnoses that were found in this study can be see in table 20.1, and are listed in order of frequency.

It is curious that such a large clinical cohort did not identify many other diagnoses identified in DM-ID; for example, adjustment disorders, post-traumatic disorders, substance-related disorders, sexual and gender identity disorder, dementia, and mental disorders due to a general medical condition not otherwise classified. It also suggests that the following diagnoses are only applied to children or by child psychiatrists: learning disorders; motor skills disorders; elimination disorders; pervasive developmental disorders (PDD); ADHD and disruptive behaviour disorders; somatoform and factitious disorders; other disorders of infancy, childhood and adolescence (attachment disorders and stereotypic movement disorders, including self-injurious behaviour); and behavioural phenotypes of genetic disorders.

One of the areas of ambiguity is that, while adult psychiatric disorders can be applied to adolescents and sometimes children (except personality disor-

Table 20.1 DSM-IV psychiatric diagnoses found in the US

Psychiatric diagnosis	*Frequency*
Impulse disorder	21%
Anxiety disorder	19%
Schizophrenia and other psychoses	18%
Depression	14%
Bipolar disorder	12%
Obsessional compulsive disorder	11%
Personality disorder	8%
Sleeping disorder	4%
Eating disorder	3%
Tourette's syndrome	2%
No psychiatric diagnosis	40%

Source: Tsiouris et al., 2008

der by definition), it is less clear to what extent child psychiatric disorders can apply to adults. Also, there is a lack of understanding of the relationship between ADHD in childhood and impulse disorder in adults. It is known that PDD is a lifelong disorder, yet it is not identified as an adult psychiatric diagnosis. It is now understood that ASD is a dimension of impairment, not solely a categorical diagnosis, but not what the relationship is between stereotypic behaviour or thinking, and obsessional compulsive disorder.

Studies in UK and by WHO

It is critical for clinicians to learn to adapt their interviewing techniques to be sensitive and understandable to someone with an intellectual disability. This necessitates specific experience, and can be aided by training in purpose-designed, reliable, and validated semistructured interviews such as the PAS-ADD 10 (Costello et al., 1997), which is the ICD-10 version of the *Psychiatric Assessment Schedule for Adults with a Developmental Disability* (PAS-ADD) (Moss et al., 1993). This instrument relies on information from a key informant to identify and rate the psychiatric symptoms to diagnose ICD-10 diagnoses with the aid of algorithms.

The *PAS-ADD checklist* (Moss et al., 1998) is a screening questionnaire, from which those with symptoms above the threshold can be assessed with the *Mini-PAS-ADD* (Moss, 2000). The Mini PAS-ADD can diagnose anxiety disorders, mood disorders, obsessive compulsive disorder, psychotic disorder, dementia, unspecified mental disorder, and autistic disorder. Cooper and colleagues (2007) provided an epidemiologically sound study of psychiatric

Table 20.2 Psychiatric diagnoses found in the UK

Psychiatric disorder	*Types of ICD-10 psychiatric disorder*
Mental ill-health of any type 40.9%	Psychotic disorder 4.4%
Problem behaviour 22.5%	Affective disorder 6.6%
Mental ill-health of any type excluding problem behaviours 28.3%	Autistic spectrum disorder 7.5%
	Anxiety disorder 3.8%
Mental ill-health of any type excluding autistic spectrum disorder 37%	Organic disorder 2.2%
	Pica 2%
	Hyperkinetic disorder 1.7%
	Personality disorder 1%
	Alcohol and substance abuse 1%
	Obsessional compulsive disorder 0.7%
	Sleep disorder 0.6%
	Other mental ill-health 1.4%

Source: Cooper et al., 2007

disorder in Scotland of a sample of 1023 adults over the age of 16 years with mild, moderate, or severe intellectual disability. They found the prevalence rates of psychiatric disorder as outlined in table 20.2.

The rates of diagnosis of different disorders in the USA and UK are strikingly different, which is a measure of methodological differences, such as sample selection and screening processes. However, the extent of the differences also indicates a lack of uniformity of diagnostic thinking and processes. This is reminiscent of discrepancies in recognising ADHD in children and adolescents on different sides of the Atlantic in the 1980s, which reflected thresholds of recognition and attitudes to such a diagnosis.

The Smiley Scottish prospective study (Smiley et al., 2008) found a two-year incidence of mental illness (new disorders) of 16.3 per cent, and 12.6 per cent excluding problem behaviours. Factors related to mental ill-health included type of accommodation (out of family care), previous mental ill-health, not having impaired mobility, urinary incontinence, more severe intellectual disability, adult abuse, parental divorce in childhood, and preceding life events.

Approaches to challenging behaviours

The concept of *challenging behaviour*, which derives from a social construction influenced by behavioural psychology, is defined as 'culturally abnormal behaviours of such an intensity, frequency, or duration that the physical safety of the person or others is likely to be placed in serious jeopardy, or behaviour which is likely to limit use of or result in the person being denied access to ordinary community facilities' (Emerson, 2001, p. 3). It is a mainstream view that unwanted or challenging behaviours need to be examined, not just by a descriptive functional analysis (Einfeld & Emerson, 2008), but with a thorough behavioural assessment by an experienced professional using a detailed approach, as characterised in applied behaviour analysis. Such a standard of intervention has been shown to lead to better outcomes (Grey & Hastings, 2005), although long-term data are lacking.

More recently, it has been proposed that causes and intervention should also be considered from multidimensional approaches to understanding. Such approaches include exploration of sensory, motor, communication, relationships, context, and cultural issues, as opposed to seeing the function of challenging behaviours solely as the need for stimulation or tangible reinforcers, or avoidance of a task or an undesired event. Neurobiological models, such as the role of endorphins (endogenous opiates) in self-injurious behaviour and measures of physical arousal, also need to be considered. Challenging behaviour can serve many functions.

Cohen and colleagues (2009) conducted a survey of aggressive behaviours and associated factors in a clinical cohort of over 2000 adults with intellectual disability. They used the *Modified Overt Aggression Scale* (MOAS) (Sorgi et al., 1991), and found four types of aggression:

1 Aggressive displays, such as shouting or breaking something (25 per cent of the variance)
2 Verbal threats (16 per cent)
3 Self-injurious behaviour (13 per cent)
4 A small group of less than 10 per cent of serious aggression.

Aggressive displays were mostly associated with environmental disruptions, such as task demands and social intrusions (such as teasing or touching other's property), more frequent in those with moderate to severe level of intellectual disability, and were more severe in people with autism (Cohen et al., 2009). Verbal threats were mostly associated with social intrusions, were more common in females, less common in autism, and highest in 'borderline' intellectual disability level. Self-injury was associated with physical discomfort (as from medical problems and environmental change), highest at the lowest intellectual disability levels, declined with age, and was higher in people with autism. Severe aggression was relatively rare, declined with age, and was marginally more common in males, but with no significant antecedent triggers.

This study suggested that most aggressive behaviours toward others in this population are avoidant, defensive, or territorial in nature. Consistent with other reports, self-injury was associated with more severe intellectual disability, and may be linked to arousal and stress. There were associations with psychiatric disorder, particularly with impulse control, psychotic, bipolar, and personality disorder in persons with mild to severe intellectual disability, and depressive and personality disorder in borderline intellectual disability. Self-injury was associated with all psychiatric disorders. Aggressive displays and threats were associated with all psychiatric disorders except anxiety and obsessional compulsive disorder. Based on this cohort, most aggressive challenging behaviours have environmental and communicative implications. However, self-injurious behaviour and severe aggression may have other more complex features.

Associated medical problems

The importance of other health problems must not be underestimated in individuals with intellectual disability. Tsiouris and colleagues (2008) found the following associated medical problems in 40 to 45 per cent of their population with psychiatric disorder (in descending order of frequency): constipation, reflux and indigestion, problems of mobility and walking, dental problems, seizures, sleep problems, heart problems, ear problems, and kidney problems. However, they also found a similar comorbid incidence of medical problems in their aggression cohort (Tsiouris et al., 2008).

Clinical experience indicates that medical problems therefore play a significant role in both challenging behaviour and psychiatric disorder, although epidemiological evidence for this causing challenging behaviour is weak. People with an intellectual disability have higher rates of a range of general health problems with significant morbidity and reduced life expectancy. These problems require routine systematised general health checks, health promotion intervention, and the use of structured assessment such as the *Comprehensive Health Assessment Program* (CHAP) (Lennox et al., 2006).

Cooper and colleagues (2006) did a randomised control trial of nurse health screening of 50 people with intellectual disability (average of 4 hours per patient, with information being passed on to the general practitioner). More than twice as many health needs were identified for the intervention group compared to the control group. The intervention group had better health benefit from a higher level of health need met of 3.56 interventions per patient, compared to 2.26 in the controls. The main interventions were dental checkups, eye tests, healthy diets, exercise, and influenza and hepatitis immunisation. With these data, it is clear that good regular general medical care is central to every person with intellectual disability. However, there was no outcome information on psychiatric disturbance.

Aggression and psychiatric disorder

Tsiouris and colleagues (2003) found that aggression was not an indicator of depression, but symptoms of depression (including irritability) were still valid in those with intellectual disability. Aggression and self-injury are the most common cause for a mental health appointment in those with an intellectual disability, but not in those with normal intellect. Aggression can be occasionally associated with any diagnosis, but frequently, despite multiple informants and comprehensive assessment, the clinician is left working in clinical and diagnostic uncertainty. Nonetheless, in practice, psychotropic medications are frequently used for severe aggression, whether this is associated with a psychiatric disorder on not.

Drugs for aggression versus psychiatric disorder?

A recent randomised control study of adults with aggression compared haloperidol, risperidone, and placebo (Tyrer et al., 2008). This study showed 58–79 per cent improvement in aggression on the MOAS (Sorgi et al., 1991), but the placebo was as effective as either major tranquilliser. This study drastically oversimplified the question of whether drugs can help aggression, in that it failed to consider whether the aggression was predatorial (for which there is agreement that psychotropics generally don't work) or affectively driven aggression (which has significant research interest). Furthermore, there was no consideration of whether aggression occurred in the context of psychiatric disorders, such as ADHD–impulse disorder, autism, depression, or psychosis, which may benefit from treatments, including psychotropic medication, that help the psychiatric disorder. Sedating medication can have a role in acute situations to help contain an individual safely, assuming it is with consent or possibly assent, or justifiable under common law or relevant mental health law.

Tsiouris and colleagues (2003) reported a study of serious self-injurious behaviour that had failed to respond to intensive behaviour management. In all 26 cases, identification and treatment of a psychiatric disorder contributed to significant improvement, although cessation of self-injury was a minority occurrence. Only in a minority was the effective medication a major tranquilliser. This observation suggests that psychiatric disorder is more likely to be found in severe behaviour disorder, and severe psychiatric disorder is more likely to benefit from psychotropic intervention.

Accordingly, there are a range of different medications that may have a role in serious behaviour disorder. There is a growing literature on drug effectiveness that focuses on treating symptoms rather than disorders, partly because of the problems of diagnostic reliability and comorbidity in intellectual disability. It can therefore be concluded that, in the context of severe challenging behaviour that fails to respond to thorough behaviour analysis and intervention, assessment by a psychiatrist is indicated, and that psychotropic medication may well have a role.

Differing rates of psychiatric disorder according to level of intellectual disability

Cooper and Bailey (2001) have looked at the rates of psychiatric diagnosis according to level of intellectual disability in adults. Some disorders were more commonly found in persons with milder levels of intellectual disability, such as psychosis and anxiety disorders. Some disorders were more commonly found in persons with more severe levels of intellectual disability, such as pica, behaviour disorder, ADHD, and autism. However, very few studies look at whether the reliability and validity of these diagnoses are different at different levels of intellectual disability.

Identifying depression in intellectual disability: experience and skill, or education and time?

The research on depression, as the most common and treatable disorder, illustrates the problems of identification and therefore access to treatment. While there is consensus that depression can be identified using DM-ID or ICD-10, in practice there are real problems with the use of these standardised criteria and with reliable identification of the critical features for diagnosis. In Scotland, Cooper and colleagues (2007) found a point prevalence of affective disorders (unipolar depression and bipolar disorder) of 6.6 per cent based on clinical diagnosis by a specialist intellectual disability mental health professional, compared with 5.7 per cent using DC-LD (Royal College of Psychiatrists, 2001), 4.8 per cent using ICD-10, and 3.6 per cent with DSM-IV-TR. The equivalent figures for unipolar depression was 4.1 per cent, 3.5 per cent, 2.8 per cent, and 2.0 per cent respectively. Smiley and colleagues (2008) also described problems with the presence of unusual features, such as lability of mood, onset of challenging behaviours, reduction in speech, social withdrawal, and increase in somatic complaints.

Hurley (2008), in a retrospective clinic population, found that most individuals with intellectual disability and depression could not meet the required number of criteria for DSM-IV or DM-ID criteria for depression. The main problem was that individuals with intellectual disability and depression do not complain of depressed thoughts. They still had depressed mood, sadness, crying and anhedonia, and withdrawal, which distinguished them from those with anxiety or bipolar disorder. Few reported suicidality. Bipolar individuals differed in having elevated mood, acute anger episodes, increase in verbalisation, pressure of speech, talk of sexual themes, increase in appetite, and poor concentration (Hurley, 2008). Anxious individuals had more fearfulness without other features of depression. Depressed individuals also had more aggression and impulsivity than anxious individuals or controls.

Torr and colleagues (2008), in an Australian study, examined general practitioners (GPs) and long-term paid carers' capacities for identifying features of depression, with the aid of a 53-item checklist for depression. The routine assessment of individuals with intellectual disability by a GP was compared with subsequent comprehensive psychiatric assessment. Carers identified many of the features that the GPs failed to identify, even with the carers present. Factor analysis identified that the consistent features of depression in individuals with intellectual disability were depressed mood (six items), loss of interest (five items), and loss of social interaction and communication (eight items). Carers were able to describe these, but they were not reliably identified by GPs. Depressed thinking was not a reliable feature of depression, reflecting the limited communication skills of many participants. GPs tended to focus more on sleep, appetite, weight control, and general functioning. It was found that 30 per cent of this clinical cohort had depression, but 25 per cent had a PDD that the study did not examine.

One case scenario study (Einfeld et al., 2007) and one clinical study (Lee et al., 2003) suggested schizophrenia can be reliably diagnosed by psychiatrists or psychologists experienced in intellectual disability. However, the findings by Torr and colleagues (2008) illustrated that diagnostic recognition is not a manualised procedure, but relies on familiarity with the field of intellectual disability as well as clinical expertise in psychiatry. In addition, diagnosis requires reliable information from a range of sources, preferably aided by specific structured questionnaires. The gravest implication is that access to mental health service provision for people with an intellectual disability is severely disadvantaged by the lack of an appropriately trained workforce, both in general practice, which is the main gateway to psychiatric services, and in psychiatry, where there is a need for psychiatrists with subspecialty skills in intellectual disability. The texts by Hassiotis and colleagues (2009) and Bernard and Turk (2009) are useful in providing the diagnostic features of the main psychiatric diagnoses and a practical framework for establishing a specialist service.

2 Child and adolescent psychiatry of intellectual disability

The development of community-based child and adolescent psychiatry in intellectual disability

The original epidemiological studies of child psychiatric disorder of the 'Isle of Wight Study' and Camberwell (Rutter et al., 1976) showed rates that were three times higher in an inner city population, at 18 per cent. This led to a bio-psycho-socio-cultural framework of risk factors and a model of multiple causal mechanisms of child psychiatric disorder. The initial emphasis of child psychiatry was on the importance of the psychosocial context, with a focus on the influence of emotional deprivation on the developing child. However Rutter and colleagues' (1976) study also demonstrated that an intellectual disability raised the risk of a comorbid psychiatric disorder fourfold.

The realisation that attachment was important for children's development led to a change in social policy in 1981 in the UK in relation to the institutionalisation of children with severe intellectual disability. Often children had been placed in hospitals or institutions from birth. Some of these environments were homely and personalised, and some were depriving and anonymous. The change in policy led to these children moving from hospitals to community-based children's homes. What was evident was that good-quality community-based care was about three times more expensive than hospitals.

Care in the community may provide opportunities for community access and belonging, but for some children with severe intellectual disability, the change in quality of life can be minimal, as community homes can risk poor and inconsistent care with greater difficulty of supervision and accountability. Furthermore, the lack of service-based residential options for most children meant that the biggest change was for mothers, who had to shoulder an inordinate burden of care (on average 7 hours a day, 7 days a week of care) at considerable personal cost. However, the normalisation of the care of children meant that they could be recognised as children first, with human needs for security and attachment. As part of the process of normalisation, it has taken time for mainstream services such as those for mental health to recognise their responsibility for the special needs of these children.

It has been contended that the medical and psychological study of delayed development has much to teach clinicians about the development of consciousness, the sense of mutual awareness (empathy and theory of mind), and the biological and social contributors to that process and its problems. This merges the biological with the psychosocial in the context of development, as illustrated in figure 20.1. This diagram illustrates the multiple factors that interact on child development and behaviour. The longitudinal aspect illustrates how earlier events influence later development, and that interactions occur between the physical environment and physical development, and between the emotional environment and social development. Both biological and social environment have big effects on the child's potential even before birth. The cross-sectional view (based on Brofenbrenner, 1979) illustrates how brain function influences intelligence, developmental skills, and relationships. The wider environment influences relationships, which in turn influence interior circles, including brain development. Recent genetic research illustrates the influence of the external environment on the internal environment (factors within the growing child). A common language of understanding behaviour has to take account of this full range of interactive factors.

Accordingly, this area of study is remarkable for its potential to reinvigorate child psychiatry (Dossetor et al., 2005) and provide a broader base from which to develop approaches to intervention. Many of the approaches come from the greater intensity of intervention required for young people with intellectual disability. The integration of the psychiatry of intellectual disability and child psychiatry also leads to a framework of developmental neuropsychiatry that takes into account developmental processes in all young people (see figure 20.2).

Evidence in psychiatry of intellectual disability

There are few epidemiological studies of ICD or DSM child psychiatric diagnoses, and minimal research on the reliability of these diagnoses specifically in children with intellectual disability, let alone the validity. One exception was the study of Dekker and colleagues (2002) of a random sample of 474

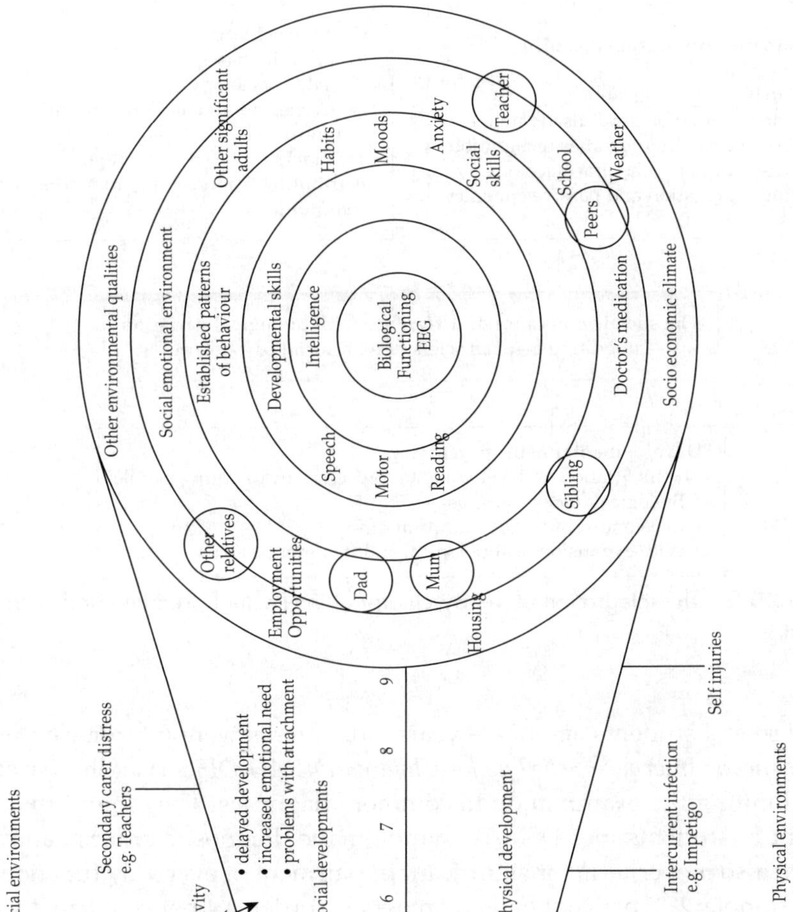

Figure 20.1 Bio-developmental-psycho-social-cultural model

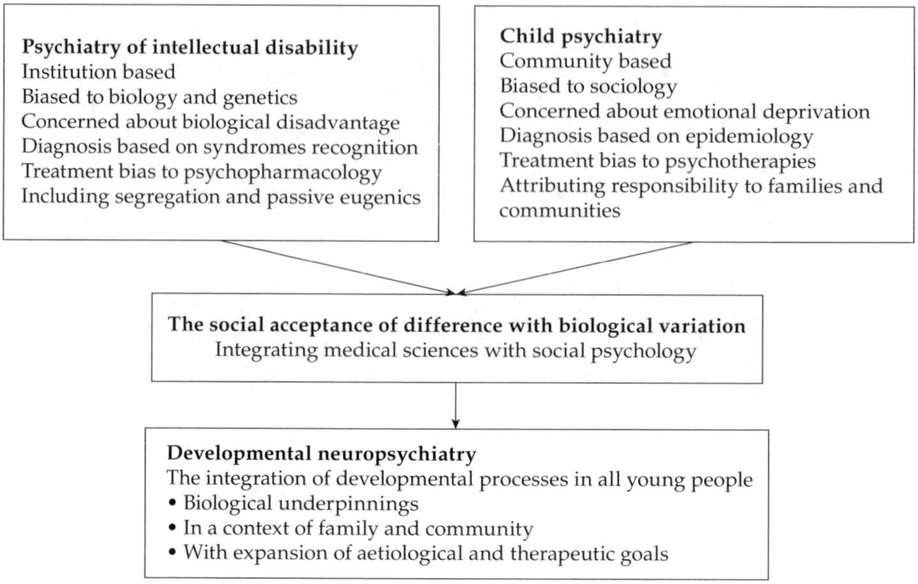

Figure 20.2 The integration of the psychiatry of intellectual disability and child psychiatry

special school students aged 7–20 years old. Parents were interviewed using the *Diagnostic Interview Schedule for Children (NIMH DISC-IV)* (Shaffer et al., 2000), limiting the examination to common diagnoses. They found that 38.6 per cent of students met DSM-IV symptomatic diagnostic criteria, and 21.7 per cent also met criteria for significant impairment of everyday functioning. Of the sample, 21.7 per cent had an anxiety disorder, 4.4 per cent had a mood disorder, 25 per cent had a disruptive behaviour disorder, and 37 per cent had more than one disorder.

Further difficulties with child psychiatric diagnoses in children with intellectual disability occur when clinicians describe problems differently; for example, one clinician may describe as a behaviour problem what another clinician sees as a psychiatric problem. There are no objective measures to distinguish the impairment associated with an intellectual disability from impairment associated with a psychiatric disorder. Child mental health researchers include any disturbance of behaviour or emotions sufficient to cause significant impairment to the child or to those caring for him or her as a significant psychiatric disorder. For older children and adolescents, mental health services start to prioritise their business for practical and pragmatic reasons. The current Australian federal and state governments' logo of 'Mental health is everyone's business' suggests that all services that deal with children have responsibilities to understand and manage mental health problems. For example, most aggression is a chronic problem that doesn't improve in psychiatric inpatient units. Most conditions are best treated in the community, and the quality of the care in the community is a shared responsibility between families, neighbourhoods, and all government departments.

The longitudinal study of young people with intellectual disability by Einfeld and Tonge (1996b), using the *Developmental Behaviour Checklist (DBC)* (Einfeld & Tonge, 1995), indicated that 40 per cent had a severe mental health disorder. The DBC provides a symptom score as a severity measure of disturbance, but it does not readily translate into psychiatric disorders, although selected items can be used to screen for autism or depression. However, whether a problem constitutes a mental illness in terms of a DSM or ICD diagnosis, or is a behaviour disturbance, is a subjective determination that is affected by the professional discipline and employing agency, which use different theoretical models, languages, and indeed priority selection criteria for service provision.

What treatments work in children with intellectual disability?

Can the problem of diagnosis be clarified by considering the evidence of the benefits of treatment? A recent literature search of the empirical evidence of effectiveness of intervention in children with intellectual disability revealed two Cochrane systematic reviews. Diggle and McConanchie (2002) found that parent training had the best evidence of being helpful. The review on behavioural intervention by Hassiotis and Hall (2008) reported short-term benefits of behavioural intervention, but there was only limited evidence of longer-term benefit.

Parent training approaches to intervention

What can the parent training approach, such as *Stepping Stones Triple P* (Sanders et al., 2003) for emotional and behavioural problems, teach clinicians? First, the program has a normalising philosophy and framework that is the same for children with intellectual disability as for those without. This framework includes the following tenets: creating a safe, engaging environment; the environment should facilitate learning of skills and positive behaviour; use of assertive discipline to shape behaviour; parental emotional adaptation to the (disabled) child; having developmentally realistic expectations; being a part of the community; and taking care of parents' wellbeing (Roberts et al., 2006).

There is evidence that promoting skill growth, independence, and self-determinism improves problem behaviour even in adults with intellectual disability (Nota et al., 2007). For parents to be emotionally and developmentally in tune is important for progress. Recognising the need to belong to a wider community is also important for both parents and children. However, this parent training approach assumes a complex understanding of behaviour problems. These include:

- *genetic factors:* including sociability, reactivity and activity levels

- *family environment factors:* including accidental rewards of undesirable behaviour, escalation traps, emotional messages, ineffective use of punishments, parents' beliefs and expectations, parents' relationships and emotions, and stress
- *influences outside of the home*, such as other relationships, including peers, school, media and technology.

The reason for working on family environment factors is they are the most accessible and easiest for parents to influence. Improving family environment factors can also influence the extent of the influence of genetic factors, and makes it easier to sort out influences outside of the home. Furthermore, the rigour of this approach is likely to have a long-term effect by improving emotional communication and attachments.

Multiplier effects of risks and disadvantage

The risk of child psychiatric disorder rises in relation to the number of social adversity risk factors, but the risk rises exponentially. The epidemiological studies of *Triple P–Positive Parenting Program* also illustrate how psychiatric problems and adverse social context have a multiplier effect. A study by Zubrick and colleagues (2005) found that children in primary schools who received intervention demonstrated improvements of both emotions and behaviour, which were sustained with associated improved parent–child relationship. Those who did not receive intervention not only did not get better, but their behaviour deteriorated and the parents' views about them got worse, leading to an even more damaging parent–child relationship. Thus change and progress are a result of complex interactive mechanisms.

Medication for ADHD shows significant improvement, but it seems likely that the long-term outcome is dependent on secondary multiplier effects, in terms of whether home and other relationships become less developmentally deleterious, and indeed developmentally enhancing. Such suggestions on multiplier effects are supported by the widespread research on the negative influence on all types of psychiatric disorder of high expressed emotion (which includes criticism and hostility or emotional over-involvement or depression) in the closest relative(s). Intervention also involves engendering hope and optimism, which in turn improves interpersonal emotional communication.

Promoting positive behaviour, limiting emotional overarousal, reducing risky behaviours, improving positive and realistic expectations, and strengthening developmentally-enhancing relationships would seem to be universal aims for interventions for all psychiatric disorders. These aims should be kept in mind also when young people are admitted to a mental health unit. The roles that are distinct for a clinician or psychiatrist are considering in greater detail the child's physical health and the possibility of intervening in the internal environment, especially through the use of medications.

ADHD and disruptive behaviour disorders: interaction of the 'internal' and 'external' environments

In child and adolescent psychiatry, clinicians are faced with the same mix of factors as described in the *Stepping Stones Triple P* (Sanders et al., 2003) parent training approach. For example, in disruptive behaviour disorders, both aetiological and treatment studies show that it is predominantly family factors that drive disruptive behaviour disorders (Scott, 2008). The final common pathway of the main genesis factors are inept parental discipline and monitoring. Yet there are also temperamental vulnerability factors, such as activity and reactivity levels, that have genetic components. Indeed these genetic factors in the child induce greater reactivity in the parents and therefore less optimal parenting.

Furthermore, ADHD is commonly associated with disruptive behaviour disorders. It has been found that 60–90 per cent of the variance of ADHD is genetic (Thapar & Rutter, 2008). This means that 60–90 per cent of the impairment of ADHD is a result of the biological factors of brain function. These factors are polygenetic, but a few of the genes have been identified. These genes then influence brain development, neurone migration, dendrite connection through proliferation and pruning, neurotrophic factors, neurotransmitters and their receptor processes, and a whole range of other largely unknown molecular processes of the brain. There is no doubt that these biological factors are affected by the environment; for example, the number of hours of non-educational TV watched by toddlers was related to the risk of having attentional problems in seven-year-olds (Zimmerman & Christakis, 2007). Also, ADHD is not a categorical disorder (either you have it or you don't), but it is a question of how much of it you have (Levy et al., 1997). Stress, abuse, and emotional deprivation make features of ADHD worse, and conversely, an improved social environment also ameliorates them. There is a large literature on the influence of these factors on the developing brain.

Interaction of genes and deprivation in childhood: pathways to adult psychopathy

It has been found that the combination of genetic vulnerability (with a reduced presence of the enzyme MAOA, an adrenaline gene) and the co-occurrence of childhood deprivation leads to lifelong violence to such a degree that it accounts for a large proportion of violent adults in the community (Caspi & Moffit, 2006). However, this is purely a research finding, which has not led to diagnosis or treatment. Nonetheless, scientists talk about the effect size in ADHD of the 'external' environment being 10–40 per cent, and the other 60–90 per cent of effects is a result of what happens at the neuromolecular and neurobiological level or the 'internal environment' (Thapar & Rutter, 2008).

Clinicians may only have a very limited understanding of the processes of the internal environment, but the interactive and multiplier effects between the internal environment and external environment are important and complex. Similar gene and early deprivation interactions have been found for anxiety, PTSD, substance abuse, and depression. Through reducing the reserves of serotonin in the brain, individuals with these disorders are less likely to respond to serotonin reuptake inhibitor antidepressants, and are more likely to get side-effects. However, in ADHD science has discovered medications that do alter the internal environment and alter behaviour. It is exploring the neurobiological and pharmacological components that are specific to medicine, particularly psychiatry.

ADHD in intellectual disability

ADHD in those with mild intellectual disability has a significant research literature, indicating reliability and predictive validity; that is, it is recognisable and it has predictive meaning (Antshel et al., 2006). However, there are significant differences, such as a prevalence of 30 per cent, equal sex ratio, possibly greater family factors, depression, and social impairment. Further, standard pharmacological treatment is not as effective and is more prone to side-effects than for those with a normal range of intelligence.

ADHD in those with severe intellectual disability lacks the same level of research for reliability and validity, and is likely to be affected by more biological and developmental factors. For example, there is an association with other developmental disorders. Both developmental coordination disorder and ADHD occur in 7 per cent of the community, but co-occur in 50 per cent (Martin et al., 2006). In clinic populations of PDD, ADHD is found in 78 per cent of cases (Lee & Ousley, 2006). In a control study of teenagers with intellectual disability with and without autism, the presence of ADHD was found in one in two of those with autism and intellectual disability versus one in seven with intellectual disability but without autism (Bradley & Isaacs, 2006). Such observations indicate that delays of different domains of development are genetically linked, as development and its delay are polygenic processes.

Genetic studies have shown linkage between autism and intellectual disability, suggesting some common pathways of development. There are reasons for considering autism as a delay of social development leading to a delay of social understanding, reciprocity, and theory of mind (Dossetor, 2004). ADHD in different (genetic) behavioural phenotypes is reported to be extraordinarily high: Smith-Magenis syndrome 90 per cent; fragile X syndrome 75 per cent; Williams' syndrome 65 per cent; Charge syndrome 50 per cent; neurofibromatosis 50 per cent; Velo Cardio facial syndrome 43 per cent; Cornelia de Lange's syndrome 40 per cent; Soto's syndrome 38 per cent; tuberose sclerosis 35 per cent; and Turner's syndrome 24 per cent. Binge drinking in pregnancy causes foetal alcohol syndrome, with a range of consequent problems, including ADHD in 49 per cent, intellectual disability in 55 per cent, learning disorders in 46 per cent, oppositional defiant and conduct disorders in 41 per cent, and anger control problems, mood disorders, and sleep disorders in 50 per cent (Bhatara et al., 2006).

Given the frequency of ADHD in these genetic syndromes associated with intellectual disability, it may be helpful to identify comorbid ADHD for the benefit of drug treatment. ADHD certainly adds to the problems of quality of life and degree of difficulty of care and parenting, but it may not be the same condition as identified in the population of children of average intellect. In the context of intellectual disability, the features of impulsivity, hyperactivity, and inattention may be more appropriately seen as elements of developmental challenge and progress affecting intellectual efficiency in the establishment of conscious processes. These are important to establish theory of mind and a sense of self and others, which are key to consciousness. It may be more appropriate to describe it as a developmental delay of these attributes of efficient mentation. Indeed, there are well-recognised developmental sequences of attention, from modulation of arousal, to selective attention, to dual tasking with attention switching. These are associated with different neurotransmitters; that is, dopamine, acetylcholine, and noradrenalin, respectively.

Accordingly, there is a dichotomy of intervention approaches. One approach supports the developmental sequence of skill building as a unifying model for improving intellectual disability and disturbance of emotions and behaviour. The other is a deconstructive approach to specific psychiatric syndromes, in the hope of identifying individual factors of causality. However, a developmental model for ADHD creates expectations of gradual improvement with support, as shown by parent training programs (AACAP, 2007). Indeed, while most treatment studies have focused on drugs versus cognitive behaviour therapy, parent skills training has been shown to be effective in ADHD (Bor et al., 2002).

Developmental models: valuable guiding principles

The universal principle of development was propounded by Heinz Werner: 'Wherever there is life there is development in a systematic sequence' (as cited by Burack, 2008). Perhaps clinicians know so little about the development of the mind, consciousness, emotions, and socialisation that developmental principles are the best guide. Piaget (1972) asserted that development involved the orderly and universal development of functioning that evolved in a consistent way. Therefore, despite the differences of every individual, the commonality of human development is the most striking feature, even for individuals whose development is distorted by genetic or biological differences.

Werner also described the orthogenetic principle that 'development progresses from relative globality and lack of differentiation to increasing differentiation, articulation, and hierarchic integration' (as cited in Hodapp & Burack, 2006, p. 237). As both the individual and context differentiates, so the process of development becomes more complex. This leads on to a development–transactional approach that recognises that real development is complex, and involves relations constantly changing or transacting with the environment. Perhaps it is not so strange that researchers of the major psychoses are raising notions that psychoses are developmental disorders, with vulnerabilities of early development leading to later crisis of adaptation, loss of well-being and quality of life, and a loss of integration of subjective consciousness.

With the progress of science, an entirely dualist approach to the mind is no longer acceptable. In some situations, clinicians' assistance to people's mental health is clearly enhanced by their understanding of and intervention in the internal environment. However, where there is no evidence of the validity of a deconstructive approach to mental health, then developmental models have face validity, and are intuitive for families and professionals alike. In many instances, delay and deviance cannot be distinguished psychometrically. A developmental framework is a good guide to clinical practice, because it is understandable intuitively, and problems of intellectual disability need to be understandable to be accepted.

This is not to say that biology isn't important in children and young people with intellectual disability. Indeed, the available research suggests that standard measures of family function account for only 4 per cent of the variance of behaviour disturbance in young people with intellectual disability over time (Tonge & Einfeld, 2000; Einfeld et al., 2006), and that the best predictor of disturbance is past disturbance. For example, even the best of family functioning can be overwhelmed by the behavioural impact of a 12-year-old with Smith-Magenis syndrome, with real risks of major harm to another member of the family, making family care no longer feasible. However, the best bet for helping young people with intellectual disability is through understanding developmental need, particularly getting in early to help these families with atunement, skills, and mitigation of the inordinate burden of care. The more it is understood how biology is manifested through developmental processes, the more parents can develop the skills that match the needs of a child with a developmental disability and promote their development in the context of loving family relationships.

Developmental approaches to understanding young people and their behaviour

In a stratified random selection of 92 12–18-year-olds with mainly severe intellectual disability, emotional and behavioural disturbance measured on the *Handicaps Behaviour Skills Schedule* (Wing & Gould, 1978) formed a single factor for analysis (Dossetor, 1991). Emotional and behaviour disturbance was not related to chronological age but to developmental age. Disturbance gradually increased from a developmental age of 1 year to 2.5 years, and then progressively declined. This concurs with developmental norms of children of normal intellect. That is, as children of normal intellect become older and more able, they show more exploratory and intrusive skills until their third year, when they develop a theory of mind. They start to realise that they have an imagination that relates to other peoples' thoughts and feelings. Accordingly, their exploratory skills focus on their internal world and they become less problematic to others. Although other developmental factors, such as adolescent hormones and life roles, also influence behaviour, the author's clinical and research experience suggests that the developmental age is most formative.

In the same way as tantrums are a normal part of development in 80 per cent of two-year-old children, it is a complex normative developmental behaviour that most children grow out of by 3–4 years, rather than a result of environmental or neuropsychiatric features. Family environmental factors are most related to severity and persistence of tantrums, but temperamental factors of the child (including significant genetic factors) predispose. Thus toddlers face a stressful challenge in integrating the meaning of the world with a growing capacity for a perspective of self and other, an internal voice, and sufficient concentration to reason. Indeed, malice of forethought or anti-social premeditated behaviour can't really be attributed before the age of 5–6 years and the development of concrete operations. Depression requires similar developmental milestones for the capacity for guilt, as an internal-cognitive means of maintaining depressive mood and its biological concomitants. Such a framework suggests that before this developmental age, psychiatric presentations are generally reactive to their environment, in keeping with a model of challenging behaviour or adjustment disorders. The exception to this would be developmental disorders, including autism and ADHD.

Dealing with moderate, severe, and profound intellectual disability focuses on the developmental processes of the under-fives. Making sense of behaviour in children with intellectual disability requires a detailed understanding of the multidimensional components of development. When development is delayed, it is likely that delay will be unequal across different developmental domains. If one domain is delayed, then it is likely that another will be delayed. For example, if language development is delayed, there is greater risk of intellectual disability or problems of social reciprocity. If you have coordination disorder, you are more likely to have enuresis. If you have delayed development, you are more likely to have ADHD. Autism is more likely in ID (confirmed by genetic linkage studies). The implication is that developmental processes vary but also are genetically linked to each other.

The main domains of development are listed below.

Sensory/visuospatial skills

Sensory processing is a source of pleasure and stimulation for individuals, but it is the primary source of physiological conscious arousal before the establishment of theory of mind and an internal imaginary world. Modulation of arousal is facilitated by adult engagement, for example, in modifying the environment and providing predictability. Once theory of mind has developed, thought, imagination, and social engagement have predominant roles influencing the control of arousal.

Motor development, activity, and coordination

Motor calmness is a prerequisite for concentration and awareness of time.

Independence skills (as for feeding, dressing, toileting)
The level of achievement in independence skills is the best clinical measure of general intelligence before the development of educational skills. It can also involve community access safety and skills.

Communication skills
- *Receptive communication*, tested functionally by response to commands, the complexity and grammar of commands, and an understanding of concepts such as time.
- *Expressive communication* again depends on its functionality.

Social development
Social development is a measure of social reciprocity and empathic understanding, and progresses from affective reciprocity to joint attention, turn taking, and reciprocal interaction to participating in group dynamics. Emotional understanding is related to social development, and is specifically delayed in ASD, which is found in 50 per cent of those with intellectual disability (Wing & Gould, 1979). It is not surprising that the presence of ASD is associated with behaviour disturbance, as social engagement is central to the social nature of humans. The author's rule of thumb is that in children with autism, social developmental level is less than 2 years, and for Asperger's it is less than 4.5 years.

These five domains relate to assessment, skill-building approaches and intervention of the allied health disciplines of occupational therapy, physiotherapy, speech pathology, and psychology. All these disciplines may be required to assess and help understand complex developmental profiles and the relationship to difficult behaviour.

A number of other child mental health clinicians working in intellectual disability have also suggested models of understanding development processes and the relationship to the development of emotions. Curran and Kyrkou (2008) developed the acronym *SPICE* for assessing the developmental dimensions of *social*, *physical* (including sensory, motor processing, other neurological impairments, and seizures), *intellectual* (including the executive function skills), *communication*, and *emotional development.*

On the other hand, Greenspan and Wieder (2008) presented a model of social development that can be applied to autistic children or typically developing children. They identified specific focus areas that equated to developmental ages: parent orientated (0–1 years: affective reciprocity); adult orientated (1–2 years: joint attention); toddler independence (2–2.5 years: parallel play); peer skill development (2.5–4 years: theory of mind); peer group association (4–8 years: second order theory of mind); pre-adolescent (9–13 years); and adolescence (13-plus years: abstract cognitive capacity). Both Curran and Kyrkou's (2008) and Greenspan and Wieder's (2008) models address similar dimensions, starting from different frameworks.

Table 20.3 Some common theoretical models and their common context

Theoretical model	*Context*
Society	Welfare, rights, cultural attitudes, and socioeconomic influences
Community	Environment, social structures, and social capital
School	Communication, other skill enhancements, and peer relationships
Family	Emotional environment and substitute care
Group	Social skills and role learning model
Individual Relationship	Attachments, intrapsychic or somatoform emotional models
Cognitions and affect	Problem solving, CBT, affect regulation, and coping skills models
Neuropsychology	Neuroanatomical function and integrity
Neuropsychiatric processes	Neurochemical and psychopharmacological models
Neurobiological risk and resilience	Genetic and neurodevelopmental and molecular biology

Clearly a developmental model is only one component of a child psychiatric assessment which also requires assessment of the medical, family environment, peer and community influences, and neuropsychiatric components. On the one hand, intensive clinical approaches, particularly in behavioural psychology, developed in intellectual disability have significantly influenced behaviour modification and skill-building approaches of mainstream child psychiatry. Conversely, disability services can no longer be restricted to thinking in a behavioural framework, and have to accept a holistic, multicausal approach where multiple factors contribute to the complexity of behaviour, emotions, and development. The secondary challenge is to look at which factors can be modified or which theoretical models provide a basis on which to intervene, as illustrated in table 20.3.

Behavioural phenotypes: intellectual disability's contribution to understanding the mind

The study of behavioural phenotypes has been described as a window into the biology of the brain. *Behavioural phenotypes* are where a behaviour or cluster of complex emotions and behaviours are associated with a genetic condition. This is a fascinating area of study, particularly when a specific gene is associated with a symptom of psychiatric concern to a wider population. For example, the association of high rates of psychotic disorder in Velo Cardio facial syndrome (22q11 gene deletion) may improve the understanding of the biological correlates of schizophrenia. Other research is linking a gene with a certain medical or neuropsychological attribute to developing certain behaviours. For example, the self-injury of Cornelia de Lange's syndrome was found to be related to unexpressed pain from oesophagal reflux or dental pain, and responded to omeprazole for reflux (Oliver et al., 2003; Oliver et al., 2008). In contrast, obsessive behaviour was related to ASD features in a range of behavioural phenotypes. Other research findings suggest that in Cornelia de Lange's syndrome anxiety was increased in social behaviour such as before speaking. Task-orientated attention switching was found to stress people with fragile X, and was associated with tantrums, whereas those with Prader Willi syndrome were only stressed by a verbal challenge to switch attention or routine (Oliver, 2008). These genetic-based differences help clinicians to understand some developmental and neuropsychological attributes that underlie maladaptive behaviour.

In some instances, the specificity of behavioural phenotypes in relation to understanding the internal environment leads to experimental biological treatments and hope of new medical treatments. Some examples include:

- fragile X syndrome, where trials with a selective antagonist for a glutamate receptor subtype 5 drug, fenobam, demonstrated a short-lived improvement in intellectual performance. This was an attempt to intervene in the neurobiology of a lack of fragile X mental retardation protein (FMRP). Fenobam and lithium can reverse a lack of methylation and a lack of FMRP that acts as a synaptic messenger, downgrading synaptic activity (Hagerman et al., 2008)
- tuberose sclerosis, where the associated intellectual disability is not purely related to the tubers in the brain, but also to the protein mTOR (target of rapamycin) (Ehninger et al., 2009). Rapamycin, an anti-transplant rejection drug, reduces tuber sizes and improves cognition and memory in animal models
- Lesch-Nynhan syndrome, which is caused by deficiency of the purine enzyme hypoxanthine-guanine phosphoribosyltransferase, with over-production of uric acid, along with mental retardation, recurrent self-injurious behaviour, and motor disability. The use of deep brain stimulation by electrode implantation, which was ethically approved to improve dystonia, also reduced severe mutilating self-injurious behaviour incidentally (Harris, 2008). Proton magnetic resonance spectroscopy showed that this was associated with improvement of the basal ganglia dopamine deficits and an increase in dopa action in meso cortical and frontal areas and better emotional regulation.

Such examples of neurobiological science could lead to future important treatments. However, Dykens and Hodapp (2001) reminded clinicians that, even though behavioural phenotypes can unlock some biological processes, these usually prove to be only one component of the behavioural phenotype, often challenging our deconstructive concepts of mental illness. Biologically driven behaviour is also still influenced by context and external environment (Dykens, 2000).

Conclusion

People with intellectual disability have raised levels of emotional and behavioural disturbance, which significantly impair quality of life for the individual and his or her family or carers. A study by Emerson and Hatton (2007) found that children with intellectual disability accounted for 14 per cent of all children in the UK with psychiatric problems, compared to 3 per cent prevalence of intellectual disability. Costello and colleagues (2007) indicated that a failure to intervene early in emotional and behavioural problems led to long-term morbidity and cost to the community. Thus, issues of equity demand that people with intellectual disability and mental health problems have access to an appropriately skilled multidisciplinary clinical workforce.

Biological forces in intellectual disability drive problems of developmental delay and disturbance. Particularly in severe intellectual disability, developmental understanding has greater relevance to understanding behaviour. The best evidence for improving disturbance, or minimising its handicap, is by promoting stimulating, supportive, and protective relationships as provided by a family. These types of intimate relationships promote a progressive sequence in independence, communication, emotional and social skills, and the development of functional consciousness.

There is a growing empirical literature on a variety of processes, theories, and interventions. Consensus suggests that multidisciplinary assessment and intervention can improve outcomes, but knowing which interventions will work in a particular child or young person with intellectual disability depends on clinical expertise.

There is need for investment in specialist parent training as one of the early universal interventions. Multidisciplinary skills in intellectual disability are needed for assessment and skill promotion. Intensive behavioural management remains a key skill, but is no longer sufficient (Carr et al., 2007). Both disability clinicians and mental health psychologists need to be trained in the modifications of cognitive behavioural therapy for people with an intellectual disability. In current practice, it has been found that family therapy knowledge and systems thinking skills are critically needed (Rhodes, 2003; Seligman & Darling, 2007). There is a self-evident need for a multidisciplinary approach to mental health in intellectual disability.

There is need for collaboration with psychiatrists. Mainstream psychiatrists are familiar with psychotropic medications and understand mainstream presentations. However, they lack experience, especially of the clinical differences in people with a severe intellectual disability, whose mental health problems are complex and have a major impact on their quality of life.

Thus, there is an imperative need to develop and recognise a psychiatric workforce in intellectual disability.

In Australia there is no specialist mental health service for people with an intellectual disability. A psychiatric workforce in intellectual disability is necessary to provide clinical expertise in areas for which other professionals cannot substitute, even as an opinion of last resort. This review has illustrated some of the reasons for needing a psychiatric workforce with specialist experience and knowledge. Such a subspecialty would be an essential source of advocacy for services and for clinical research for this special population, but would also enrich mainstream mental health and psychiatry.

21

Promoting resolution and safety: A case study example

Lesley Whatson, Debra Corfield, and Brett Owens

Introduction

The prevalence of emotional and behavioural difficulties in children and adolescents with intellectual disability has been reported to be between 30 and 50 per cent (Einfeld & Tonge, 1996b; Molteno et al., 2001). These difficulties may present in various ways, including emotional outbursts, physical aggression, property damage, and self-injury. Regardless of these differences in presentation and/or underlying causality, the issue of risk and risk management is inherent in each.

Risk is described as action(s) that jeopardise something of value (Reber, 1995). There are risks of physical harm to the child or young person, to others, and to the environment. There are also risks of harm to relationships and the emotional and psychological well-being of those involved, including feelings of anger, resentment, sadness, and the potential for longer term development of mood or anxiety disorders, and disrupted attachment (Nugent, 2005). All of these risks necessitate careful consideration and response.

The challenge of balancing risk management with quality of life and least restrictive, least intrusive care is one that must be carefully negotiated. Risk management is of particular importance during crisis, when the child's emotional or behavioural difficulties are at their most extreme. Reber (1995) described crisis as a condition of instability or danger, a dramatic emotional or circumstantial upheaval, a point at which sudden change occurs, leading to sudden improvement or further deterioration of a situation. At these times, the goal is simply to promote safety and the resolution of the crisis situation. *Crisis management strategies*, also known as *reactive strategies* or *situational management strategies*, are developed to achieve this end. While they may be devised to stand alone, crisis management strategies are more commonly developed as part of a broader approach. They are necessary for as long as it takes for the proactive components of a plan to show some benefit. As Osgood (2004) states, 'Reactive strategies are not aimed at teaching, but at stopping things with dignity and safety, so because they are not inherently constructive, they must never be used on their own but alongside proactive interventions' (p. 6).

The case study example that follows illustrates the benefits of a multidisciplinary approach to the management of crisis and the risks associated with it. It highlights how the varied perspectives of members of a team can collectively offer useful insight in shaping a more holistic intervention for a child with complex needs.

Case study: John

John is 12 years old and has a moderate intellectual disability and autism spectrum disorder (ASD). He is highly mobile, is 135 centimetres tall and weighs 64 kilograms. While John has a few spoken words, his primary means of communication is key word sign and natural gesture. He also uses photographs and pictographs at school.

John lives in the inner city with his mother Marnie, and his younger sister Olivia, who is four years old. The family has no contact with John's father, who left the family home soon after Olivia was born. Marnie says that being a single mother is stressful, and finds that no matter how much time and attention she gives John, he seems to need more. Marnie reports feeling frightened of John when he is in a rage and worries about Olivia's safety. She also reports feeling concerned about how much damage John might do as he gets bigger and stronger. Marnie recently told her disability case manager that she didn't know how long she could keep caring for John, and wondered whether someone else might do a better job.

For the past two years, John has been receiving increasing amounts of care at a children's respite unit. The family's allocation is now Monday to Wednesday each week and one weekend per month. John is in Year 6 at a special school, 15 minutes from home.

All settings are finding it difficult to manage John's challenging behaviours. These challenging behaviours are described as:

- screaming and crying
- hitting, pinching, and pulling hair of adults and other children
- eye gouging of other children, causing injury
- grabbing at reading glasses being worn by adults and children
- breaking and throwing objects.

Sometimes there will be a slow escalation of John's agitation and arousal. At other times, John will appear to move rapidly from a relatively calm state to crisis. John will sometimes use several of the listed behaviours in combination, or he will use one in isolation.

In the respite unit, John prefers to interact with staff rather than peers. When other children attempt to interact with him, they are usually ignored or hit by him. Staff are worried about the risk that John poses to other children, particularly those he has targeted before. It can be difficult to predict who John will attack, but children who seem frightened, move slowly, or who wear glasses are more vulnerable. Staff have noticed that John seems bothered by children who squeal or cry. The respite unit manager is liaising with the disability case manager about which children requiring respite care are compatible with John.

At school, John has similar difficulties with peers, particularly in the playground. He requires close supervision around other children at all times. Assaults on peers and staff have led to two previous (two-day) suspensions from school. These suspensions complicate the respite situation, as the unit is not staffed during the day and cannot provide support to John. This means that John returns home and spends the days he is excluded from school with Marnie.

John becomes stressed when there are changes to his routine, such as staff changes at respite, school holidays, his teacher's aide being away, medical appointments, and school transport being late. John finds it easiest to manage his behaviour when boundaries and limits are clear. John becomes concerned when he is told 'no', or is punished or criticised.

John likes to be busy and enjoys cooking, watching selected DVDs (such as *Ice Age*), and activities involving drawing. He particularly likes drawing with chalk on the driveway. John enjoys outdoor activities, such as going for a drive, walking, shopping, and riding a three-wheel bike. At the respite unit, John is happy to participate in household activities, such as setting the table (place mats), hanging out the washing, and making his bed (pulling up the doona). John highly values positive feedback, and enjoys sharing the news of his day at school. He loves to show off his merit awards and stickers for work well done.

The support system

Perspectives of the presenting issues

Each person in John's family and service system is affected differently by his challenging behaviour. Socio/genograms (see figure 21.1) help bring all the key elements of John's network into view. Each has a different role and set of responsibilities in relation to John's development and behavioural support. Perceptions will have been shaped by each person's understanding of John (based on assessment information and his or her experience of him), his or her own social history, professional background or discipline, role in the case, and relationship(s) with others in the system. While it would be impossible to represent the entire range of insights generated by those in a system such as John's, a summary of the various perspectives makes a useful foundation for the exploration of a response/reactive strategy.

John's perspective

When John went to school a few weeks ago and found that his teacher was away sick, he became very upset. His routine was different, and he didn't get

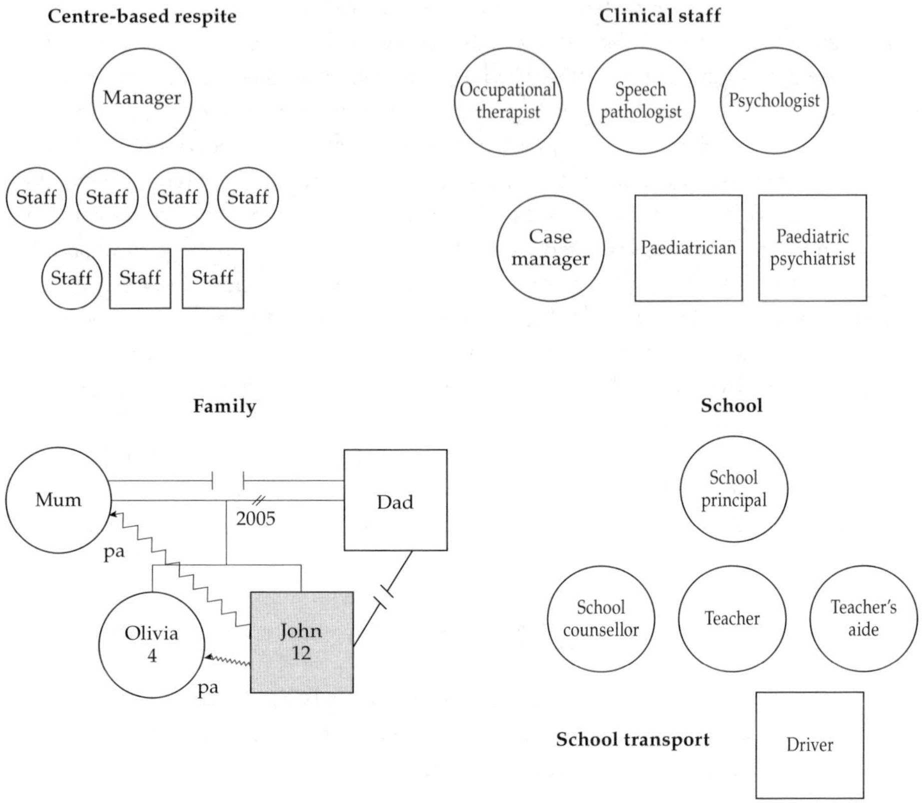

Figure 21.1 John's support system

to clean the board or help take books to the library. When the casual teacher told John he needed to stop drawing and come to circle time, he began to scream, picking up his chair, and throwing it. He continued to escalate, throwing himself on the floor, and kicking out at peers. The others in the class had to be removed to the playground. While the teacher's aide was trying to prevent John from striking another child, he managed to forcibly pull her glasses off and strike her in the face.

After taking John home, at the request of the school, Marnie asked John about the incident. He shrugged his shoulders and walked away. Further attempts to discuss the issue only led to him crying and pinching his sister, so Marnie decided not to discuss the event further with John. It was only later that she realised that John's teacher had been away and that he'd probably found the change of routine confusing and unsettling.

Marnie's (Mum's) perspective

Marnie explained that she is 'living in constant fear that John will go off'. She worries about Olivia being so much smaller and so vulnerable. She worries that John doesn't know his own strength, and that one day he will really hurt either

Olivia or herself. Marnie also worries about her ability to manage John's behaviours. She realises that, as John's behaviour escalates, she finds herself winding up too. After smacking John on one occasion, Marnie recalls the tremendous guilt and distress she felt. She didn't want to smack John—she just wanted him to stop. The potential for her to lose control again scares Marnie, and she has started to doubt whether she can give John the care he needs. Marnie understands that John's ability to cope and her own ability to cope are intertwined. This dynamic is discussed by the psychologist at a later point in the chapter.

The respite team's perspective

The issues raised by staff working in the respite setting suggest a growing apprehension about working with John. Although most members of the team have several years' experience in the field, there has been animated discussion at team meetings about the risks involved in managing John, particularly when the male staff are not on duty. Staff report being fearful that John will 'go off' at any moment, and are worried that another child, a staff person, or John himself will be hurt.

Team members report trying a range of approaches and strategies to diffuse escalating behaviour. There is little consistency in their responses to crisis. Some feel strongly that John should be punished for attacking others and breaking items around the house. They believe consequences should be applied to John's actions as a way of teaching him that he can't hurt others or damage things that don't belong to him. Some of the suggestions include exclusion from swimming on Saturday mornings and no DVDs after dinner. These staff feel that 'if John is given an inch, he'll take a mile', in other words, that he'll learn that he can get away with unacceptable behaviour.

Other support staff believe that the challenging behaviour is John's way of telling them that his needs are not being met. They feel that the team should work to understand and enable him, rather than punish him. They are concerned that attempts to restrict his lifestyle might exacerbate the challenging behaviour and lead to further punishment. Some staff are worried that John has only limited control of his behaviour when he is highly agitated, and feel that he needs more support to calm himself; they also doubt that John will connect the behaviour to the punishment.

This team clearly needs assistance to develop a consistent approach to the management of John's challenging behaviour. It is likely that team members will need opportunity to discuss and debate the strategies included in the response plan, to ensure that they understand the strengths and weaknesses of the various options, and commit to implementing them as prescribed. The strategies should be designed in a way that ensures the least confident, least powerful staff member can implement them, as this will promote consistent implementation. Staff will require training and opportunities to practise the new procedures. Given the stressful nature of shifts, the team will need regular opportunities to reflect on events and progress, vent, and debrief.

The respite manager's perspective

The manager of the respite unit has become increasingly concerned about the risk of injury to children and staff. She recognises that staff are finding their shifts stressful and demanding. The families of two children who regularly access respite with John have asked that their respite allocation be changed, as they are not confident their children will be kept safe if John's stay coincides with their children's.

In processing leave forms, the manager has noticed a significant increase in the amount of leave taken by several staff. She wonders whether these leave patterns and the stress generated by John's behaviour are linked. Vacant shifts are becoming difficult to fill as casual staff are reluctant to work in the unit. Her greater concern is that staff employed at the house will resign and that staff turnover will become an issue.

Incident reports are being filled out as required, though the language in some accounts has become emotive. Staff describe John's behaviour as 'vicious' and 'manipulating'. The manager suspects that some staff are personalising John's behaviour, and are finding it difficult to feel positive about working with him. She recognises the need to maintain team meetings, and thinks that staff might also benefit from debriefing sessions. The manager is keen to have the respite team participate in any training offered by the psychologist and therapists, and is happy to liaise with the family and school.

The paediatric psychiatrist's perspective

Referral to a paediatric psychiatrist was made by John's paediatrician. The paediatrician cited challenging behaviour as the primary reason for the referral and queried the potential usefulness of PRN medication (*pro re nata*—according to circumstances) as part of the overall response to John's situation.

Following consultation, both doctors agreed that there were problems in medicating John's aggression for a number of reasons. First, medication for aggression itself is seldom helpful. The value of oral PRN medication is limited by the time it takes to be digested and reach the blood stream (approximately 50 minutes). However, the two practitioners noted that PRN is sometimes helpful in anticipation of stressful situations, particularly to reduce the need for a regular medication that might have a problematic side-effect (such as weight gain from increased appetite).

The psychiatrist described the necessity to check for a psychiatric disorder or vulnerability that might predispose John to aggression and the loss of emotional regulation. The psychiatrist reflected that aggression that is intentionally malicious seldom responds to medication, but that intellectually disabled young people, such as John, do not generally have capacity for malevolent intent or moral judgment of behaviour. Accordingly, John's aggression is expected to be affect driven, and likely to have associated developmental or mental disorders.

The two practitioners confirmed that John's profile and history indicate an autistic spectrum disorder (ASD). They explored the possibility that aggression because of intense stereotypic behaviour or thinking might be helped by selective serotonin reuptake inhibitors (SSRI antidepressants). Also, given John's ASD diagnosis, the 50 per cent chance of comorbid attention deficit hyperactive disorder (ADHD) and its associated vulnerabilities (non-compliance and anger dysregulation) should be considered as a focus for treatment (Bradley & Isaacs, 2006).

The doctors discussed pharmacological options, including trials of stimulants, daytime clonidine, antidepressants that benefit ADHD (such as amitriptyline, mirtazapine, or strattera), atypical antipsychotics (such as risperidone, olanzapine, or aripiprazole), and perhaps conventional antipsychotics. Unstable or labile mood, which some psychiatrists compare with bipolar disorders or cyclothymia, might benefit from mood stabilisers such as carbamazepine, sodium valproate and lithium carbonate. Other medications, such as beta adrenergic blockers, could help with affectively driven aggression, as could antipsychotics.

The two agreed that it is always important to look carefully for evidence of depression, panic disorder, post-traumatic stress disorder (PTSD), obsessive compulsive disorder (OCD), generalised anxiety disorder (GAD), and psychotic disorders. Dissociation is seldom a good target for medication. Organic mental states causing acute confusion or cognitive decline need consideration. In pharmacological treatment of those with intellectual difficulty there may be less frequent positive results, and more frequent side-effects from medications such as stimulants. This necessitates caution: starting low and going slow, and being available to consider side-effects if they arise. Often, more than one comorbid mental health disorder may be present, and more than one medication may be required, with due caution about interactions and side-effects. Finding an optimal medication regime may take patient trialling of drugs in sequence. This is best done in the child's normal environment, and seldom can a hospital inpatient admission be used for this purpose (Bhaumik & Branford, 2008; Dossetor, 2003; Lask et al., 2003).

The consultation excluded evidence of major psychiatric disorder. The paediatrician and psychiatrist agreed to trial amitriptyline in response to John's longstanding features of ADHD; this decision was made in the hope that the medication might make John more receptive to other interventions. As some outbursts were lasting for up two hours, the psychiatrist made PRN risperidone available, in an attempt to reduce the risk of injury to John and others. The psychiatrist agreed to liaise with the psychologist in documenting a PRN protocol for inclusion in the reactive strategy, as part of the broader *behaviour support plan*.

The psychiatrist flagged one last concern: in a situation such as this, there is a high risk that Marnie will be suffering an anxiety or depressive disorder requiring assessment and treatment. Attention to this possibility is critical for both John and Marnie, as it determines, to a great extent, Marnie's capacity for warmth, responsiveness, and affective regulation.

The teacher's perspective

The primary concerns raised by John's teacher and the school principal were those of safety and duty of care: the difficulty of managing John's behaviour while ensuring the safety of other students, staff, and John. In the past, the school has resorted to suspending him, but staff feel that previous suspensions have only served to exacerbate the problem on his return to the classroom. Staff see John's potential and want to support him in developing skills for life.

In their endeavour to find a way to manage the presenting risks in the school environment, John's school made a number of important discoveries. The teacher observed that giving John errands when he appeared to be escalating (such as returning some heavy books to the library) was helpful in averting crises. During crisis, however, she felt John was virtually impossible to redirect: 'He just gets so worked up. It's like he can't hear you.' So, rather than focusing on John at these times, John's teacher redirected her attention to helping the other students remain safe and protecting the physical environment.

When John began to escalate, the teacher's aide began calmly to evacuate the five other students from the classroom and engage them in outdoor activities. Inside the classroom, John's teacher would calmly and quietly move around the room, removing potential missiles, pulling down blinds to protect windows, and pushing desks against a vulnerable gyprock wall. At times she would try to explain to John that she needed him to calm down and that she wanted him to stay safe. However, this rarely seemed to help. John would grab at her hair and attempt to pull her glasses from her face, so for the most part, she would give him space.

These strategies were particularly helpful when they could see John's behaviour gradually escalating. However, on some occasions he seemed to move from being calm to a crisis state in a matter of seconds. In these scenarios the school felt at a loss. Several of the students had mobility issues, and the process of evacuating them from the classroom was slow. There was insufficient time when John escalated quickly. John's teacher wondered why John could be so volatile and what could be done to manage the risks at these times.

The psychologist's perspective

The psychologist involved expressed concerns regarding John's emotional reactivity, with relatively small things triggering rapid escalation and 'fight or flight' behaviours. In considering the stress response system, the psychologist hypothesised that changes in brain and physiological functioning during crisis could explain part of John's presenting difficulties. When John perceives a situation as threatening, an alarm is sent to his hypothalamus, which activates his sympathetic nervous system. Hormones such as adrenaline,

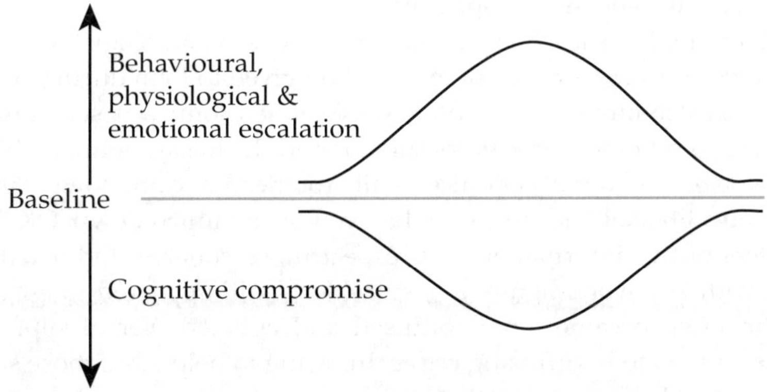

Figure 21.2 Behavioural, physiological, emotional, and cognitive changes across the crisis cycle

Source: adapted from Holden et al., 2001

noradrenaline, and cortisol are released and a range of bodily responses are triggered, including increased heart and respiration rate, dilated pupils, increased sweating, and increased blood clotting ability (Benson, 2000; Davis et al., 2000; Kalat, 2009). This short-term, survival-orientated response prepares John's body to mobilise, hence enabling the individual to either confront or flee from the perceived source of danger (whether real or imagined). In John's case, this hyperarousal might present as an assault on a peer or running from the classroom after being brushed against or touched unexpectedly.

Changes in John's brain activity also occur at these times, as blood is redirected away from the cerebral cortex to more primitive and survival-orientated parts of the brain (Perry & Szalavitz, 2006). This means that during crisis (when in a state of hyperarousal) John has reduced capacity for higher order reasoning, abstract thinking, and problem solving (see figure 21.2). Not surprisingly, then, crisis is not the optimal time for teaching new skills. The focus must be resolution and promotion of safety. The strategies employed during crisis must take into account John's reduced capacity for planning and reasoning.

The psychologist also wondered whether any parallel processes were occurring. After reflecting on how John's challenging behaviour had had an impact on her own levels of arousal during a home visit, she wondered whether a stress response was simultaneously being triggered in others. John is not the only person experiencing a crisis situation, but his mother, teacher, carers, peers, and clinicians do as well. As illustrated in figure 21.3, it is reasonable to suggest that during crisis, changes in the caregiver's behaviour, physiology, emotions, and cognitions can be expected, albeit to varying degrees. This led the psychologist to realise that the reactive strategy component of John's multi-element behaviour support plan would need to be tailored to both the interactive and parallel processes occurring between John and his caregivers (and/or peers) during crises.

The speech pathologist's perspective

After observing John at school and home, the speech pathologist was particularly interested in the amount of information given to John during crisis and how this was communicated. For example, when John was screaming and attempting to hit others, it was common for adults to say, 'John, no hitting. I can see you're mad but it's not nice to hit. You need to calm down. I'm going to give you a break. I'll come back when you have calmed down. OK?' While the content of this information was respectful, reasonable, and usually augmented with key word sign and gesture, John still appeared to escalate. In fact, John often became more confused and agitated. Verbal support just didn't seem to help in diffusing crises. In trying to help John, those supporting him seemed to be making things worse.

Drawing on the information presented in figure 21.2, the speech pathologist suggested that John's capacity to comprehend and process language was being compromised during crisis. Similarly, his ability to produce speech, or formulate a response, would be significantly reduced compared to his typical communication skills (when calm at baseline) (Cross, 2004). As the regions of the brain involved in language are located in the cerebral cortex, they become increasingly inhibited as the intensity and/or duration of the perceived threat increases. As previously discussed, this is a result of the redirection of blood flow to the more primitive centres of the brain, which focus on safety and survival.

Thus, the amount of information conveyed during crisis should be limited, and draw on the individual's communication strengths. In John's case, his proficiency in key word sign means that this is the most helpful mode of communication for others to use as his behaviour and level of emotional arousal escalates. At the peak of a crisis, however, the absence of communication and interactions with others might actually assist in promoting resolution and safety.

The speech pathologist also highlighted that the use of challenging behaviour during crisis might be John's way of telling others something about his

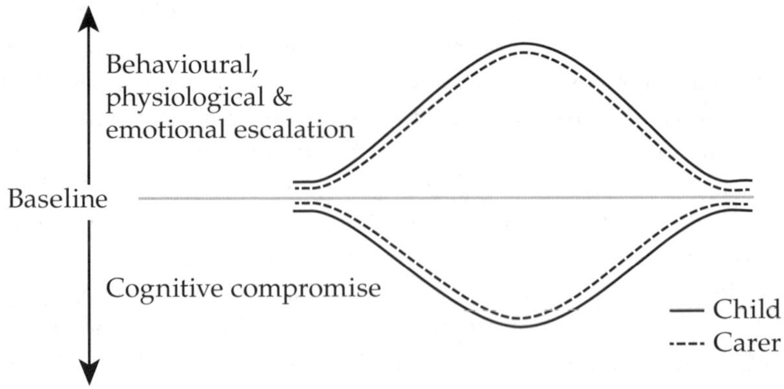

Figure 21.3 Parallel processes between child and caregiver across the crisis cycle
Source: adapted from Holden et al., 2001

needs; for example, 'This is what I want or don't want to happen' (Emerson, 2000; Gardner, 2002; Prendergast, 2000). Understanding this communicative intent, and ensuring that John's communication partners have a good understanding of his skills, is essential to enhance everyday interactions, respond to early indicators of distress, and, ultimately, reduce the risk of incidents of challenging behaviour. The speech pathologist wondered how skilled John's communication partners were in using his augmentative communication strategies, and whether they might benefit from additional training. She recognised the importance of consistent use of strategies across environments.

The occupational therapist's perspective

After observing John in the classroom and school playground, the occupational therapist (OT) suspected that an underlying sensory processing disorder may be contributing to John's emotional and behavioural difficulties. Further assessment revealed that John is hypersensitive to light touch and noise (Brown & Dunn, 2002), which are considered to be sensory and arousal modulation problems. This means that John experiences this type of sensory information as distressing. The OT was interested in John's level of arousal, which contributed to his heightened emotional state. She considered arousal in a functional way, and described it as a state of alertness that matched the environmental and task demands for the child. She noticed John was frequently hyper or highly aroused, which interferes with his ability to remain calm, attend, learn, and participate in daily activities (Kimball, 1999). In the classroom, these difficulties may present as difficulty screening out irrelevant information, high levels of distractibility, poor levels of work completion, and rapid behavioural escalation or overreaction when touched by others and/or exposed to high-pitched and loud noises (such as kids squealing in the playground). It is important to note that heightened arousal (hyperarousal) is associated with the activation of the sympathetic nervous system: the fight, flight, freeze response, as previously discussed (Kimball, 1999).

The OT also identified John's processing of visual information as an area of personal strength. Thus visual support strategies could be very helpful in communicating information and teaching him new skills. Firm pressure (which is the proprioceptive sense in action) was also found to be very calming and organising for John. This could partly explain the enjoyment he receives from completing 'heavy work activities', such as helping to hang out the washing, pushing the trolley at the shops, and riding his bike. This type of sensory input assists John to maintain an optimal level of calmness, interact with others, and participate in activities.

As previously discussed (see figure 21.2), the cognitive processing capabilities of the brain alter during crisis. The parts of the brain that remain in working order play a significant role in the processing of sensory-based information. Therefore sensory-orientated strategies, such as visual, firm pressure or proprioceptive input in John's case, can be effective intervention options at these times. That said, John would need to be taught these strategies systematically when he is calm, rather than in the midst of a crisis situation. Finally, the OT acknowledged the need to build sensory-based activities (sensory diet) into John's routine so that he receives the necessary input to assist him in modulating his level of arousal and to be calm enough to attend to lessons in the classroom, and develop prosocial skills.

The disability case manager's perspective

The disability case manager has established a relationship with Marnie and John over 18 months. During this time she has watched John increase in size and strength, and frighten Marnie with his aggressive outbursts. She is concerned that Marnie has begun making statements about John living outside the home. The case manager isn't sure whether this stems more from Marnie's genuine fear for Olivia's safety, as well as her own, or her loss of confidence in managing John. She suspects it is a combination of both. The case manager is aware that there is no support provided by extended family, and that Marnie has become increasingly isolated from her social network as John has become more difficult to take out. Thus, the centre-based respite is critical.

The case manager is aware of the requirement to make a report to child protection services because Olivia is at risk of harm from John. John too may become homeless should Marnie cease to cope. She knows this will mean an open discussion with Marnie about the mandatory reporting responsibilities in relation to child protection issues, and her intention to do everything possible to keep the family safe and intact. The case manager is also conscious of the number of service providers involved with John and his family, and is very keen that all services work collaboratively. She realises that she has a key role in bringing everyone together.

Multidisciplinary collaboration

The case manager's concern for the safety of Marnie and Olivia prompted her to contact other service providers and suggest a meeting in order to develop a standard response to critical incidents. All agreed it was important to involve Marnie.

The agenda for the meeting

The group came together, and included Marnie, the case manager, the respite unit manager, a support worker from the respite unit, John's teacher, the psychologist, the speech pathologist, and occupational therapist. John's paediatric psychiatrist offered to provide feedback on the approach developed in the meeting. After some initial information sharing regarding the current situation, the group set about verifying what the behaviour(s) of concern looked like in each context. With the behaviour described, they then planned to pool their ideas about critical inclusions in the reactive strategy, and collectively develop the strategy and a means of monitoring its implementation.

Defining the behaviour

The group developed a working definition of the behaviour. Participants did this in a way that would assist them in measuring the behaviour and identifying points for intervention. This portion of the meeting was led by the psychologist, who drew on the collective knowledge of the group to map John's escalation cycle, including early warning signs of difficulties, escalation, crisis, de-escalation, and recovery (see figure 21.4).

Drawing on the insights of all involved

The whiteboard summary of issues and ideas for the development of a strategy (as drawn from individual perspectives) is summarised in table 21.2.

Development of the strategies

The group discussed the various strategy options and their potential usefulness as part of the reactive strategy. Each was examined in terms of its strengths and weaknesses. This discussion was influenced by the understanding that responses needed to be individualised to meet the needs, abilities, and resources of both John and those supporting him. The group realised that the strategies selected would be most robust if they were viable for the smallest, least confident, and least experienced implementer. Additionally, all agreed that according to the policies of all agencies represented, strategies needed to be:

- focused on ending the crisis as quickly and safely as possible
- legal and ethical (all necessary consents and approvals obtained)
- represent the least intrusive, least restrictive options available at the time. This does not preclude the implementation of strategies that are significantly restrictive if a potentially dangerous situation requires it (such as physical restraint, support from emergency services, acute care admission) (Hassiotis et al., 2009)
- respectful of the dignity of all involved
- realistic, given the resources available, physical, financial, and emotional.

The group debated and agreed on a response, then recorded it below the escalation cycle already mapped on the board (see table 21.1). In recognition of the importance of keeping the support mechanisms in optimal order, they also agreed on response strategies for those managing the crises. These decisions were also mapped onto the escalation cycle, given the likelihood that a parallel process of escalation might happen for those trying to manage the situation (see table 21.1).

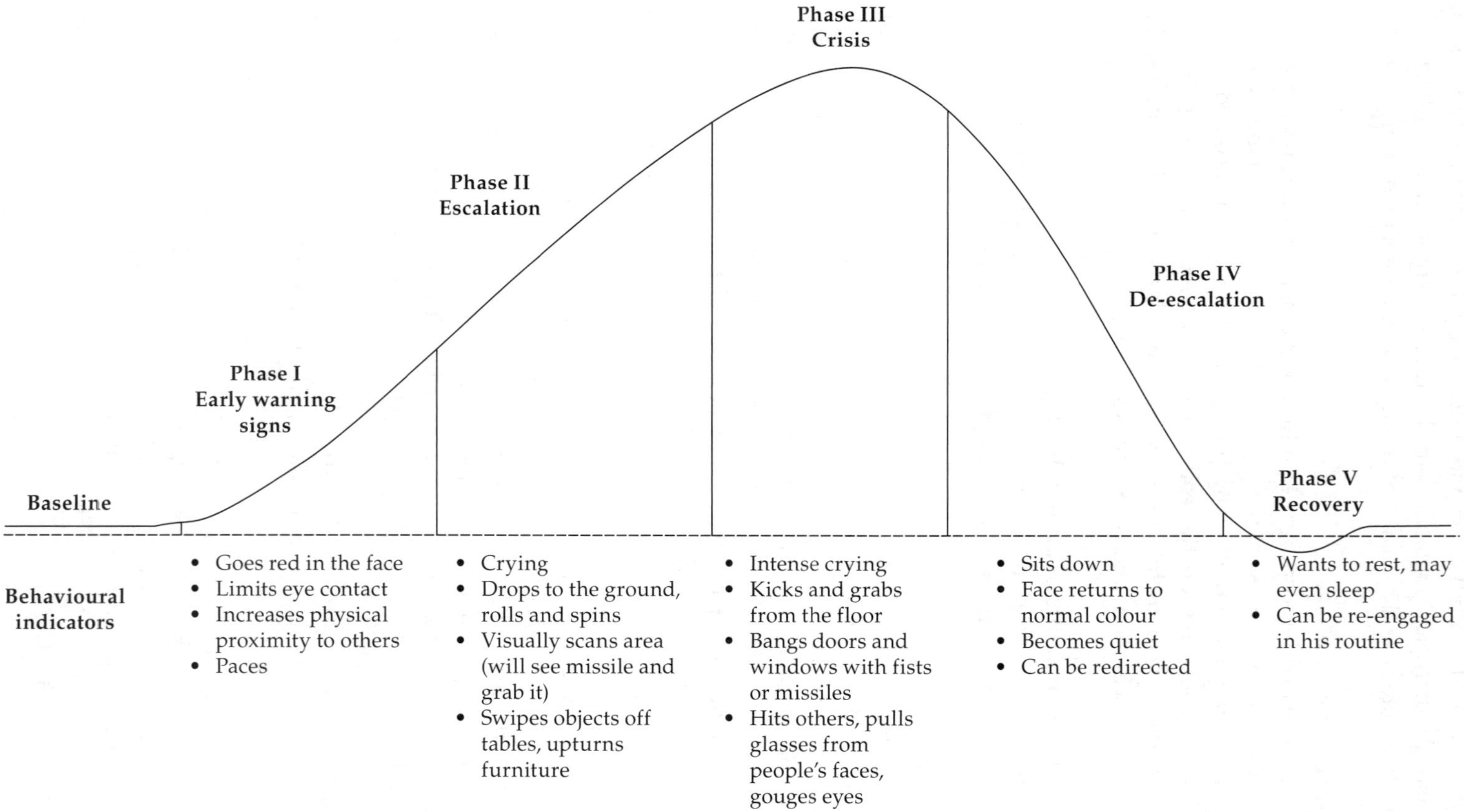

Figure 21.4 Summary of crisis management strategy

Table 21.1 Reactive strategies

	Phase I	*Phase II*	*Phase III*	*Phase IV*	*Phase V*
Child focused	• Make eye contact with John. Call his name. • Redirect John to his routine or a job that provides calming sensory input (see list on file) • Provide descriptive praise if he engages in his routine or job • Draw his attention to his increasing arousal, e.g. 'John, I can see your engine is really revving. What's up?' • Attempt to resolve the issue by naming the problem and exploring options • Remind him of the rules and rewards • Allow him some extra time to respond	*First staff member:* • Reduce stimuli, e.g., turn off music, pull down blinds or turn down lights • Remove unnecessary demands • Reduce 'talk'. Use simple language augmented with keyword sign • Provide low-key positive feedback if John attempts to calm himself, e.g. 'Good John. You're slowing down', or a smile • Consider administration of PRN (as per protocol) *Second staff member:* • Discretely remove others from area • Remove objects that could be used as missiles	• Supervise and monitor from a safe distance • Remain available • Prompt John to use soothing and calming sensory-based strategies or techniques (which have been taught to him when calm)	• Allow him some space and time to rest: direct him to his beanbag	• Allow him to restore his relationship with you • Redirect to his routine and praise attempts to participate • Gradually increase level of stimuli and demands • Move on
Carer focused	• Check readiness for action. Consider clothing, shoes, and hair • Be calm and confident and 'fake it' • Alert the second staff member discretely that there has been some escalation in behaviour. Agree who will manage the situation	• Scan the environment for risks • Be aware of your physical positioning within a room, e.g. access to exits • Be aware of tone of voice and body language • Be aware of your own fight-or-flight response. Use calming strategies as required	• Prioritise your own safety. Maintain a safe distance while monitoring John • Tag team through this period if first staff member needs a break • Implement evasion and breakaway techniques, as trained	• Continue to tag team supporting John, as required	• Report and record the event • Provide feedback about the efficiency of the strategies • Seek debriefing or additional support if necessary

Table 21.2 Summary of issues and proposed strategies

Issues and ideas	*Implications for the reactive strategies*
Manage John's hypersensitivity to light, (gentle) touch and noise	• Physical intervention likely to be unhelpful • Decrease arousal by turning off lights, pulling down blinds or closing curtains, turning down/off music, offering reassurance using an even and low tone, e.g., 'You're safe', offering a weighted blanket
Help John to recognise his escalating arousal	• Use a child-chosen metaphor in the very early stages of escalation, e.g., 'John you're like a fast horse now, its time for …'
Provide John with information and support regarding change	• Try to recognise growing agitation as soon as possible and provide information that might help resolve the issue for John • Use key word sign to provide information
Promote the safety of John, family, peers, and staff	• Consider PRN • Remove others, as to remove John is likely to fuel his agitation and increase risk • Ensure appropriate clothing and footwear; limit jewellery • Teach self-protection strategies as part of the broader plan
Emotional reactivity of Marnie and staff	• Be aware of any parallel escalation process—use tag team, debriefing
Modify the physical environment to reduce risk	• Move or secure anything that can be thrown, tipped over, or smashed • Maintain a safe physical distance (to prevent John reaching for the glasses) • Provide a door behind which family or staff can withdraw • Ensure garden is securely fenced to prevent John running off in a distressed state
Respond to John's reduced capacity for higher order reasoning, abstract thinking, or problem solving during crisis	• Reduce demands and expectations
Respond to John's reduced capacity to process and understand verbal language	• Reduce complexity and quantity of *verbal* support • Explore use of a small number of critical key word signs and natural gestures • Remain aware of body language and tone: stay available, at a safe distance, and present as calmly as possible
Respond positively to John's attempts to calm himself	• Provide low-key positive feedback: a smile, a gentle 'Good John, you're slowing down'
Assist John's recovery (and prevent re-escalation)	• Allow John to rest briefly if he appears exhausted post incident • As soon as reasonable, reorientate John by encouraging him to re-engage in activities according to his scheduled routine
Address the confidence issues of family and staff	• Train, provide opportunities for practice, opportunities to review progress, and to modify strategies • Use accurate reporting and recording to enable the review of the strategies
Teach opportunities outside crises; ensure best possible match between John and his environment	• Integrate the above into a broader multielement plan

Outcomes

At a recent case review, all agreed that forming collaborative partnerships across John's support system was an essential first step in better understanding John and the risks associated with his challenging behaviour. This collaboration also underpinned the design and implementation of the agreed reactive strategies to support John during crisis. The implementation and revision of John's individualised behaviour support plan over time has also led to significant improvements in John's emotional and behavioural well-being. The number of reported incidents has reduced significantly across settings and, generally speaking, incidents are of shorter duration and are less severe. John's participation in his daily routines and his interactions with others are continuing to improve.

Marnie reports that she is no longer 'just trying to survive the day', but is enjoying spending time with John and is feeling positive about life for all family members. John will start high school in the next year, and his current school has commenced transition planning in partnership with John and Marnie. Staff report feeling less apprehensive about working with John, and also confirm feeling better prepared to support John during crisis. While crises occur from time to time, the impact on John and those around him has reduced. Consequently, his relationships with others have improved.

A last thought

The notion of early intervention and prevention is central to a positive approach to challenging behaviour and the promotion of emotional well-being in children and adolescents with intellectual disability. The emphasis is on system-wide change and prevention through the management of environments rather than people (Sigafoos et al., 2003). In effect, the quality of life of the child or adolescent with an intellectual disability is enhanced through early intervention. In John's case, without the development and implementation of positive supports, and proactive and preventative interventions, the underlying function of his presenting difficulties would have been neither identified nor addressed. The positive outcomes achieved reflect the joint efforts of John's support system and the broader intervention strategies applied systemwide.

Acknowledgments

The authors would like to acknowledge members of the Statewide Behaviour Intervention (SBIS) and Department of Psychological Medicine (CHW) teams for their contributions; and also Frances Roberts, Manager (SBIS), for reviewing this chapter.

22

Modifications of cognitive behaviour therapy and counselling for individuals with intellectual disabilities

Victoria Grahame

Introduction

Individual psychotherapeutic interventions for children and young people with intellectual disabilities have traditionally focused on using behavioural strategies to reduce psychological distress and maladaptive behaviours. Recently, however, there has been increasing interest among clinicians in the application of cognitive behaviour therapy (CBT) for this client group. Despite this interest, there is a lack of research evidence to support CBT as an effective intervention for children with intellectual disabilities, and many clinicians have had to rely on the adult literature for useful information. This chapter will therefore discuss how applicable CBT is for children and adolescents with intellectual disabilities, and the modifications necessary for adapting any kind of individual therapy for this client group. It will also provide some practical ideas for clinicians who may be considering using CBT.

What is cognitive behaviour therapy (CBT)?

Cognitive behaviour therapy (CBT) is based on the theory that psychological issues (such as anxiety and depression) or behavioural problems arise as a result of cognitive deficits and cognitive distortions (Stallard, 2002). The aim of CBT is to identify and correct these deficits and distorted patterns of thinking, to alleviate the psychological or behavioural problem (Dagnan & Lindsay, 2004).

What skills are needed for cognitive behaviour therapy (CBT)?

In considering the suitability of CBT for children and young people with intellectual disabilities it is important to ask: (a) what skills are needed in order to engage in CBT? and (b) do children with intellectual disabilities have these skills? CBT requires an ability to systematically identify, challenge, and generate alternative ways of thinking (Stallard, 2002). Do children with intellectual disabilities have this degree of cognitive maturity?

Theory of mind research indicates that by age four to six years children start to take into account others' desires and beliefs when predicting how a particular situation affects emotions (Howlin et al., 1999); for example, Katie knows her sister wants a doll for her birthday but believes she is getting a car and will be sad. This is also true for children with intellectual disabilities who at age five years (nonverbal mental age 38 months) have been shown to predict the emotion of a character in a story, if they have been given the character's belief (Phillips et al., 1995). Similarly, theories of cognitive development suggest that by middle childhood (7–12 years) children enter the *concrete operational stage*, which means their understanding of their own and others' emotional states improves, although they still have difficulty with abstract reasoning (Vernon, 1989). However, during adolescence children gradually shift into the *formal operational thinking stage* (11–15 years), in which they are able to think more abstractly, and are better at predicting logical consequences (Vernon, 1989).

Despite the slower cognitive progress of the child with intellectual disabilities, there is, nevertheless, a progress in adolescence into the formal operational thinking stage. This suggests that CBT may be more suitable for adolescents with intellectual disabilities than for younger children. In support, Durlak and colleagues (1991), in their meta-analytic review of CBT for children, found that the child's age is an important factor in relation to efficacy of treatment. Results indicated that CBT was more effective with children in the formal operation stage (aged 11 years plus). However, it was not clear whether younger children struggled because they lacked the cognitive skills, or if the intervention was not pitched at the right developmental level.

What are the developmental considerations when using CBT?

In adapting CBT for children with or without an intellectual disability, there are a number of developmental issues that should be considered. This is particularly important because childhood is a period of skills acquisition, and there will be times when the child will not have acquired the required skills to engage in CBT (as discussed above). In reviewing the literature, it appears that developmental considerations are often overlooked, with the assumption that children at all stages of development can be catered for within a single treatment approach.

A further developmental consideration that is often overlooked is the context of the child and the impact that this has on the development of cognitions and beliefs, as well as variations in the manifestation of problems. This includes the possible influence of families, peers, and schools. It is likely that these contextual factors will have more relevance when working with children with intellectual disabilities compared to typically developing children, because such children and their families are often involved with a range of agencies from a young age.

The role of parents is also important. Parents have the potential to act as facilitators, helping their children with intellectual disabilities apply the skills learnt in therapy to the home environment. It is therefore crucial that any CBT approach includes collaboration with the child's family. However, therapists need to be aware that parental beliefs (how they understand their child's difficulties) will have an impact on how they manage their child's psychological and behavioural problems (Drinkwater & Stewart, 2002). Research has begun to identify the links between how parental beliefs influence the development of a child's cognitions (Garber & Robinson, 1997). A number of CBT studies include a family component in the treatment, such as *The Cool Kids* (Rapee et al., 2005) program for anxiety, discussed later in the resource section.

Assessing suitability of CBT for individuals with an intellectual disability

Clinicians' approach to assessing whether a child or young person is suitable for CBT varies, ranging from highly standardised assessments to clinical judgment (Haddock & Jones, 2006). The difficulty for clinicians is in deciding whether their client has the basic intellectual skills necessary to grasp the core concepts of CBT. Dagnan and colleagues (2000) developed a protocol of five tasks, which progressively assess an individual's ability to identify different emotions and discriminate among thoughts, feelings, and behaviours. This protocol, outlined in table 22.1, may be useful to clinicians wishing to undertake a structured assessment.

As a minimum standard it is suggested that clinicians assess their client's overall intellectual functioning and his or her receptive and expressive language abilities. Research indicates that people with learning disabilities who have higher intellectual functioning and a good receptive vocabulary are more likely to understand the cognitive model, based on their ability to

Table 22.1 Measures for assessing suitability for cognitive behaviour therapy

Measure	*What the assessment involves*
The British Picture Vocabulary Scale (BPVS-II) (Dunn et al., 1997)	Receptive language ability
Emotion recognition (Dagnan & Proudlove, 1997)	Individuals are presented with five pictorial facial expressions, and asked to indicate which face represents a stated emotion
Differentiating emotions and events (Reed & Clements, 1989)	Six simple scenarios are described and individuals are asked to identify whether in that situation they would feel happy or sad. Responses are verbal or by pointing to either a happy or sad face
Differentiating emotion, given a scenario and belief, using *Evaluative Beliefs Scale* (Chadwick et al., 1999)	Five scenarios are presented twice, once with a positive belief and once with a negative belief, and clients are asked, 'Do you feel happy or sad?'
Identifying the belief (Dagnan et al., 2000)	Five scenarios are presented twice, with the associated emotion, and individuals are asked to choose the belief

Source: adapted from Dagnan et al., 2000

identify different emotions and to discriminate thoughts, feelings, and behaviours (Swanson, 2001). When working with adolescents it may be helpful to pay particular attention to how they perform on verbal abstract reasoning and visual reasoning tasks; for example, the *Similarities* subtest from the *Wechsler Intelligence Scale for Children (WISC-IV)* (Weshler, 2003).

Stallard (2002), in his book *Think Good—Feel Good,* discussed a less standardised approach for assessing the basic skills required for children to engage in CBT. This approach relied heavily on clinical judgment and can be flexibly applied (see table 22.2). Haddock and Jones (2006) consulted with a group of expert clinicians using CBT with clients with intellectual disabilities. The main exclusion criteria identified were limited or no language skills, lack of willingness to participate, autism, and psychosis.

How to adapt therapy for individuals with intellectual disabilities

When adapting CBT for children and adolescents with intellectual disabilities, the components and style of CBT needs to be appropriate to the developmental level of the child. Obviously, individual differences will play a large role in treatment outcome. The difficulty for clinicians is that researchers rarely report how they have adapted the components of CBT for children and young people. However, the ideas outlined in table 22.3 may be useful.

Table 22.2 Assessing the basic skills required to engage in CBT

Key task	*Method*	*Example*
Accessing and communicating thoughts	Direct questioning	Interviewing the child about his or her thoughts. For example, ask the child to describe 'What were you thinking?' or 'What thoughts were running through your head at the time?'
	Indirect approach	Children can be asked to describe a recent difficult situation, or draw it. Clinicians should note whether the child is able to describe what happened and some of his or her thoughts about the event
	What might someone else be thinking?	Children can be provided with a set of situational scenarios, such as a birthday party, from which they can choose what the thoughts might be, such as, 'I love cake'
	Thought bubbles	In this approach the child is presented with cartoons or pictures and asked to suggest what the characters may be thinking
Generating alternative attributions	Hypothetical situations	The child is presented with a set of hypothetical situations to assess whether he or she is able to identify explanations for events (Doherr et al., 1999). For example, a child in the playground shouts 'Hello' at his friend, but his friend just runs past. The child is then asked to think of as many different explanations as possible for what has happened
	Generative cartoons	The child can be given a set of cartoons and asked to write or draw as many ideas as possible about what the characters may be thinking
	Puppets and play	A difficult situation can be acted out, and the child asked to suggest what each of the puppets may be thinking about the situation
Awareness of emotions	Identify and express emotions	If children are unable to provide a verbal description of how they are feeling, they may be able to draw instead. Quizzes and games can also be used to assess whether the child can identify how others feel
Thoughts, feelings, and events	Linking thoughts, feelings and events	This could be a card task where different feelings have to be matched with different thoughts, or acted out using puppets

Source: adapted from Stallard, 2002

First, there are some general principles that should always be considered when counselling a child or young person with an intellectual disability. It is important that clinicians adjust their vocabulary appropriately, and tailor their interventions according to the child's or young person's level of comprehension—avoid jargon and psychological wording (Barrett, 2000). The use of puppetry or hands-on materials (such as balloons or art supplies), rather than purely verbal strategies, will reduce the language demands.

Table 22.3 Adaptations of psychotherapy techniques

Adaptation	*Definition and example*
Simplification	Reduce usual technique in complexity; break down interventions into smaller chunks, shorter length of sessions
Language	Reduce level of vocabulary, sentence structure, and length of thought. Use short sentences; use simple words
Activities	Augment typical techniques with activities to deepen change and learning. Add drawings, homework assignments
Developmental level	Integrate developmental level into presentation of techniques and material. Use games; assess development into relevant social issues
Directive methods	Because of cognitive limitations, one must be more direct. Outline treatment goals, progress, and give extra 'visual' guides
Flexible methods	Adjust usual techniques to suit cognitive level and lack of progress. Draw from other modalities
Involve caregivers	Use family, support staff, to help with change. Assign homework or rehearsals at home with the help of staff or family
Disability and rehabilitation approaches	Issue of disability must be addressed within treatment; therapist must raise issues and support positive self-view

Source: adapted from Hurley, 1989; Whitehouse et al., 2006

When using CBT with individuals with intellectual disabilities, one of the main difficulties for clinicians is how to present abstract concepts using more understandable examples. Haddock and Jones (2006), in an attempt to reach practitioner consensus in the use of CBT for individuals with a learning disability, noted that overcoming such a difficulty was reported to be complex by all of the clinicians interviewed. They found that some practitioners often tried to avoid abstractions completely, whereas others tried to explain abstract concepts with concrete examples, or used visual aids, role-plays, vignettes, and puppets to support the explanation of abstract concepts.

The use of comic strip conversations (Gray, 1994) has also proved a useful technique for visually presenting an abstract concept. Comic strip conversations are a way of illustrating an interaction between two or more people that would otherwise be difficult to explain. They may be used instead of, or in combination with, social story telling. Comic strip conversations can be used to help define social terms and/or identify what people might be thinking or feeling in different situations. In comic strip conversations, verbal information and explanation is enhanced by simple stick men drawings and colour.

When working with younger children, it is important that concepts and strategies are presented at an appropriate developmental level. For example, anger could be described as a volcano that builds up and erupts, or the metaphor of a MP3 player playing in the child's head to describe automatic thoughts. However, when working psychotherapeutically with younger children, the focus is more likely to be on the behavioural component of CBT.

The literature suggests a need for key modifications to ensure children with learning difficulties are taught effectively. These learning strategies include the use of behavioural techniques, and augmentative and alternative communication (AAC) strategies, to help an individual learn new skills. Behavioural techniques include modelling, rehearsal, feedback and reinforcement as key approaches. AAC strategies refer to supplementary methods or visuals tools that are used to support or extend an individual's existing communication system (Beukelman & Mirenda, 2005).

CBT typically involves asking clients to undertake 'homework' tasks, to gather information outside of clinical sessions. Clinicians should ask themselves whether the homework task is really necessary, as young people often fail to complete such tasks, even if you call it something else! If the task is necessary—for example, if it helps to generalise skills learnt in therapy to the home situation—the importance of the task should be openly discussed in the session. A careful explanation of the rationale of the task may help, focusing on how the task will be used in therapy when completed. If there are difficulties completing the task it may be useful to explore any automatic thoughts associated with the homework. Haddock and Jones (2006) reported that 'homework' had very negative connotations for people who often had a very difficult educational background.

What CBT resources are available?

There are unfortunately no specific CBT resources available to clinicians interested in using cognitive behaviour techniques with children who have intellectual disabilities. However, there are a number of excellent manual-based programs and books that experienced clinicians may find useful as a guide to adapting therapy for children with intellectual disabilities. These are outlined in the following sections.

Anxiety disorders

The *Cool Kids Anxiety Program* (Rapee et al., 2005) is a 10-session CBT program that is available from the Emotional Health Clinic (formerly the Macquarie University Anxiety Research Unit) in Sydney. The program is designed to help children aged 7–16 years manage their anxiety, and can be conducted either in a group or individual format. The program includes parent and child workbooks to accompany all of the sessions. It also includes a manual for therapists, describing in detail how to conduct each session of the program. However, Macquarie University strongly recommends that clinicians who wish to conduct the program attend one of their training workshops.

There is also a *Cool Kids Anxiety Program (School Version)*, which is designed to be run in school by school counsellors and related mental health workers.

The book *OCD in Children and Adolescents: A Cognitive-Behavioural Treatment Manual* (March & Mulle, 1998) is designed to help clinicians treat children and adolescents with obsessive compulsive disorder using CBT, specifically in relation to exposure plus response prevention. It is the result of over 15 years of research exploring how CBT can be used effectively to treat OCD. It has been used with children aged four-plus years, and has been shown to be applicable across a broad range of ages and abilities. There is an accompanying book *Talking Back to OCD: The Program That Helps Kids and Teens Say 'No Way' and Parents Say 'Way to Go'* (March & Benton, 2007), which is a guide for parents who are comfortable in the self-help mode.

For very young children the book *Up and Down the Worry Hill: A Children's Book about Obsessive-Compulsive Disorder and Its Treatment* (Wagner, 2004) may be a more developmentally appropriate resource. The book emphasises that many people experience OCD, and discusses its causes, effects, and treatment options. It may also help prepare children to engage in treatment, as it describes CBT in a child-friendly manner.

Building positive self-esteem

The book *Cool Connections with Cognitive Behavioural Therapy: Encouraging Self-esteem, Resilience and Well-being in Children and Young People Using CBT Approaches* (Seiler, 2008) can be used by a range of mental health professionals. It is designed to modify positively the everyday thoughts and behaviours (reduce feelings of anxiety and depression) of young people aged 9 to 14. The workbook includes step-by-step guidelines on how to use the materials appropriately, with a mixture of games, handouts, home activities, and therapeutic exercises.

Friends for Life (Barrett, 2004, 2005), for school-aged children and young people, and *Fun Friends* (Barrett, 2007a, 2007b), for young children, are designed to help children and young people deal with feelings of fear, worry, and depression by building resilience and self-esteem. The program is designed to be used in schools but can easily be used with individual clients. It teaches cognitive and emotional skills in an easily understood child-friendly format. It is the only childhood anxiety prevention program acknowledged by the World Health Organization (WHO), and has eight years of comprehensive validation across several countries and languages using rigorous randomised control studies (WHO, 2004).

Anger management

The book *Exploring Feelings: Cognitive Behaviour Therapy to Manage Anger* (Attwood, 2004) is one of two *Exploring Feelings* programs. One program was designed to explore and manage anxiety, the other to explore and manage anger. The original program was developed to be delivered in a small group to children with Asperger's syndrome aged 9–12 years, and to be delivered in a small group. However, the workbooks can easily be modified to be used with individual children with developmental disabilities.

Understanding own and other people's feelings

Think Good, Feel Good (Stallard, 2002) is a practical CBT workbook for young people. The materials have been developed by a consultant clinical psychologist, and have been trialled extensively in clinical work with young people presenting with a wide range of psychological problems. This resource is also helpful for clinicians, as it explains the basic theory and rationale behind CBT and how the workbook should be used. The book is available in print and as a downloadable resource (as an eBook) on the internet. There are 10 modules, which can be used as a complete program, or adapted for individual use.

What Works When With Children and Adolescents: A Handbook of Individual Counselling Techniques (Vernon, 2002) is a practical handbook designed for counsellors, social workers, and psychologists in schools and mental health settings. It offers over 100 creative activities and effective interventions for clinicians undertaking individual counselling with children.

My Book Full of Feelings: How to Control and React to the Size of your Emotions (Jaffe & Gardner, 2006) is an interactive workbook for children with social disabilities, including autism spectrum disorders. It is designed as a teaching tool for parents and professionals to help the child become more aware of his or her own emotions, and then learn how to manage those feelings. The book uses a pyramid graphic that children can easily use to point out how they are feeling, and the intensity of that feeling.

Conclusion

There are a number of reviews that provide encouraging evidence for the efficacy of CBT in adults with intellectual disabilities (Taylor et al., 2008), and for the value of CBT as a therapy for use in children and young people who have a range of disorders (Christie & Wilson, 2005). However, there is still considerable work to be done to evaluate CBT's effectiveness for children and young people with intellectual disabilities.

The language and cognitive skills required to engage with CBT suggest that it may not be suitable for young people with moderate to severe intellectual disabilities. However, clinicians wishing to use CBT should undertake a detailed assessment of the individual's abilities, and consider the necessary modifications to therapy, such as developmental considerations. This will ensure that many of the therapeutic challenges can be addressed, thus making CBT a promising treatment option for individuals with intellectual disabilities.

23

The regulation of arousal in intellectual disability

Bruce W. Chenoweth

Introduction

Dysregulation of affect is commonly found in people with an intellectual disability, and in particular in those with autistic traits. This chapter emphasises the relevance of early experience in the establishment of the capacity to self-regulate emotions, and to highlight the importance of enduring and consistent good quality relationships in the maintenance of affective stability. This emphasis is not to be considered to be at the expense of the many other contributions to emotional instability found in this population (which are acknowledged) but to expand the field of enquiry when seeking to be helpful.

The neurobiology of experience

When a baby is born, the brain weighs about 400 grams. By the time the infant is 15 months old, the brain may have doubled or even trebled in weight. In that critical time, the process of neural genesis and migration has been accompanied by a process of bundling and parcellation of neural networks, and through apoptosis, the planned pruning of redundant neurons (Schore, 1994). Thus functional processes, which have been useful at an earlier time, become superseded and are replaced by processes and functions of a higher order of hierarchical complexity (Jackson, 1931).

Late-maturing cortical areas of the brain are particularly sensitive to post-natal influences. Among the many functions established in this period of the first year of life are the beginnings of the capacity for regulation of one's emotional world later in life. It is clear that the reciprocal dyadic process called *empathic attunement* between mother (or primary carer) and infant over many hours, days, weeks, and months is critical for the formation of these neural pathways. This attunement is the foundation of a lifelong sense of security that one's needs will be met, and also establishes the mechanisms for affect regulation. Thus, there is a dyadic origin of the adaptive capacity to self-regulate affect. Conversely, the absence of well-modulated socioaffective stimulation leaves the infant unable to neurobiologically mediate self-regulatory functions (Schore, 1994).

This latter capacity for emotional regulation may not be fully apparent until mid adolescence or beyond. The lack of this ability may lead to increased vulnerability to traumatic events and even to psychiatric morbidity in the form of a personality disorder (Grotstein, 1987). People with an intellectual disability statistically are more vulnerable to experience serious abuse or traumatic events (Balogh et al., 2001). They also may have an increased vulnerability to the long-term consequences of that trauma if there is an unstable sense of self and a lack of internalised imagery or memories as a source of self-soothing.

Perhaps fear and apprehension, even panic that their needs may not be met may drive people in this population into unsafe or unwise situations in adolescence or later. This vulnerability may expose them to predatory exploitation. There is some good evidence that they are more prone to complex post-traumatic stress disorder (PTSD) than those more fortunate in their earlier secure attachments. Nijenhuis and colleagues (2004) label these people *emotional personalities (EPs)*, whose vulnerability to trauma is different to *apparently normal personalities (ANPs)* in a wide number of neuro- and psychobiological ways.

It is important to acknowledge at this point Winnicott's notion of the *good-enough parent* (Winnicott, 1960). Most parents anxiously review their parenting skills wondering if they in fact had been empathically attuned enough, particularly during the more difficult moments of infancy. However, most parenting is deemed 'good enough' for the purpose of establishing eventually a modicum of emotional regulation and an adequate sense of self.

In neurobiological terms, the modulation of unruly feelings comes from a well-functioning orbitofrontal cortex, which is the thinking, anticipating, judging, and conscience-ridden higher centres of the brain. These regulatory mechanisms are slowly acquired over childhood and adolescence. The prefrontal cortex continues to develop this modulating and regulating function of behaviours until people are well into their twenties, earlier for women than for men (Schore, 1996). Attachment is mediated intrinsically as a right hemisphere function. Lateralisation of hemispheric functions occurs much earlier than two years of age (Mento et al., 2009).

What can go wrong?

In the more primitive areas of the brain—those areas more concerned about survival—lurk the vestigial remnants of the 'fight,' 'flight,' 'rage,' and immobilising fear responses. Such areas are in the amygdaloid nuclei and periaquaductal grey matter, as well as in other limbic structures. These structures were from an evolutionary perspective extremely important when our small furry forebears were hopping around in some primeval forest, which also harboured sabre-toothed tigers! Life is now somewhat safer, and consequently the well-tempered prefrontal cortex has limited the necessity for, and the activity of, these survival functions. The hippocampus has the task of integrating memory and affect. It is extremely sensitive to the effects of stress of all kinds, a phenomenon that can be demonstrated anatomically by volumetric changes.

The nature of dissociation

Dissociation is a psychological defence wherein the overwhelmed individual cannot take meaningful action or successful flight, and escapes by altering internal organisation (Kluft, 1985). Dissociation is described as a failure to synthesise and personify terrifying experiences (Kluft, 1985). From the perspective of evolutionary biology, and even evolutionary psychology, responses to extreme life-threatening events are varied and frequently specific to the species. Understanding of dissociative states has been clouded by the great disparity, in the form of clinical presentation of dissociation between individuals, and even in an individual at different times, and in different circumstances.

Individuals with dissociative states can present with a spectrum of behaviours, including states of fugue or absence, a withdrawal, and seeming oblivion to surroundings. A parallel could be drawn with a gazelle on the Serengeti being pulled down by a lion: glazed eyes, passively awaiting fate, immobilised, and apparently unfeeling. Victims of sexual assault or other violence frequently describe such responses at the time, and perhaps subsequently, following the event. Frozen immobility is a variation of this, with the preservation of appropriate affect.

A state of dissociative rage may be ascribed to a cornered animal, such as a Tasmanian devil fighting blindly and indiscriminately, impervious to changes in circumstance. Clinically, people demonstrate this in some states of *episodic dyscontrol* or *intermittent explosive disorder*. At some stage in the escalation of anger, a point can occur where the rage takes on a life of its own, and efforts at distraction or diversion are ineffective. At such times the neural connections between the prefrontal cortex and these primitive structures are not functioning.

The chaotic and pointless panic and milling of a flock of sheep that have been attacked may have a survival advantage for the flock if not the individual. *Blind panic*, however, has been easier to study in humans with elegant PET scans of Vietnam veterans with complex PTSD who are suddenly exposed to the sound of the Bell Ranger helicopter. This can immediately cause a flurry of neural activity in the areas of the amygdaloid nuclei and related structures with an almost complete collapse of all prefrontal cortical activity (Shin, et al., 2004). At such times, the veterans were inaccessible to reason or reassurance. It was as if such reassurance was being given to a non-functioning part of the brain, seemingly remote from the actual regions of activity. Likewise, *blind flight* has a clinical correlate in the frantic efforts to escape crowds in supermarkets by someone suffering an acute panic.

Nijenhuis and colleagues (2004) have contributed a neural model of dissociation based on ethological observations as described above. They suggest that all humans have these latent and vestigial behavioural capacities. Severe attachment traumas may establish a permanent reactivity in the limbic areas of the right brain, thereby inhibiting its capacity to deal with future stress. This right-sided lateralisation may account for the nonverbal encoding of traumatic memory in PTSD subjects (Schiffer et al., 1995).

Post-traumatic stress disorder

Acute and chronic stress cause structural brain changes, notably in the hippocampus and prefrontal cortex (Schiffer et al., 1995). This is in response to increased glucocorticoid and noradrenalin exposure as well as to proinflammatory cytokines and other peptide regulators. There can be a loss of integrative hippocampal volume, and hence loss of functional capacity. The emotional person re-experiences unintegrated trauma as though it is happening now, and these 'hallucinatory, solitary, and involuntary experiences consist of visual images, sensations, and motor actions, which engross the entire perceptual field' (Nijenhuis et al., 2004, 'Theory of structural dissociation of the personality' section, ¶ 2). Personality variables, personal vulnerabilities, and some genetic predispositions all determine the form that dissociation takes given sufficient stress.

The Dunedin Study (Nada Raja et al., 1992), which has followed a large cohort of children for over 30 years, has recently highlighted individual vulnerabilities, which may contribute to an ongoing underlying substrate of anxiety or depression. Importantly, poor attachment, deprivation, or trauma have been associated with lower serotonin levels as mediated by serotonin transporter gene variation, deficits of which may predict subsequent suicidality and poor response to antidepressants. Conversely, early good attachments are protective, contributing to the formation of an 'apparently normal personality' with the concomitant neuroprotective structures.

Affect regulation and intellectual disability

Intellectual disability is rarely a simple deficit of ability or capacity. There may be some major disruption of neural architecture that predisposes the individual to perceptual, communicative, emotional, or behavioural difficulties. Sometimes these difficulties or challenging behaviours are predictable, as in the case of a specific behavioural phenotype associated with a known genetic syndrome. For example, those behaviours typically associated with Prader Willi or the Fragile X syndromes are well known. Also, despite some limitations to this generally deterministic approach, it is often useful to start with, and apply, what we know about the responses of the more neurotypical populations in attempting to understand some of the more distressing and challenging behaviours of those with an intellectual disability.

Empathic attunement and intellectual disability

All experience is encoded architecturally in our brain in some form. *Attunement* is such an experience, and occurs, not as a one-way street, but as dyadic reciprocity over time. Changes occur in the brain of both mother and carer and infant, and in a sense, the mother is, metaphorically speaking, the prefrontal cortex for the infant for many years until her influence becomes embedded in the child's cortical function. In the situation where the infant has an intellectual disability and the mother receives little response from the infant, or if the infant is dysmorphic or autistic, empathic attunement may be very difficult to establish. Maternal depression, marriage failure, cultural alienation, and excessive demands of a sick or very demanding child – all can take their toll on the process of reciprocal attachment. Many parents are devoted to the disabled child but exhausted by the task of caring for that child.

In a previous era, many disabled children went into care at a very young age and remained in care all of their lives. Many of these who are now adults may have had several primary caregivers each year of their lives. In that less enlightened time, their parents and families were encouraged to give them into care and to forget them. Many of these people have demonstrated a lifetime of emotional dysregulation, poor sense of self, fears of abandonment, self-harming behaviour, and other symptoms of attachment failure. The natural development of mechanisms regulating emotional responses through bonding and secure attachments may not have occurred.

Clinical presentation: what do we see?

First, a high level of *generalised anxiety* can prevail, for many reasons, in those with intellectual disability. For this population, the world can be a harsh, uncomprehended and uncomprehending place, with real and perceived threat. As children with disability develop, parents can no longer interpret their world for them. The child becomes aware of 'differentness'. Relationships can be tortured and tortuous. Depression and anxiety may follow.

Autism

The state of autism confers a particular level of dismay, frustration, mistrust, and generalised anxiety, with recurrent episodes of panic. People with autism may lack the flexibility to switch their focus of attention rapidly. Allen and colleagues (1997) regard this partly as a consequence of cerebellar dysfunction.

Transitions of all types are therefore difficult for people with autism. This may include transitions from one activity to another, such as from bed to bath, from home to school, from class to playground, from primary to secondary school, and to work placement. All of these transitions may need slow and adequate preparation if anxious protest is to be averted. Gualtieri (2002) noted that 'no anxiety state is quite as dramatic in all of psychiatry as that of an autistic child whose routine is changed or whose environment is disrupted' (p. 244). Likewise, people with autism can be overwhelmed by complex simultaneous stimuli or by crises of intimacy when emotional demands are excessive. Sensory hypersensitivity, particularly auditory hyperacusis, can create intolerable anxiety in people with autism.

Mechanisms for coping with anxiety by those with intellectual disability

Intellectually disabled people use many and varied attempted strategies for coping with anxiety; some are helpful and some not. Some behaviour could be interpreted as anxiety-relieving strategies, or can be interpreted in less helpful ways. Descriptive terms such as *attention-seeking behaviour* are often best replaced by the description *care-eliciting behaviour.* Some of these anxiety-reducing strategies include school refusal, ritualistic behaviour, some compulsions, self-stimulating behaviour, relentless and remorseless verbal onslaughts, stereotypic behaviour, oppositional and defiant behaviour, somatic preoccupation, self-injurious behaviour, masturbation, and hyperphagia. The list is long. These behaviours may also occur for other reasons, which could be explored through a detailed *functional analysis of behaviour* by a skilled psychologist. However, the clinician can do well to regard aroused or challenging behaviour initially as anxiety driven once physical causation has been eliminated.

Episodes of heightened arousal or challenging behaviours may be seen as an indication that the individual still retains some sense of agency, or has some executive or imperative functionality, in relating to their circumstances; that is, they retain the capacity for hippocampal integration of past experience with the present stress (Nijenhuis et al., 2004). When this sense of agency evaporates, dissociative episodes may occur. Unreachable rage, panic, or flight may occur, with the episode itself taking on a life of its own, and during which there can be great risk to persons and property. In the past, a diagnosis of psychosis was frequently made. Gualtieri (2002) noted, 'No skills are available for self-reflection or to describe an inner state for the clinician to utilize' (pp. 170–1). More often now, a diagnosis of an anxiety disorder will be made.

Assessment of challenging behaviour

Physical causes and pain

Discussion here will be limited to the obvious medical causes of emotional dysregulation or challenging behaviours. Beange and colleagues (1995) documented the most common medical causes of distress in those with an intellectual disability. Some of these included dental pain, otitis media, constipation, chest infections, urinary tract infections, gastro-oesophageal reflux, arthralgias, and headaches.

Domiciliary dynamics and relational issues: the right to enduring quality relationships

Most people have some degree of choice about with whom they live. For those in group homes and residential care, this is not the case. Not only can they be accommodated in situations of misfit, with disparate persons with disparate abilities and with less than complementary behavioural patterns and demands, but they have to accept instability of staffing placements, with many changes of attachment figures. It is curious that in the statements outlining Vision, Purpose, Values, Client focus, Equity, Integrity, and Performance, government departments and agencies charged with the care of those with disabilities make no mention of an individual's right to enduring, sustained, consistent, and rewarding relationships.

Conversely!

After a lifetime of failed attachments, sometimes of abuse or neglect, people with intellectual disabilities might find themselves in a caring, professional setting. All may go well for a 'honeymoon period'. However, once a bond with a carer or significant level of trust develops, the relationship could predictably be tested, often to a degree where the placement breaks down.

It is paradoxical that extremely challenging behaviour may in fact be a milestone of success in the establishment of a trusting relationship, and that the behaviour may reflect some crisis of intimacy, or perhaps an expectation at a non-conscious level of further abandonment. Any attachment could lead to an innate sense of immanence of threat or loss. It is encouraging that in some jurisdictions and agencies, there is now an emphasis on consistent and stable staffing for children entrusted to care. The policy of moving carers at regular intervals to avoid entrenched practices is being questioned.

Functional analysis of behaviour

In situations where the origin of distress and emotional dysregulation is puzzling, a trained psychologist may be engaged to tease out the relevant causal elements as part of a comprehensive functional analysis of those behaviours. This investigation would usually emphasise basic needs, such as physiological comfort, security within the residential setting, issues of communication, and the presence or absence of sociopsychological satisfaction (see figure 23.1).

Exploration too, may focus on obtaining a profile of sensory functions and an assessment of thresholds of distress for a number of sensory stimuli.

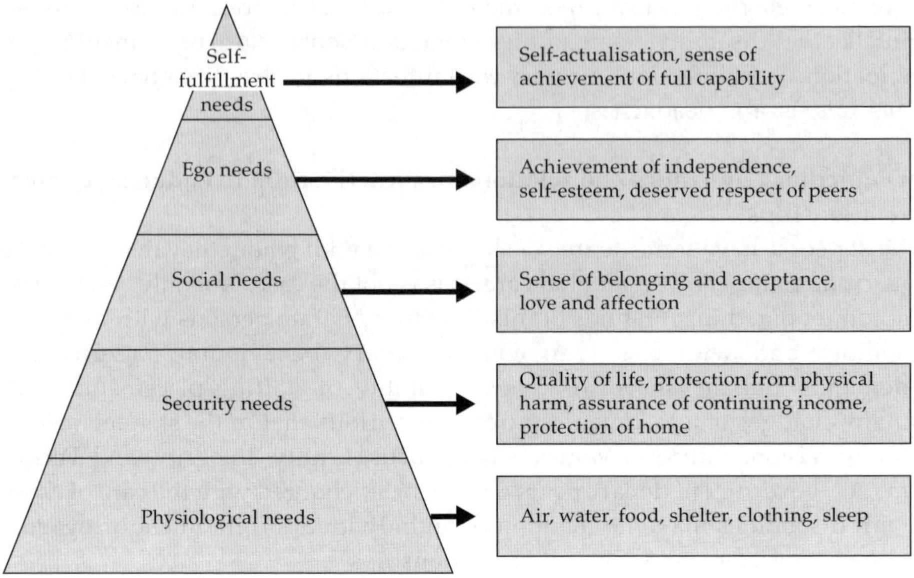

Figure 23.1 Maslow's hierarchy of needs
Source: Maslow, 1954, 1970; from <www.businessballs.com/maslow>

Hypersensitivity to multiple intercurrent sensations may overwhelm an individual. Conversely, other high-threshold inputs, which are better tolerated, may offer alternative modalities of contact, communication, and reassurance. Recourse to a multiaxial psychiatric diagnostic formulation could then follow according to the protocol of the text revision of the fourth edition of the *Diagnostic and Statistical Manual of Mental Disorders* (DSM-IV-TR) (APA, 2000). There are many useful tools to elucidate functional capacity as well as assist in psychiatric diagnosis. Of these, the *Developmental Behavioural Checklist (DBC)* (Einfeld & Tonge, 1995) is perhaps one of the most useful in terms of assessing the presence of psychopathology.

A *behavioural intervention strategy* or set of protocols can be developed from such a comprehensive analysis. Appropriate training of parents or staff should follow to assist them to better understand the child or client and to sensitise them to specific and required needs. Careful analysis, if done well, may lead to the empowerment of staff, the avoidance of pejorative judgments, and renewed enthusiasm for an albeit difficult management task.

What of DSM-IV?

By its nature, much of DSM-IV-TR (APA, 2000) is a set of descriptors, which tend to cluster together on multivariate factor analysis into predictable diagnostic groupings. These are useful tools to utilise in people with mild to upper moderate disability, but of limited value for those with moderate to severe and profound disability.

Medication

Increasingly in intellectual disability, there is a move to identify the underlying neurobiology of behaviour. The pathways and receptor sites subserving emotional states are rapidly declaring themselves. Multiaxial DSM-IV-TR (APA, 2000) formulations can assist in decision-making about the place of medication in the redressing of supposed up-regulated or down-regulated neural activity. Limbic and mesocortical overactivity can be regulated, prefrontal underachievement can be stimulated, amygdaloid and periaqueductal grey matter arousal can be modulated, more efficiency can be extracted from the nucleus accumbens and other association nuclei, and so on.

The crude hypothesis is that anxiety and depression have, as a final common pathway, some paucity of serotonergic activity. Conceptualising anxiety and depression in this narrow and oversimplified manner can initially be a productive way of achieving an entry point in dealing with a very complex problem. Selective serotonin reuptake inhibitors (SSRIs) may have a place in the management of these conditions, and should be used within the broader contexts discussed above. Caution is required in prescribing their use in children, especially in those with intellectual disability, because of the exquisite sensitivity to side-effects often encountered in this population.

The repair of affect dysregulation

The mechanism of affect regulation is of intense interest to researchers and clinicians across a converging range of disciplines. These disciplines include medical, biological, psychological, and social sciences, as well as clinicians in psychiatry, psychology, and social work. The emphasis in these endeavors has progressively shifted from the study of conscious to non-conscious processes.

The model of down-regulating affect through conscious effort or through the imposition of strategies is the central theme of cognitive psychology. However, most affective responses occur intuitively, spontaneously, and instantaneously; they are nonverbal and preconscious. Efforts are now being focused on nonverbal, noninterpretive components, responses mediated through the right prefrontal cortex. This area is dominant in dealing with the stress and uncertainty of life. This part of the cortex is also engaged in the interpretation of facial, prosodic, and bodily communication, in the recognition and maintenance of empathy, and the response to stress. Homeostatic mechanisms occur here that maintain a coherent, continuous, implicit sense of self. Bowlby (1969) held to the centrality of a non-conscious internal working model for which good early attachment was essential.

As the psychotherapeutic alliance reflects the infant–mother dyad, so too does the benign respectful and enduring relationship between carer or parent and the disabled child work its magic in altering the internal structural brain systems that non-consciously and consciously process and regulate external and internal information (Schore, 2003). As in a therapeutic alliance, the prime variables affecting positive change can be independent of the theoretical model employed. Similarly, the stability of relationships for those with intellectual disability is a critical factor in alleviating anxiety and dissociative episodes. The brain responds architecturally to all input.

Conclusion

The process of 'good enough' empathic attunement in the first 15 months of life confers a neurobiological advantage in the generation of the capacity for appropriate affective regulation later in life. Failure of this process can lead to high anxiety and dissociative states when stressed. This can be particularly prominent in those with intellectual disability, where obstacles in the way of the attainment of such attunement abound, amplifying any inherent lack of higher cortical modulatory functioning.

Dissociation is described within bioevolutionary and evolutionary psychology frameworks. The way in which anxiety and dissociative states present is described through assessment of those states. Particular emphasis is placed on the quality, security, and enduring nature of relationships in such an assessment, and on the imperative for these basic needs to be met if repair of affective dysregulation is to occur. The repair of affect regulation can and does occur within stable caring relationships if those relationships can withstand some strenuous testing.

24

Psychopharmacology: The use of medication to treat challenging behaviour in children and adolescents

Anthony A. Zehetner

Introduction

The prominence of psychopharmacology and its evidence in treating severe psychiatric disorders supports the importance of neuropsychiatric brain processes. This chapter examines the six major neurotransmitters (glutamate, gamma-amino butyric acid (GABA), acetylcholine, serotonin, noradrenaline, and dopamine) in the human brain, and the available drugs that target them. Newer atypical neuroleptic agents, attention-deficit hyperactivity disorder (ADHD) medications, and an approach to managing self-injurious behaviour are covered in greater detail. When prescribing medication to modulate behaviour in children and adolescents, the clinician must be cognisant of the neurotransmitter targeted. The complex interplay between drug, neuronal circuitry, and internal environment must be evaluated, and the child monitored for any adverse effects. Guidelines for psychopharmacotherapeutic drug prescribing are provided.

The advent of multiple novel psychotropic medications has meant that the contemporary clinician must adopt the role of a pharmacologist when prescribing. All medications have differing target receptors, and many have been poorly studied in children. This chapter aims to outline the main neurotransmitters of interest in mental health and their neuronal mechanisms and pathways. The various mechanisms through which drug classes act and expected potential adverse effects guide the selection of medication when targeting treatment for specific challenging behaviours.

It must be cautioned that this is a potted précis, which is provided to illustrate some of the mechanisms of an individual's internal environment. Remember: for every neurotransmitter action (agonist effect) there are feedback systems that activate the opposite counterbalancing effect (antagonism). In mental health, clinicians are primarily concerned with altering the environment to improve mental health. In more severe cases of behaviour disturbance, clinicians necessarily have to consider the patient's *internal environment* as a means of environmental manipulation. Genetic studies, for example, comparing monozygotic (identical) twins with dizygotic (fraternal) twins, and twins reared together versus twins reared in different families, enable us to determine to what extent components of patterns of behaviour are genetic or environmental (Thapar & Rutter, 2008). For example, ADHD, autism, and anorexia nervosa are all highly genetic, with genetic factors accounting for 80 per cent or more of the variance of behaviour. This genetic factor is often described as the *internal environment*, because it is not so much which specific genes matter but how those genes influence brain development, neuronal connectedness, and molecular and neurotransmitter capacity. The genetic, or internal environmental, component of depression and panic disorder is moderate, and its influence on conduct disorder in the absence of ADHD is less. However, if 85 per cent of the environmental effect on a type of severe behaviour pattern is from the internal (or neurochemical) and other molecular biology components of the brain environment, that leaves only 15 per cent for external environmental influences, such as relationships, communication, stimulation, and thoughts. It may be that clinicians only understand 15 per cent of the internal environment, but this knowledge has had a huge influence on reducing suffering and disability in mental illness. This chapter is an introduction to some landmarks and topography of what is known of the internal world.

After detailing the major and most clinically significant neurotransmitters in the brain that govern behaviour, this chapter then examines two specific conditions, attention-deficit hyperactivity disorder (ADHD) and self-injurious behaviour, in closer detail. A summary of new atypical neuroleptic agents and their rationale for use is also provided.

Neuronal activity of the brain

Modulation of neuronal activity via neurotransmitters is a fundamental mechanism of brain function. The elegant model is the neuronal synapse (see figure 24.1). Psychopharmacology works to facilitate or inhibit neurotransmitter release, stimulate or hinder synaptic uptake of the neurotransmitter, and/or modulate the number of postsynaptic receptors (Stahl, 2008). Drugs achieve this usually after binding to specific receptors on the neurone, which then cause changes in the electrical activity, or conversely increase the resting

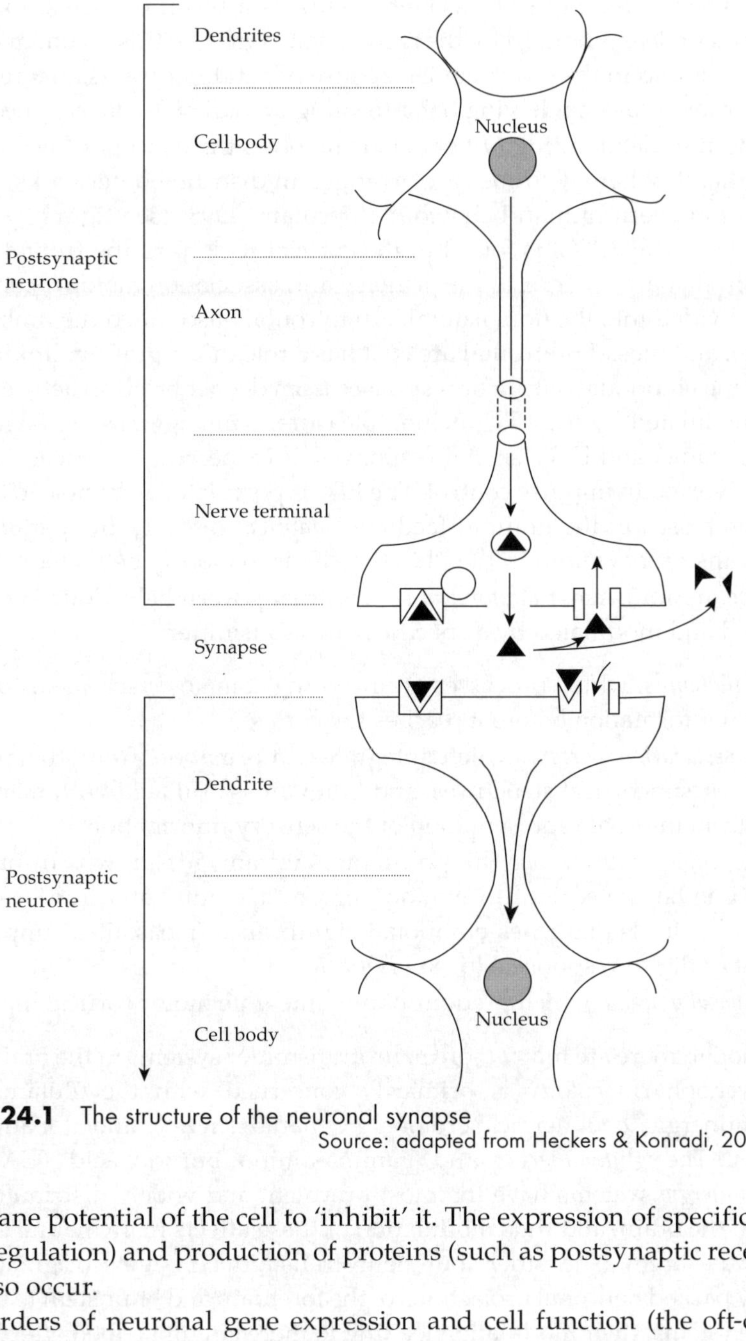

Figure 24.1 The structure of the neuronal synapse
Source: adapted from Heckers & Konradi, 2000, p. 2

membrane potential of the cell to 'inhibit' it. The expression of specific genes (gene regulation) and production of proteins (such as postsynaptic receptors) may also occur.

Disorders of neuronal gene expression and cell function (the oft-quoted 'chemical imbalance') are believed to underlie the deficit in neurodevelopmental and psychoaffective disorders, such as depression (Siever & Davis, 1985; Stahl, 2008). The use of psychotropic drugs aims to correct this imbalance. Frequently the delay in the effect observed after administering psychotropic drugs is the result of a secondary effect, such as a change in the number of postsynaptic receptors. This often occurs as a result of increased neurotransmitter release induced by the medication. It may be this secondary effect, such as is found in the therapeutic response of antidepressants, that results in psychotropic drugs not having habit-forming or addictive consequences.

Modern understanding of behaviour involves the concept of *neuronal circuitry*; that is, where neurones are arranged in distributed networks of brain regions to govern human behaviour (Mesulam, 1998) (see figure 24.2). The prefrontal cortex (PFC) is found in the cortical regions of the frontal lobe of the brain that are anterior to the primary and association motor cortices. The PFC is divided into the dorsolateral, orbitofrontal (also called the limbic frontal lobe), and mesial prefrontal areas. It has a role in integrating, linking, and regulating emotional output or responses from deeper brain structures. Emotions modulated by the PFC include pleasure, pain, aggression, anger, fear, reward, panic, and basic sexual responses. It is the body's 'decision-maker', and is involved in impulse control. The PFC is postulated to be able to 'recruit' other processes in the brain to facilitate *adaptive reasoning*. By manipulating neurotransmitters found in the PFC, the aim is to modify behaviour.

There are four major *anatomical systems* that govern behaviour, each characterised and modulated by a specific neurotransmitter:

1 The *thalamus*, which processes all incoming somatosensory, auditory, and visual information before it reaches the cortex
2 The *association cortex*, which integrates information from the primary cortices, subcortical structures, and brain areas affiliated with memory to create an internal representation of the sensory information
3 The *medial temporal lobe* (hippocampus and amygdala), which integrates multimodal sensory information for storage into and retrieval from memory. It also attaches emotional significance (pleasant or unpleasant, 'fight or flight' responses) to experiences
4 The *basal ganglia*, which predominantly integrate motor cortical input.

Although there are many more neurotransmitter systems in the brain, clinical psychopharmacology is primarily concerned with the glutaminergic, GABAminergic, cholinergic, serotonergic, noradrenergic, and dopaminergic systems. The *glutaminergic* and gamma-amino butyric acid (GABA) or *GABAminergic* systems have the most prevalent and widely distributed neurones in the brain, and thus modulation of these affects many neural systems within the brain. The other four neurotransmitter systems originate from densely packed neuronal projections of the forebrain and brainstem to selected neural systems, their modulation leading to more circumscribed effects.

In simplified terms, the main neuroanatomical origins of these neurotransmitters to the forebrain and cerebrum are:

- *cholinergic neurones:* a network that mainly originates in the basal forebrain and brainstem and connects to the hippocampus

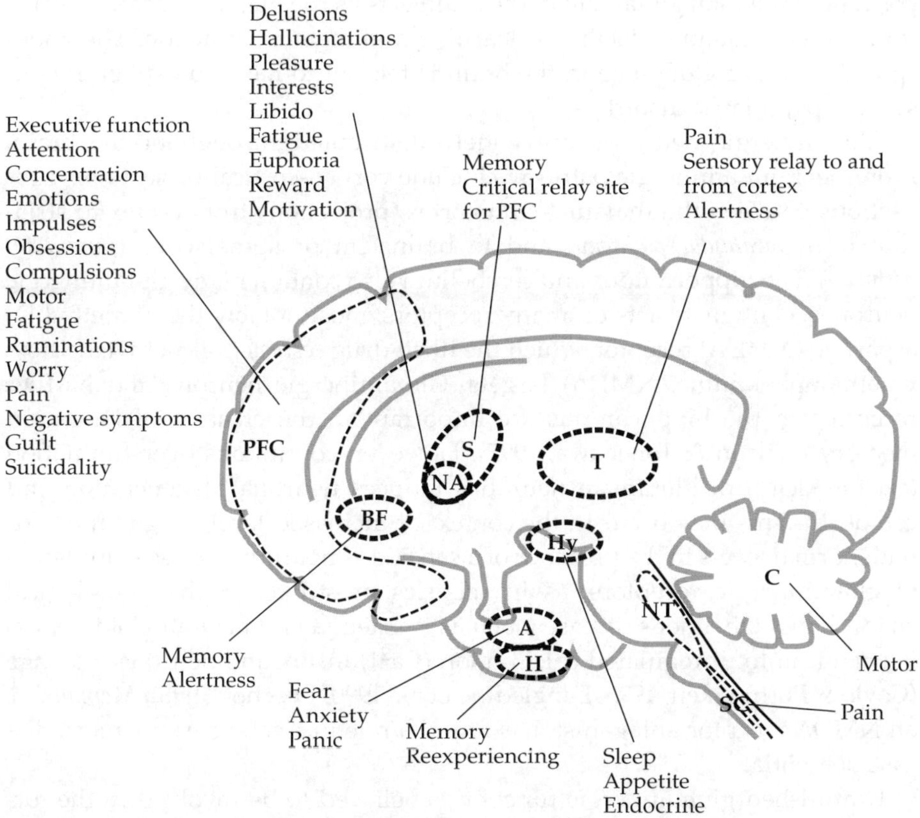

Figure 24.2 Behaviours linked to specific brain regions: PFC: prefrontal and association cortices; BF: basal forebrain; S: striatum; NA: nucleus accumbens; T: thalamus; HY: hypothalamus; A: amygdala; H: hippocampus; NT: brainstem neurotransmitter centres (containing substantia nigra, ventral tegmental area, locus coeruleus, and raphe nuclei); SC: spinal cord; C: cerebellum. (For clarity, the basal ganglia, containing and spanning the striatum (S), and substantia nigra within the brainstem neurotransmitter centres (NT), are not shown.)

Source: adapted from Stahl, 2008, p. 203

- *dopaminergic neurones:* originate in the substantia nigra and ventral tegmental area
- *noradrenergic neurones:* originate in the locus coeruleus
- *serotonergic neurones:* originate in the raphe nuclei.

Glutaminergic neurotransmission

Glutamate is the most abundant neurotransmitter in the *central nervous system (CNS)*. It also functions as an intermediate in neurotransmitter metabolism, being a precursor for gamma-amino butyric acid (GABA). Approximately 30 per cent of the total glutamate in the brain acts as the major excitatory neurotransmitter. Glutamate facilitates learning and memory function. The widespread action of glutamate in the brain is felt not to have an explicit role in specific psychiatric disorders.

Glutaminergic neurones are widely distributed throughout the brain. Prominent glutaminergic pathways include cortico-cortical projections, connections between the thalamus and cortex, projections from cortex to striatum (*extrapyramidal pathway*) and to brainstem or spinal cord (*pyramidal pathway*). The hippocampus and cerebellum also contain many glutaminergic neurones. Glutamate acts on many receptors, most notably the N-methyl-D-aspartate (NMDA) receptor, which the illicit drug *ecstasy* (3,4-methylenedioxymethamphetamine, NMDA) targets. Glutaminergic neurons and NMDA receptors in the hippocampus are important in the creation of long-term memory (Wilson & Tonegawa, 1997). However, continuous overstimulation (excitotoxicity) of glutamate neurones induces neuronal degeneration and cell death. This may occur in the context of increased levels of glutamate or with normal levels in the presence of a sensitised neurone. Excess stimulation of glutaminergic receptors, as in seizures or stroke, or the pathological changes in Alzheimer's disease (such as ischaemia and beta-amyloid deposits) can lead to unregulated calcium ion (Ca^{2+}) influx and neuronal damage (Coyle & Puttfarcken, 1993; Dingledine et al., 1990; Loscher, 1998). *Memantine*, an NMDA receptor antagonist, has found a role in treating Alzheimer's disease dementia.

Diminished glutaminergic function is believed to be involved in the formation of psychotic symptoms. Potent NMDA receptor antagonists, phencyclidine (found in the illicit drug *angel dust*) and the anaesthetic *ketamine*, can induce psychotic symptoms. Additionally *glycine*, an inhibitory amino acid, can decrease psychotic or negative symptoms in schizophrenia, although it is reported to not be therapeutically useful (Farber et al., 1999). *Acamprosate*, used to treat alcohol addiction, is a derivative of the amino acid taurine. Like alcohol (ethanol), it both reduces excitatory glutaminergic neurotransmission and enhances inhibitory GABAminergic neurotransmission.

GABAminergic neurotransmission

Gamma-amino butyric acid (GABA) is the major inhibitory neurotransmitter in the CNS. Cortical and thalamic GABAminergic neurones are crucial for the inhibition of excitatory (glutaminergic) neurones. Aside from local circuit neurones (*interneurones*) in the cortex, striatum (part of the basal ganglia), cerebellum, and spinal cord, GABAminergic neurones radiate from the caudate/putamen, via the globus pallidus, to the thalamus and substantia nigra (and back to the thalamus and superior colliculus), and from the septum pallucidum to hippocampus.

GABA acts on two receptors, $GABA_A$ and $GABA_B$. Benzodiazepines, such as *diazepam*, bind to the α-subunit of the $GABA_A$ receptor, opening a chloride channel to decrease the excitability of the cell. Barbiturates (such as phenobarbitone) and alcohol (ethanol) bind near the chloride channel (independent to the presence of GABA) to increase channel opening time and cause cell inhibition, which manifests as drowsiness and sedation. Thus, benzodiazepines and barbiturates are efficacious in the treatment and prevention of seizures. The similar mechanism of benzodiazepines and ethanol on $GABA_A$ receptors is the basis for utilising benzodiazepines in alcohol detoxification (Grobin et al., 1998). Modulation of $GABA_A$ receptors is beneficial in the treatment of anxiety disorders, insomnia, and agitation, most likely because of a generalised inhibition of neuronal activity (Olsen & Tobin, 1990; Stahl, 2008). *Baclofen* is an agonist at presynaptic (reducing neurotransmitter release) and postsynaptic (causing decreased excitability) $GABA_B$ receptors (Dutar & Nicoll, 1988; Stahl, 2008). It is primarily used as a muscle relaxant in cerebral palsy to treat spasticity.

Cholinergic neurotransmission

Cholinergic neurones project from the basal forebrain to the entire cortex, hippocampus, and amygdala, as well as from the brainstem to thalamus. Cholinergic interneurones in the striatum modulate the activity of striatal GABAminergic neurones. In the *peripheral nervous system (PNS)*, acetylcholine (ACh) is the neurotransmitter in the autonomic ganglia, parasympathetic postganglionic synapse (modulating heart rate via the vagal nerve), and the neuromuscular endplate. This accounts for anticholinergic drugs' adverse effects and potential toxicities. ACh acts at *muscarinic* and *nicotinic* (mostly PNS) receptors. Presynaptic cholinergic receptors may modulate the release of several neurotransmitters (Wonnacott, 1997). ACh is removed from the synapse through hydrolysis into acetyl-CoA and choline by the enzyme acetylcholinesterase (AChE). Removal of ACh from the synapse may be blocked irreversibly by organophosphosphate compounds (such as toxic pesticides) and botulinum toxin (*Botox*), and in a reversible fashion by AChE-blocking drugs such as *physostigmine*, used in myasthenia gravis.

Cholinergic neurotransmission modulates attention, novelty seeking and memory via forebrain projections to the cortex and limbic structures. Alzheimer's disease (AD) and anticholinergic delirium are examples of an ACh-deficient state. Enhancing synaptic levels of ACh via blocking AChE function strengthens cognitive function in AD, and has yielded a whole new class of drugs (*anticholinesterase inhibitors*) used to treat dementia, such as *rivastigmine* (Geula, 1998; Giacobini, 1998). Brainstem cholinergic neurones are essential for the regulation of sleep–wake cycles via projections to the thalamus. Cholinergic interneurones modulate striatal neurones by opposing the effects of dopamine. Parkinson's disease is a disorder of dopamine deficiency with effects modulated by acetylcholine (ACh). Increased cholinergic tone in Parkinson's disease and decreased cholinergic tone in patients treated with neuroleptics highlight an imbalance of these two systems in the striatum.

Serotonergic neurotransmission

Serotonergic (or 5-hydroxytryptamine, 5-HT) neurones project from the midline brainstem (raphe nuclei) to the thalamus, hypothalamus, amygdala, striatum, and cortex. Other fibres project to neurones within the brainstem, to the cerebellum and spinal cord. Peripherally, serotonin acts as a vasoconstrictor (as in migraines) and a vasoactive procoagulant. Blockade of 5-HT receptors in the area postrema by drugs, such as *ondansetron*, decreases nausea and vomiting. These widespread serotonergic projections and the heterogeneity of serotonergic receptors modulate many brain functions, including mood (anxiety, depression), behaviour (obsessive-compulsive actions, motivation), and the concept of self (schizophrenia). Hallucinogens, such as *lysergic acid diethylamide* (LSD), modulate serotonergic neurones via serotonergic autoreceptors. The concept of *theory of mind,* often deficient in individuals with autistic spectrum disorders, has been postulated to be a result of loss of the integrity of serotonergic and dopaminergic neurotransmitter pathways (Abu-Akel, 2003).

Serotonin deficiency within the brain is known to predispose to depression, anxiety, suicidality, violent behaviour, and migraine headaches. Links have also been made between low serotonin levels and premenstrual stress, obesity, compulsive gambling, insomnia, seasonal affective disorder (SAD), and alcoholism. Long-term psychosocial stress causes atrophy in the size and number of hippocampal astrocytes (neurones) seen in a variety of psychiatric and neurological disorders, including recurrent depression, schizophrenia, bipolar disorder, post-traumatic stress disorder, epilepsy, head injury, and Alzheimer's disease (Dhikav & Anand, 2007). This may be an underlying aetiology for the increased mortality seen in such conditions as depression following cardiac infarction. Studies have shown that lithium and selective serotonin reuptake inhibitors (SSRIs), such as *fluoxetine,* are neuroprotective in preventing hippocampal atrophy and cell death (apoptosis) (Boldizsar et al., 2006).

Repetitive behaviours that are often found in individuals with autism (such as head banging, hand flapping, and body rocking) have been likened to the stereotypies of obsessive compulsive disorder (OCD), and the notion that autism is a serotonin-deficient state (Whitaker-Azmita, 2001; Herault et al., 1996). Serotonin reuptake inhibitors, including *clomipramine* and SSRIs, may be useful for reducing stereotypical repetitive behaviour in autism and other pervasive developmental disorders. They may also reduce aggression and improve aspects of social relatedness, particularly reduced echolalia and repetitive questioning. It should be noted that *haloperidol* (blocking dopaminergic neurotransmission) has also been found to reduce stereotypical behaviour and activation, though, because of sedative side-effects, is less tolerated (Malone et al., 2001).

Noradrenergic neurotransmission

Approximately half of all noradrenergic neurones are located in the locus coeruleus, innervating the cortex, hippocampus, thalamus, cerebellum, and spinal cord. The remainder are distributed in the tegmentum innervating the hypothalamus, basal forebrain, and spinal cord. In the PNS, noradrenaline is the neurotransmitter of the sympathetic postganglionic synapse, and contributes to hypertension and the adrenal glands' fight-or-flight crisis response of affective-driven aggression or panic. β-adrenergic blocking agents (*beta-blockers*), such as *propranolol*, are used to antagonise adrenergic and noradrenergic effects both peripherally and centrally.

Noradrenergic projections in the thalamus, limbic structures, and cortex modulate sleep cycles, appetite, mood, and cognition. These functions are targeted by antidepressant drugs. The great number of noradrenergic neurones (receiving afferent stimuli from both internal and external environments) in the locus coeruleus is believed to be crucial to the fine-tuning of attention function of the cerebral cortex, such that perturbations of this system may result in feelings of anxiety (Svensson, 1987). Locus coeruleus neurones express a variety of autoreceptors. The firing of these may be reduced by *clonidine* (Buccafusco, 1992), which has been used in ADHD and as an anxiolytic and to control explosive outbursts. Clonidine acts to reduce synaptic levels of noradrenaline by binding (as an agonist) to presynaptic α_2-receptors, which inhibit noradrenaline release. Parents should be advised to avoid abruptly discontinuing clonidine to prevent rebound increases in blood pressure, tics, and anxiety (Leckman et al., 1986). Opioids, such as *morphine*, decrease locus coeruleus firing, and opioid withdrawal leads to increased firing. This is the rationale for clonidine use in the treatment of opioid withdrawal syndrome.

Reboxetine is a selective noradrenaline reuptake inhibitor that is effective and used clinically as an antidepressant. It may also have a role in attention-deficit hyperactivity disorder (ADHD). *Mirtazapine*, another atypical antidepressant, is less selective. It acts primarily through α_2-noradrenaline presynaptic and 5-$HT_{2A/3}$ postsynaptic antagonism respectively, leading to increases in noradrenaline and 5-HT_{1A} activity. The antidepressant *venlafaxine* is a selective serotonin and noradrenaline reuptake inhibitor (SSNRI). *Atomoxetine* (discussed below), a drug used in ADHD, increases both noradrenaline and serotonin synaptic concentrations. The tricyclic antidepressant *amitriptyline* increases synaptic concentrations of noradrenaline and dopamine greater than that of SSRIs, and may be useful in treating aggression.

Dopaminergic neurotransmission

Dopaminergic neurones are significantly found in the substantia nigra (SN), radiating to the caudate, putamen, and ventral tegmental area (VTA). VTA neurones project to limbic regions (nucleus accumbens and amygdala) to form the *mesolimbic system*, and to frontal, cingulated, and entorhinal areas of the cortex to comprise the *mesocortical system*. Dopaminergic neurones also project from the hypothalamus (including the pituitary gland), and are found in the retina and olfactory bulb. Dopaminergic projections from the hypothalamus to the pituitary gland tonically inhibit the production and release of prolactin via D_2-receptors. Blockade of these receptors, such as with neuroleptic drugs, leads to *hyperprolactinaemia* and *galactorrhoea*, a common and unwanted adverse effect. SN dopaminergic neurones modulate the function of striatal GABAminergic neurones. Parkinson's disease and extrapyramidal side-effects (discussed further below) following treatment with neuroleptics are examples of decreased dopaminergic function.

The mesolimbic system is known to be involved with *reward behaviour* and in the development of *addiction* to drugs such as ethanol, cocaine, nicotine, and opiates (Diana, 1998; Koob, 1998). The mesocortical system's role is to fine-tune memory and cognition (Goldman-Rakic, 1998). *Dopamine* is an intermediate monoamine in the synthesis of noradrenaline and adrenaline, as well as being a neurotransmitter in its own right. Dopamine is synthesised by the enzyme *L-aromatic amino acid decarboxylase* from 3,4-dihyroxyphenylalamine (L-DOPA). Dopamine levels can be elevated if extra DOPA is supplied to the brain, such as *L-DOPA* administration in Parkinson's disease. Dopamine is released into the synapse from vesicles, a process facilitated by *amphetamines*, such as *dexamphetamine* or *methylphenidate* (Ritalin). Amphetamines may precipitate psychosis. *Tetrabenazine* is a non-neuroleptic that depletes presynaptic dopamine and has weak post-synaptic dopamine-blocking properties. It has found a role in reducing motor tics in Tourette's syndrome.

Pergolide is a mixed D_2/D_1 agonist developed for the treatment of Parkinson's disease. The rationale of using a dopamine agonist to treat tics is its postulated function in 'balancing out' dopaminergic neurotransmission. In conditions such as Tourette's syndrome with heightened dopaminergic tone, pergolide acts as a dopamine antagonist. By contrast, in Parkinson's disease with decreased dopaminergic activity, pergolide acts as a dopamine agonist. Pergolide's formal role in the treatment of Tourette's syndrome is yet to be defined (Lipinski et al., 1997). *Amantadine*, an antiviral agent used in Parkinson's disease, potentiates dopaminergic neurotransmission by means of blocking dopamine reuptake into presynaptic neurones and stimulating CNS dopamine release.

Attention-deficit hyperactivity disorder

The pattern of neuropsychological deficits found in children with *attention-deficit hyperactivity disorder (ADHD)* implicates deficits in executive function and working memory (Barkley, 1997). This pattern is similar to that found among adults with frontal lobe damage, suggesting dysfunction of the frontal lobe or regions projecting to it. It has been postulated that ADHD consists of deficits in noradrenergic inhibitory influences of frontal cortical activity, driven by dopamine agonists acting on lower striatal structures (Zametkin & Rapoport, 1987). In several studies, stimulants appear to 'normalise' ADHD behaviour in children (Whalen, 1989), including an increased ability to perceive peer communications, self-perceptions, and situational cues. These children show improved modulation of the intensity of behaviour, improved communication, and greater responsiveness (Whalen et al., 1990). Additionally, stimulant-associated improvements in social interactions positively influence the social behaviour of others in the child's environment (Whalen & Henker, 1992; Cunningham et al., 1991). Parents, teachers, siblings, and peers are more positive and less critical of the child with ADHD who is receiving stimulant medication. Studies have also indicated that both behaviour and cognitive performance improve with stimulant treatment in a dose-dependent manner (Douglas et al., 1988; Rapport et al., 1989; DuPaul et al., 1989). Doses that improve behaviour rarely constrict attention or lead to *over-focusing* (Douglas et al., 1995; Solanto & Wender, 1989). When negative social behaviour and deficits are associated with ADHD-type symptoms, pharmacotherapy is a useful treatment modality. However, improvement of the internal environment by stimulants should be used to potentiate the external environment, in terms of enhancing developmental promotion in the family, school, and community.

Atomoxetine blocks presynaptic reuptake transporters in the prefrontal cortex, creating an equivalent increase in noradrenaline and serotonin there. It does not increase dopamine within the nucleus accumbens, so lacks euphoric effects, reinforcing properties, and the potential for drug abuse. It also does not increase dopamine within the striatum, so is not associated with motor or vocal tic adverse effects that stimulant treatment of ADHD may cause. As atomoxetine acts specifically on noradrenergic rather than cholinergic neurotransmission, it has no effect on cardiac conduction and the potential for cardiac arrhythmia side-effects, unlike tricyclic antidepressants.

Monoamine oxidase inhibitors

Monoamine oxidase inhibitors (MAOIs) block the function of the intracellular catabolic enzyme *monoamine oxidase*. Both types, MAO-A and MAO-B, metabolise tyramine and dopamine. Additionally, MAO-A preferentially metabolises noradrenaline, adrenaline, and serotonin. *Irreversible* MAOIs (such as *phenelzine* and *tranylcypromine*), traditionally used to treat depression in adults, have the potential for hypertensive crisis, should the patient concomitantly ingest tyramine-rich foods (such as aged or cheddar cheeses, broad or fava beans, fish, especially pickled herring, alcohol (such as red or Chianti wine, beer, and some liqueurs), meat, such as pepperoni sausage, yeast products, and banana peel). A hypertensive reaction may also occur if the patient concurrently takes sympathomimetic drugs or amphetamines. A *serotonergic syndrome* of neurotransmitter excess may develop when MAOIs are combined with SSRIs. (The clinical features of serotonergic syndrome are described in table 24.1 (p. 302)). These dietetic restrictions and potential drug interactions limit the use of irreversible MAOIs in children. Preliminary studies have however suggested that MAOIs are effective in ADHD (Zametkin et al., 1985). Notably, the non-selective reversible MAOI *moclobemide* does not possess this risk, and provides for greater safety when used in children. Its role in the treatment of ADHD is yet to be elucidated.

Buspirone

Buspirone is a non-benzodiazepine anxiolytic with a high affinity for serotonin 5-HT_{1A} receptors, as well as having a modest effect on dopaminergic neurotransmission and α-adrenergic activity. Its anxiolytic effect is believed to result from inhibiting the spontaneous firing of serotonergic neurones in the dorsal raphe nucleus of the hypothalamus by binding to presynaptic 5-HT_{1A} receptors. It reportedly improves disruptive behaviour and psychosocial function, with only mild side-effects (such as dizziness, nausea, and agitation) in children with ADHD (Malhotra & Santosh, 1998). In comparison to benzodiazepines, buspirone has a lower incidence of side-effects, no risk of dependence, and no withdrawal syndrome.

Melatonin

Melatonin is the neurotransmitter secreted by the pineal gland. It acts on specific melatonin receptors in the suprachiasmatic nucleus of the hypothalamus to affect sleep onset and regulate circadian rhythm. Administration of melatonin as a pharmacological preparation may be of benefit in childhood sleep disorders or altered sleep–wake cycles, albeit these may be inherently altered in the child with cortical dysplasia or neurodevelopmental dysfunction. Individuals with *Smith-Magenis syndrome* have an inverted circadian sleep–wake cycle, with more melatonin produced in the early hours of the day and less at night. Beta-blockers administered in the morning halt the body's production of melatonin, whilst melatonin medication is supplemented at night, thus correcting the normal physiological cycle (Cardinali & Pandi-Perumal, 2005; Elsea & Girirajan, 2008; De Leersnyder et al., 2006; De Leersnyder et al., 2001).

Atypical neuroleptics

Atypical neuroleptic drugs possess potent D_2- and 5-HT_2-blocking properties. This latter activity is believed to account for their ability to improve the negative symptoms of schizophrenia and be protective against extrapyramidal side-effects (EPSEs). EPSEs include the loss of fluidity of movement, flattening of emotional expression, fine tremor (drug-induced parkinsonism), increased muscle tone and muscular spasms (dystonia), as well as restlessness of the limbs (akathisia). The onset of tardive dyskinesia, repetitive involuntary purposeless movements, is also possibly reduced. These putative 'safety' features of atypical neuroleptics make them attractive alternatives to traditional neuroleptic agents, such as haloperidol, especially if the child with a behavioural disorder is to be medicated over several years.

Clozapine

Clozapine, the original atypical neuroleptic, is a potent 5-HT_2 blocker with lesser D_2-antagonism. It has not been associated with significant extrapyramidal symptoms or tardive dyskinesia. Clozapine appears effective in reducing aggressive behaviour (Glazer & Dickson, 1998) and improving quality of life for those with chronic schizophrenia resistant to other antipsychotics. Clozapine's major drawback is its 1 per cent risk of potentially fatal agranulocytosis.

Olanzapine

Olanzapine acts similarly to clozapine, however with greater D_2-blockade and much lower risk of agranulocytosis. Like clozapine, it also acts at 5-HT_{2A}, 5-HT_{2C}, D_1, D_2, D_4, muscarinic M1, α_1-adrenergic and H_1-receptors. Olanzapine's most significant side-effects are sedation and weight gain (Pottenza et al., 1999). Every antipsychotic acts uniquely on a varied dopamine receptor subtype, which is an explanation why drugs in the same group may have subtle but different clinical outcomes. Such differences are difficult to predict in any individual case.

Risperidone

By improving the negative signs and symptoms of schizophrenia, *risperidone* has been trialled in adolescents with autism to treat similar withdrawn behaviour, with varying degrees of success. Improvements in aggression, self-injury, explosiveness, overactivity, and poor sleep have also been observed with risperidone (Horrigan & Barnhill, 1997). In a head-to-head study with haloperidol, risperidone has been shown to be superior in improving patient hostility independent from reducing psychosis (Czobor et al., 1995). The most common side-effect associated with risperidone use is weight gain (proposed to be via H_1 and 5-HT_{2C} receptor blockade). *Quetiapine* has been reported to be less efficacious and less tolerable than risperidone when used in pervasive developmental disorders. Though weight gain is also associated with its use, this is to a lesser extent than with olanzapine and risperidone.

Ziprasidone

Although similar to risperidone and olanzapine in blocking D_2 and 5-HT_2 receptors, *ziprasidone* has additional 5-HT_{1A}-agonist properties and modest noradrenaline and serotonin reuptake blocking action. These may contribute to anxiolytic and antidepressant effects (Chappell et al., 1997).

Aripiprazole

Aripiprazole is a partial dopamine D_2 receptor and 5-HT_{1A} agonist, in addition to being a 5-HT_{2A} antagonist (Burris et al., 2002). Significant improvements have been noted with its use in reducing aggression, self-injury, and irritability (Stigler et al., 2004). It generally causes less weight gain than olanzapine and risperidone. Aripiprazole causes minimal cardiovascular side-effects.

Mood stabilisers

Lithium and *anticonvulsant drugs* have not been found to be effective in treating ADHD, but have been found helpful in treating aggression in individuals with developmental disabilities. They have also been used in the management of intermittent explosive disorder (Trimble, 1990). *Carbamazepine* has proved effective in treating lithium-resistant mania.

Selection of an anticonvulsant to treat disruptive behaviour must involve consideration of each drug's potential toxicity and patient tolerability; for example, *valproate*-induced hirsutism in adolescent girls. Newer antiepileptic agents, such as *lamotrigine*, may be candidates for novel mood-stabilising agents so long as their significant potential toxicities, including Steven-Johnson syndrome, a severe allergic effect, are considered (Folgelson & Sternbach, 1997; Kotler & Matar, 1998; Sporn & Sachs, 1997; Calabrese et al., 1996). *Topiramate* has been trialled as a treatment for eating disorders and alcoholism, with promising results (McElroy et al., 2007; Johnson et al., 2007).

Self-injurious behaviour

Individuals with intellectual disabilities are more likely to develop psychiatric disorders than the general population (Hardan & Sahl, 1997). Maladaptive and disruptive behaviours, such as aggression, self-injury, and stereotypical mannerisms, are common. The presence of any of these symptoms compromises an already limited capacity for adaptive functioning, and in some cases this will improve with pharmacological therapy.

The appearance of *self-injurious behaviour* in an individual with severe impairment is non-specific. It may be the result of acute medical illness or related to mood, psychosis, anxiety, or impulse-control disorders. An attempt to identify the antecedents of the behaviour should be made. Common causes may include dysphoria from loneliness, depression, and physical pain. Difficulties may arise from hypersensitivities to sensory experiences and the individual's preferences. Often the formulation of a personal 'sensory profile' by a specialised psychologist experienced in modulating arousal is of immense benefit.

Self-injurious behaviour should be characterised in terms of precipitating factors, frequency, duration, and severity. If the behaviour is of recent and acute onset, the search for any underlying physiological pathology is essential. If there is an associated change in appetite or level of activity, an underlying mood disorder may be the cause. Avoidant or highly situational behaviours may indicate anxiety, while poor self-restraint proposes an impulse control disorder.

The consequences of the self-injurious behaviour should be identified. Carers may inadvertently reinforce the behaviour by providing attention, undue support, and permitting misbehaviour. An objective functional analysis of the behaviour by the clinician may identify more suitable caregiver interventions, which do not reinforce the behaviour, but do provide appropriate coping mechanisms to the carer. Atypical antipsychotics and SSRIs are the mainstay of treatment for self-injurious behaviour.

Dopamine D_1-receptor sensitivity appears to provoke self-injurious behaviour in both animal and human models (Aman, 1993). Congenital dopamine deficiency of *Lesch-Nyhan syndrome* is thought to underlie the associated self-injurious behaviour. Propranolol, a β-adrenergic blocking agent, has been reported to be effective in treating refractory aggression in brain-injured patients (Kuperman & Stewart, 1987; Grizenko & Vida, 1988). Interest in the role played by endogenous opiates (endorphins) in the pathogenesis of self-injury has led to the use of opioid-receptor antagonists, such as *naltrexone* and *naloxone*, to treat this condition. Studies to date have offered inconclusive results (Barrett et al., 1989; Sandman et al., 1990). Clinical algorithms for a multitude of psychoaffective disorders have been proposed, including maladaptive aggression (see figure 24.3).

The notion of a *behavioural phenotype*—the attribution of a specific set of behavioural or psychiatric expressions to an underlying genotype—is popular. This has arisen in part by advances in molecular genetics and neuroimaging. Nevertheless, the clinician should be familiar with specific syndromic diagnostic possibilities, such as Fragile X, Williams, Prader-Willi, Smith-Magenis and Down syndromes.

Violent behaviour may also be linked to genetic conditions or genetically determined enzymatic activity. An association between increased violent

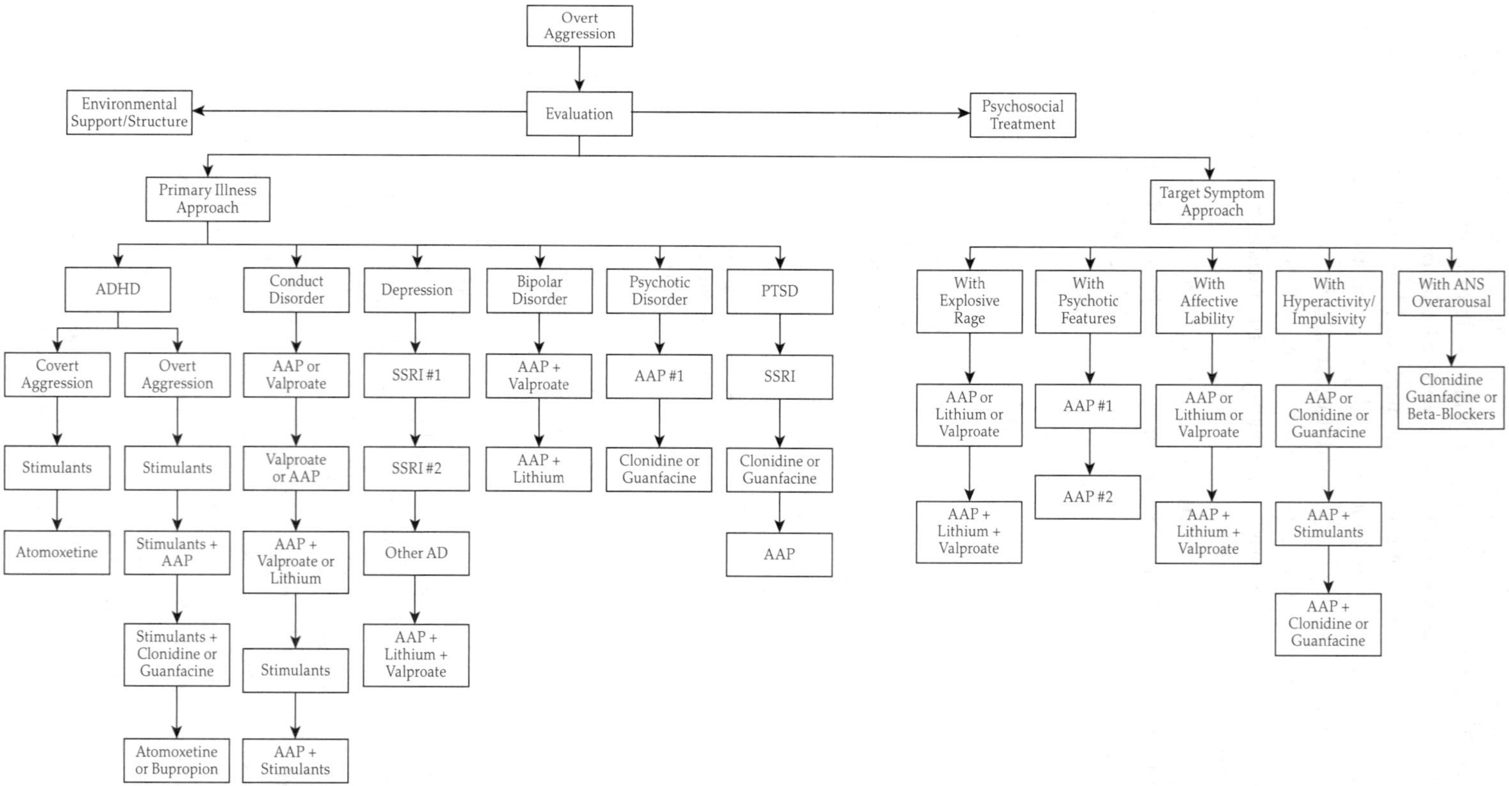

Figure 24.3 A clinical algorithm for the medical treatment of maladaptive aggression in children: AAP: atypical antipsychotics; SSRI: selective serotonin reuptake inhibitor; AD: antidepressant; PTSD: post-traumatic stress disorder; ANS: autonomic nervous system.

Source: reproduced from Connor & Meltzer, 2006, p. 333, with permission behaviour and reduced activity of the catabolic *catechol-O-methyltransferase (COMT)* enzyme, leading to higher concentrations of synaptic L-DOPA, has been found (Lachman et al., 1998). The use of pharmacological COMT inhibitors, *tolcapone* and *entacapone* (as in Parkinson's disease), has similarly been found to induce aggression. Social deprivation in the early years of a child's life has been found to have an interactive gene–environment multiplier effect leading to higher rates of antisocial behaviour (Henry et al., 1996). Psychosocial stimulation plays a vital part in neurodevelopment. Prolonged deprivation is associated with a proportional stunting of brain growth (observed as microcephaly on centile growth charts), lower IQ, and increased mental health problems, independent of nutrition (Sonuga-Barke et al., 2008).

In general, psychopharmacological treatments for disorders of maladaptive aggression are adjunctive to psychosocial, psychoeducational, and community treatment plans. Comorbid paediatric neurodevelopmental and psychoaffective disorders with aggression, as a significant associated symptom, should be diagnosed and treated. These include ADHD, anxiety, depression, adolescent bipolar disorder, post-traumatic stress disorder (PTSD), and psychosis, which must be assessed in the context of the child's developmental age.

Pharmacogenomics

Drug response within a patient, as determined by its genetic expression, such as enzyme concentration, is termed *pharmacogenomics*. This may be particularly important in the cytochrome P450 pathways of hepatic metabolism of psychotropic medication. A few centres are already testing a patient's cytochrome P450 genotypic expression with the aim of selecting a personalised therapeutic dose and avoiding potential dose-related side-effects.

Process of psychopharmacotherapy

1. *Select* an appropriate pharmacological *agent* and dose *form*. Be alert for drug–drug interactions.
2. Determine an initial *target dose*, ideally once a day, according to lean body weight or surface area.
3. *Start low and go slow:* gradually escalate the dose to an optimum level.
4. *Wait* an expected length of time for the therapeutic effect to occur.
5. *Assess* the *response*, ideally using an objective rating scale.
6. Be *alert* for *adverse effects*.
7. Consider *augmentation* (adding another agent) or *substitution* (using a different compound with the same therapeutic indication).

8 *Step down ineffective medication doses* and allow an appropriate *washout* period (4–5 half-lives of the drug).
9 If all else fails, *review the diagnosis*.

CONCLUSION

Psychopharmacology uses drugs to modulate neurotransmission within anatomical systems to influence behaviour. Our current understanding of these complex networks is rudimentary, and fraught with unwanted adverse effects (see table 24.1). Psychopharmacology attempts to match a targeted behaviour with an appropriate medication in order to modulate that behaviour (see figure 24.4).

The field of psychopharmacology currently contains a multitude of medications, with few accompanying studies to guide their prescription and use in children. Drug development involves extensive research and testing (phase I–III trials). Long-term safety data (from phase IV post-marketing surveillance data) are customarily the last to be collected. More recently,

Table 24.1 Summary of major neurotransmitters and their respective adverse effects

Neurotransmitter	*Agonist example*	*Antagonist example*	*Adverse effect*
Glutamate	Monosodium glutamate, ecstasy (not clinically used)	NMDA antagonists (e.g. memantine)	Seizures, encephalopathy, excitation
GABA	Benzodiazepines (e.g. diazepam), barbiturates, gabapentin	Flumazenil ('benzodiazepine antidote')	Disinhibition, somnolescence, ataxia, dependence (withdrawal seizures)
Acetylcholine (muscarinic)	AChEs (e.g. rivastigmine), nicotine, bethanecol	Anticholinergic drugs*, TCAs (e.g. amitriptyline), benztropine	Salivation, sweating, diarrhoea, urinary incontinence
Serotonin (5-HT)	SSRIs (e.g. fluoxetine)	Cyproheptadine	Hypertension, tachycardia, hyperthermia, myoclonus, sweating
Noradrenaline	SNRIs (e.g. reboxetine)	Beta-blockers (e.g. propranolol)	Hypertension, tachycardia, wakefulness
Dopamine	L-DOPA, dexamphetamine, methylphenidate	Neuroleptics (e.g. haloperidol)	Stereotypies, mania, exacerbation of tics and movement disorders

* Anticholinergic side-effects include dry mouth, urinary hesitancy, blurred vision, constipation, confusion, pupillary dilatation.

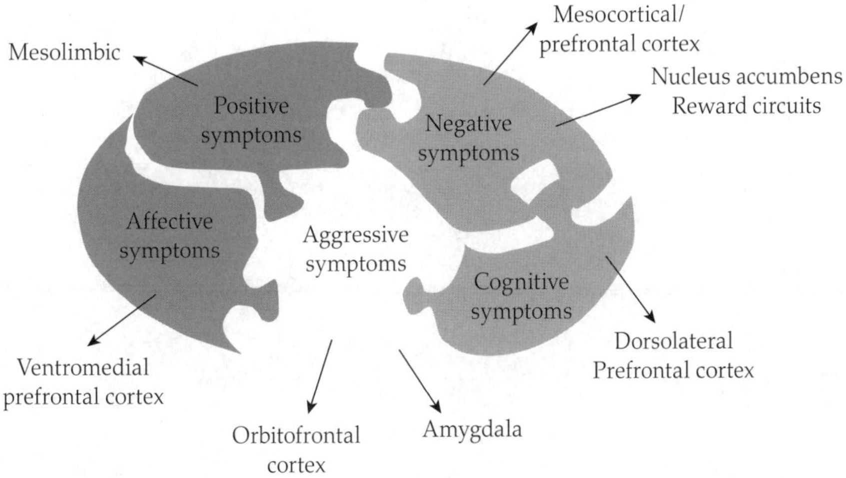

Figure 24.4 Symptoms (of schizophrenia) matched to malfunctioning brain regional neural circuits

Source: reproduced from Stahl, 2008, p. 203, permission pending

these include safety data in children. Though drugs generally have strong levels of evidence of effectiveness, changing the internal environment of the child and young person is not without risk. Vigilance and the proper management of side-effects form part of best practice. Over time, designer drugs will be developed to target specifically localised neuronal receptors and behavioural objectives.

Acknowledgments

The author would like to acknowledge Dr David Dossetor for his clinical experience and opinion in the field of psychopharmacology; and Judith Longworth, pharmacist, Department of Psychological Medicine, The Children's Hospital at Westmead, for her assistance in reviewing this chapter.

Part 5

Integration of service systems

25

A service model for the mental health needs of children and adolescents with intellectual disability

David Dossetor

Introduction

In Australia and many other parts of the world, health services lack designated specialist mental health services for individuals with intellectual disability. This presents a challenge to provide such a service, using the combined efforts of separate specialist intellectual disability services, and health and mental health services.

The decline of institutional provision of care for people with intellectual disability and mental health problems has depended on a change in community and political attitudes, backed up with significant additional funding for community support and accommodation. The focus therefore, has been on intervention for adults who had been institutionalised, with little planning for what was needed for the new generation of young people with intellectual disability and mental health problems, and their carers. There is growing evidence of the inadequacy of community-based service provision for this population. A study of carers by Cummins and colleagues (2007) showed that the mental well-being of carers of people with an intellectual disability was significantly worse than other carer groups, with 50 per cent suffering depression. Additionally, the Australian longitudinal study of people with an intellectual disability (Einfeld & Tonge, 1996b) demonstrated the level of persisting severe psychiatric morbidity (40 per cent) and lack of adequate access to specialist mental health services (9 per cent). If mental health services were to provide for this level of need, it has been estimated that this would require an investment equivalent to all services provided for schizophrenia! Similarly, Beange and Lennox (1988) highlighted the lack of attention and identification of general health problems of this population in general practice.

In Australia, specialist service provision for people with an intellectual disability has been transferred from state health departments to welfare departments over the years, and it was assumed that equity of access to generic state health services would meet their health and mental health needs. Unfortunately the generic mental health services have been seen to provide poorly for this special need group. Indeed, the state specialist mental health services provide for severe mental illness, and the federally funded Medicare is expected to provide the community-based services for general practice and subsidise private mental health services. The economics and epidemiology of mental health need make clear the deficits. For example, in New South Wales (NSW), Child and Adolescent Mental Health Services is responsible for 30 per cent of the mental health burden of health, but receives only 6 per cent of the funding. In the UK, it has been shown that although children and adolescents with an intellectual disability constitute between 2 and 3 per cent of the population, they constitute 14 per cent of the mental health burden of care (Emerson & Hatton, 2007). In NSW, this is not reflected in the service provision, and indeed, it is a commonly reported experience that having an intellectual disability is grounds for exclusion from a mental health service. For young people with intellectual disability, a gap between mental health need and service provision is evident in each Australian state and territory. Furthermore, in the absence of a capacity to communicate information on mainstream abnormal mental phenomena, young people presenting with an intellectual disability are likely to be seen as mentally disordered or having challenging behaviour rather than having a mental illness, although to the lay person this might seem to be using semantics to limit access to overstretched services.

Proposed service model

In order to alleviate some of the difficulties in the provision of mental health services to young people with intellectual disability within a limited system, a tiered service model is proposed. This model is based on the holistic model of bio-developmental-psycho-socio-cultural mental health and well-being, along with problem-solving and collaborative approaches across clinicians and organisations.

Assumptions

The proposed service structure is based on a number of assumptions. These are outlined below:

1 Mental health problems of young people are complex and persisting. Parents have always had complex explanations for the behaviour of their child.
2 There is limited funding for mental health services, which means that other health and human services are essential to meeting the need.
3 There should be a spectrum of services, ranging from prevention to early intervention, to specialist intervention, rehabilitation and community support, and accommodation. Accordingly, common problems should be managed with preventative and universal approaches.
4 A tiered structure of specialist service provision provides a problem-solving framework for more challenging cases, with increased involvement of different professionals for assessment and intervention as the complexity and severity of these cases increases. These then have to be couched in a humane and community-based system of service provision and care.
5 The specialised skills of different disciplines for the mental health needs of young people with intellectual disability are not found in any one agency, which therefore requires protocols for interagency collaboration.
6 This book provides an empirically based holistic bio-developmental-psycho-social-cultural model framework that can enable all disciplines to work together for the needs of the children and adolescents.
7 Recognition of the rights and special mental health needs of young people with an intellectual disability necessitates access to subspecialty multidisciplinary psychiatry services. The critical role of pharmacology in community mental health care requires the inclusion of psychiatrists with special expertise in intellectual disability.
8 While it is evident that clinicians' explanations for mental health problems are often limited, complex, and uncertain, it is essential to support the development of expert clinicians with subspecialty skills who pursue clinical research to advance the evidence base.
9 These clinical academic subspecialty clinicians contribute to a *learning institution*, which shares new knowledge with less specialised and more generic services over time. Such a framework can accommodate the advance of knowledge in a way that not only improves the services for people with intellectual disability but enriches mainstream health and mental health services.

A tiered service structure

The proposed tiered service structure is described below and in figure 25.1. The tiers are explained using examples from the current service system in NSW.

Tier 1: Generic health provision

Tier 1 involves service integration of the mental health needs in general health, education, and community services. This is in keeping with the community acceptance of 'mild and moderate' mental health problems, and

Tier 5: Acute short/medium term interventions that inform Tier 4
Includes: Emergency departments, MH in-patients assessments, other residential behaviour servies; and **Specialist/tertiary MH in ID clinicians** from mental health and disability services.

The Tier 4 circle: The final common pathway
Complex ease management decision making; 'best endeavour' obligations including decisions about out-of-family community placements.

Tier 3: Multidisciplinary and multi-agency collaboration
Disability service: behaviour clinician, speech pathologist, OT, other specialist psychology service;
Health: GP, paediatrician or neurologist; MH psychologist, social worker, family therapist, psychiatrist; and
Education: teacher, aide, school counsellor, principal, behaviour support specialist.

Tier 2: Community disability services providing case management and specialist parent training. Mainly from Disability Services but can be MH or other agency or non-government organisations.

Tier 1: Generic health provision for families
Includes: GPs, comunity nurses, community health teams, selective prevention initiatives and special education provision

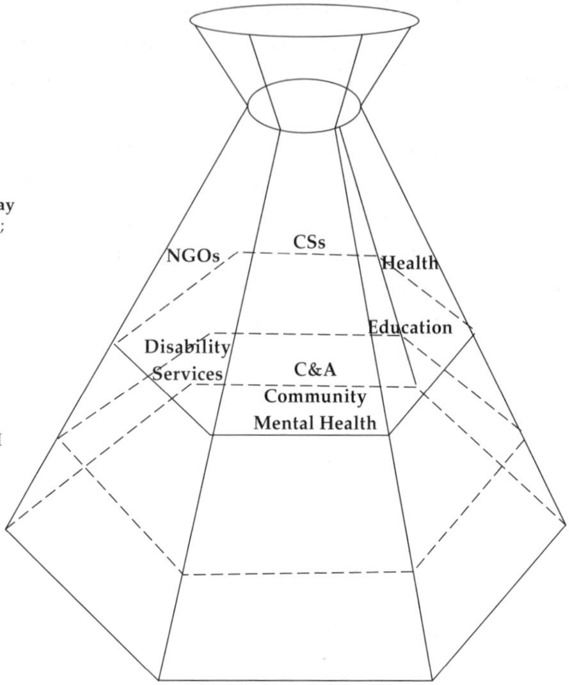

*3D Model provides for **all other human services** to be part of the pyramid*

Figure 25.1 Tiered pyramid of services for children and adolescents with intellectual disability and mental health problems

recognised under the rubric that 'mental health is everyone's business'. This tier would include general practitioners (GPs), community nurses, community health teams, and special education provision, including that provided in a mainstream setting.

Tier 2: Community disability service: case management and targeted prevention interventions (for example, specialist parent training)

Tier 2 involves a first level of specialist disability or mental health clinician, with responsibility for case management for the individual and family. Disability case managers are often in a better position to access other intellectual disability resources, such as various forms of respite, to tackle the inordinate burden of care. However, GPs and general paediatricians frequently take on the case-coordination role, acting as gatekeepers to more specialist services.

Case managers should have a defined range of generic holistic clinical skills. Given the evidence base, the case managers should be trained in specialist parent training programs that could be provided in conjunction with special education resources. This would build the relationship between parents and schools, and strengthen community connectedness and access for families and schools. Other prevention, promotion, and early intervention approaches for mental health would need to be developed and validated in specialist educational services.

Tier 3: Multidisciplinary and multiagency collaboration

In NSW, collaborative services for a young person with an intellectual disability may include such agencies as Ageing, Disability and Home Care (ADHC, Department of Human Services), Department of Education and Training (DET), Department of Health, possibly Mental Health, Community Services (CS, which provides social and welfare services) and other non-government services. In other states of Australia, and in other countries, tier 3 of the proposed service structure would involve a multidisciplinary team, which may or may not include a paediatrician, and access to a psychiatrist from the public or private health system. The multidisciplinary team may include a behaviour clinician, a speech pathologist, an occupational therapist, a social worker, a family therapist, a psychologist, a GP, a paediatrician, a psychiatrist, and a neurologist.

The multidisciplinary team works on collaborative good intent, guided by the best interests of the young person with intellectual disability, as viewed by his or her parents or carers. Any of the above child-orientated agencies could initiate the multiagency process, but the individual's presentation may guide which agency has the primary role. Disability services may have the lead role for challenging behaviours or externalising disorders, paediatrics may have the lead role for developmental psychiatric disorders such as autism spectrum disorders or attention-deficit hyperactive disorders, and mental health services may have the lead role for severe mental health problems, such as depression and psychosis.

Tier 4: Complex case management decision-making model

Tier 4 must have a cross-agency, multidisciplinary management decision-making capacity that involves both intellectual disability and mental health specialist expertise. This tier of service integrates the best available clinical opinion with the individual's environmental needs (whether this is within or outside of a family setting) to provide complex clinical insight. This process drives the business case for funding.

Tier 4 would provide a common language and mechanism for establishing priority of need, both for short-term interventions and long-term placements. This level of decision-making should ensure that all available expert clinical perspectives are taken into account. Such a *complex case conference* should have a mechanism for each agency to make requests of other agencies for professional assessments of the individual, or assistance as required. Provision of assistance across agencies and government departments should be afforded priority, consistent with 'best endeavours'. Monitoring the frequency and outcome of such best-endeavours requests would provide a centralised measure of the success of interagency collaboration.

Tier 5: Acute short-term psychiatry model

Tier 5 is emergency mental health involvement, mental health inpatient assessment and treatment, and the input of specialist mental health services of intellectual disability. In short, this tier tests out what neuropsychiatry and inpatient assessment can contribute. However, this service tier is necessarily short term, as is the case for all acute psychiatry services, and longer term management would necessitate services from tier 4 to be engaged to manage the multifaceted nature of community-based care.

The need for specialist mental health in intellectual disability services

It is a widely held view that chronic mental health comorbidity is the greatest reversible handicap in people with an intellectual disability. This leads to great costs to the individuals with intellectual disability, their families, and the wider community, including the services that are provided, in terms of the financial costs, the impact on quality of life, and standards of humanity. The bio-developmental-psycho-socio-cultural model leads to the division of mental health problems into (a) challenging behaviour, (b) developmental problems, and (c) psychiatric problems, which places a primary responsibility on disability services, paediatric services, and child and adolescent mental health services. There are a range of other services and professions involved in these problems, as illustrated in figure 25.2.

The biggest failure of this system is for young people with dangerous or complex challenging behaviour who have a high of risk of unrecognised severe mental health problems or disorders. These young people often do not receive adequate early intervention in the education system, which results in threats of harm to self or public safety. Failure of treatment and reduced access to generic child and adolescent mental health services, through lack of 'intent' or insufficient verbal skills, threaten the child's or adolescent's placement in the family, predispose to abuse, and may lead to the need for long-term out-of-home placement. The latter may result in major costs and service challenges (such as blocked beds in respite care placements).

It is this group of young people who need an empirically orientated specialist mental health and multidisciplinary intellectual disability subspecialty team. Equity of access to appropriate services and standards for relief of distress and chronic impairment demand the availability of such a service. Such a clinically expert team could also provide education and training to generic services, and take account of the special needs of this group; for example, enabling admissions to general hospitals for other health issues. A clinical

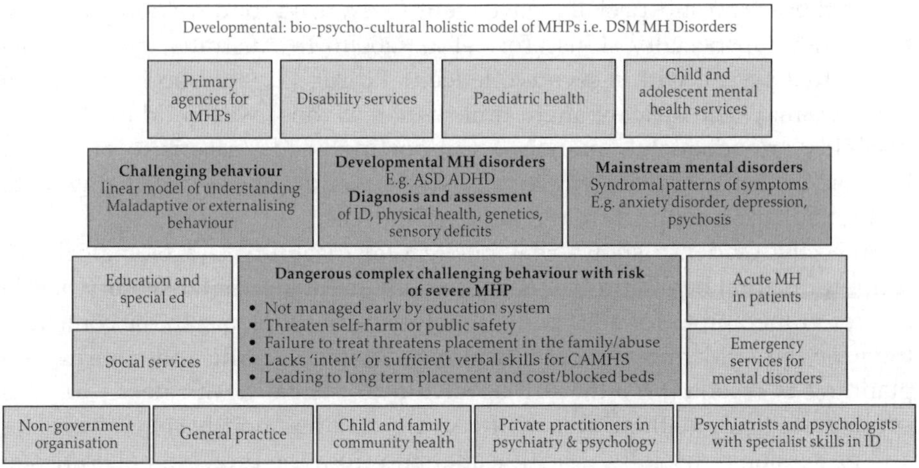

Figure 25.2 Understanding the pathways to care?

expert group can keep pace with the knowledge revolution for this population. This would enable a learning culture for the entire health system in this growing area of specialist knowledge.

Conclusion

The service development of the last generation has seen improvements in the capacity of professions and services to cure conditions, improve disabling problems, build compensatory skills, minimise handicap, improve the quality of care, and humanise support. Harnessing the advance of knowledge is the least costly intervention to continue the betterment of the quality of life of children and adolescents with intellectual disability, which is the basis of the proposed service model.

In the UK, the Royal College of Psychiatrists has set out service standards for a specialised comprehensive mental health service for children and adolescents with intellectual disability. This set of standards describes four tiers of specialist psychiatric service (Dugmore & Hurcombe, 2007). It sets a gold standard for benchmarking such psychiatric services internationally, and the UK has embarked on the road of providing separate specialist mental health services for this population. The literature indicates that subspecialty skills are required for an adequate service structure. The debate for professionals is: how much should these skills be mainstreamed into generic child and adolescent mental health services versus developing and maintaining separate subspecialty mental health services?

Psychiatrists in the UK, where they have a significant subspecialty in intellectual disability in children and adolescents, support an increase in mainstreaming of the specialty skills. On the other hand, psychiatrists in Australia, where there is no subspecialty, have identified a need for developing a workforce with subspecialty skills (Torr et al., 2008). In Australia, psychiatrists report that people with a severe intellectual disability are poorly treated in mainstream psychiatric inpatient units, whereas those with mild intellectual disability are adequately managed. Supporting paediatricians to provide a key role in these services will require strengthening the service pathway to and consultation support from child psychiatrists.

Since the evidence shows that intellectual disability is a biological risk factor for mental health problems, those with an intellectual disability have a greater vulnerability for all types of mental health problems. In the context of the growing epidemic of mental health problems, specific and coordinated planning is essential for the full spectrum of mental health needs for this special need population. This will require collaboration between agencies and professional disciplines, with leadership from the professional bodies to recognise the special clinical knowledge, skills, and programs. Thus, proactive political will is required to provide equitable services to meet the mental health needs of young people with intellectual disability.

26

A special school community: An inclusive setting for addressing the mental health needs of students with an intellectual disability

Jodie A. Caruana, Barbara Fleming, Hebah Saleh, Helen Goltzoff, and David Dossetor

Introduction

A collaborative framework that includes education, health, disability, and other service areas is critical for mental health promotion, prevention, and early intervention for students with an intellectual disability. Most students attend primary and secondary school for a cumulative total of approximately 15 000 hours, and public funding for education is the greatest financial investment that a society makes in terms of the future potential and well-being of children (Rutter et al., 1980). Research suggests that almost half (40.7 per cent) of the number of children and adolescents with an intellectual disability will experience mental health problems and disorders (Einfeld & Tonge, 1996b). This constitutes 14 per cent of the mental health burden for children and adolescents in our society (Emerson & Hatton, 2007). Special purpose schools provide a unique opportunity for collaboration between education, health, and disability professionals to ensure that students with an intellectual disability meet their full potential. Schools are a vital setting to promote mental health and well-being for students. Students with an intellectual disability, however, are often not well catered for. This chapter will focus on schools as mental health settings and the importance of prevention, promotion, and early intervention programs to address mental health problems and disorders for students with an intellectual disability.

Schools as mental health settings

Schools can promote positive mental health outcomes for students and, in turn, their school performance. Students' behaviour and attitudes are influenced by their experiences at school and by the characteristics of the school itself (Rutter et al., 1980). Research suggests that the school has an important impact on students' development, with a strong indication that the positive social features of a school afford success (Rutter et al., 1980).

As schools have such an influence on students, they are in a special position to intervene to promote the mental health and well-being of children and adolescents. Hendren and colleagues (1994) reported that the World Health Organization (WHO) had identified that schools were the best place to promote mental health universally, as almost all children and adolescents attend school. They described schools as strong social bodies that can be safety nets for protecting a child's or adolescent's psychological well-being, but can build or undermine a student's capacity and self-esteem (Hendren et al., 1994). Similarly, findings from the *National Survey of Mental Health in Australia* discussed how access to schools provided the opportunity to target large numbers of students with various interventions. This is especially important, as many mental health problems emerge during the school years (Sawyer et al., 2001). Although there is substantial evidence to suggest that mental health promotion, prevention, and early intervention are likely to have some effect on students in general, there is little research on the effects of such interventions in special schools that cater for students with an intellectual disability.

Mental health promotion, prevention, and early intervention programs for students with an intellectual disability

Mental health promotion, prevention, and early intervention programs are imperative for students with an intellectual disability for three main reasons. First, successful interventions may lead to a reduction in the incidence of new cases of mental health problems and disorders for students with an intellectual disability. Second, successful interventions may lead to a reduction in prevalence rates; that is, the number of students with intellectual disability presenting with mental health problems and disorders at any point in time. Finally, early intervention may reduce the social and financial burden of mental health; if left untreated during childhood or adolescence, mental health problems and disorders can become acute in early adulthood and may develop into serious and chronic psychiatric disorders (Hurley, 1996).

Approximately 70 per cent of all secondary schools in Australia currently utilise *MindMatters*, a whole school mental health promotion, prevention, and early intervention program (Rowling, 2007). Unfortunately, there are a lack of resources that are suitable for use with students with an intellectual disability. This is reflected in a much lower utilisation rate (less than 10 per cent) of similar programs by specific schools that cater for students with intellectual disability (Dossetor et al., 2009).

A recent literature review by Dossetor and colleagues (2009) highlighted the paucity of mental health promotion, prevention, and early intervention programs available to schools that cater for students with an intellectual disability. They examined 103 programs or resources recommended by two national whole-school mental health promotion programs that were aimed at general primary (KidsMatter Primary, Commonwealth Department of Health and Ageing, CDHA, n.d.) and secondary schools (MindMatters, CDHA, n.d). Only 10 programs were identified as being suitable for students with special needs, and only five of these programs were for students with a mild intellectual disability. These programs included: *Stop Think Do, Triple P Stepping Stones, PATHS, Social Decision Making/Social Problem Making Program,* and *Alert Program,* which will be discussed later in this chapter.

The *KidsMatter* (CDHA, n.d) program is a whole-school mental health promotion and prevention program, aimed at primary school students. This program has recently undergone a two-year trial and evaluation. The program contains four dimensions of intervention: (a) a positive school community; (b) social and emotional learning for students; (c) parenting support and education; and (d) early intervention for students experiencing mental health difficulties. These four dimensions provide an excellent framework and supportive structure for mental health promotion in schools.

The final evaluation of the two-year trial reported that the *KidsMatter* program reduced mental health difficulties and increased mental health strengths, particularly for those students who displayed higher levels of mental health difficulties at the start of the program (Slee et al., 2009). However, results were not reported by specific school or for students with an intellectual disability. The four components of the mental health framework utilised by *KidsMatter* will be further explored in relation to special schools that cater for students with an intellectual disability and the role of interagency collaboration in this process.

A positive school community

Various protective factors have been identified as influencing the development of mental health problems and disorders in children (see table 26.1). The majority of mental health promotion, prevention, and early intervention programs attempt to address the various individual, family, school, and

Table 26.1 Protective factors potentially influencing the development of mental health problems and mental disorders in individuals, particularly children

Individual factors	*Family factors*	*School context*	*Life events and situations*	*Community and cultural factors*
• Easy temperament • Adequate nutrition • Attachment to family • Above-average intelligence • School achievement • Problem-solving skills • Internal locus of control • Social competence • Social skills • Good coping style • Optimism • Moral beliefs • Values • Positive self-related cognitions	• Supportive caring parents • Family harmony • Secure and stable family • Small family size • More than two years between siblings • Responsibility within the family (for child or adult) • Supportive relationship with other adult (for a child or adult) • Strong family norms and morality	• Sense of belonging • Positive school climate • Prosocial peer group • Required responsibility and helpfulness • Opportunities for some success and recognition of achievement • School norms against violence	• Involvement with significant other person (partner or mentor) • Availability of opportunities at critical turning points or major life transitions • Economic security • Good physical health	• Sense of connectedness • Attachment to and networks within the community • Participation in church or other community group • Strong cultural identity and ethnic pride • Access to support services • Community/cultural norms against violence

Source: Commonwealth Department of Health and Aged Care (CDHAC, 2000). Reproduced with permission from the Commonwealth of Australia

community-related protective factors. Schools are a vital element in any broad-based mental health promotion strategy. It is crucial that programs and materials are available for teachers in special schools to enable them to develop and enhance protective factors of students regardless of their level of intellectual disability.

Positive behaviour for learning

In Australia, *Positive Behaviour for Learning (PBL)* is derived from the *Positive Behaviour Interventions and Supports (PBIS)* (TA Center, n.d.) program developed in the United States (Mooney, Dobia, Barker et al., 2008; Mooney, Dobia, Yeung et al., 2008). There are four main elements to PBIS: (a) supporting student behaviour; (b) supporting staff behaviour; (c) supporting decision-making; and (d) supporting social confidence and academic achievement. These elements are underpinned by behavioural science, practical interventions, lifestyle outcomes, and a systems perspective (PBIS) (TA Center, n.d.; Sugai et al., 2000).

More generally, PBIS is used to attain socially significant behaviour change (Sugai et al, 2000). For example, a study by Hetzroni (2003) focused on the effect of communication techniques on behaviour in a special school where the majority of the 67 students had a moderate intellectual disability. The study concluded that, while the student's communication abilities increased, the behaviour problems (such as hitting and biting) decreased. Additionally, a meta-analysis of interventions for challenging behaviours by Harvey and colleagues (2009) highlighted the effectiveness of PBIS. They found that behavioural treatments reduced challenging behaviours in children and youth with developmental disabilities. They noted that interventions that changed whole systems (schools) were mostly used in combination with other interventions, and therefore could not be evaluated on their own. Harvey and colleagues (2009) also reported that, in combination with other intervention types, systems change was moderately effective with self-injurious and aggressive behaviour, and highly effective with inappropriate social and destructive behaviour.

PBL is an emerging whole-school intervention that supports building a positive school community, addresses numerous protective factors in the school context, and has been linked to improved behaviour outcomes. Internationally, schools are utilising a positive behaviour framework to create a supportive school environment to improve academic and behaviour outcomes for students. A critical component of PBL, especially for students with complex needs, is the active involvement and training of the whole school community in developing and implementing strategies. Behaviour management is planned collaboratively with parents and other agencies where possible, explicitly taught, and reviewed regularly. Core values and agreed behaviours are also made explicit by using a common language within the school community and augmentative and alternative communication strategies (such as pictures and symbols).

A practical example of PBL in an Australian context is at a special school in South Western Sydney for students with an intellectual disability, where the school rules 'We learn, we are safe, we care' have been implemented. This whole-school system has included strategies for defining, teaching, and supporting appropriate behaviours and creating positive school environments. Following PBL implementation at the beginning of 2008 (term 1), data on specific problem behaviours (such as kicking, spitting, and throwing objects) were collected over approximately 18 months (until term 3, 2009). Analyses of the data indicated that problem behaviours significantly declined over this period; for example, throwing objects declined by 80 per cent, spitting and kicking declined by 75 per cent, and hair pulling declined by 72 per cent (Fleming, 2010). In addition, there was a significant increase in staff using PBL materials noticing and rewarding appropriate student behaviours.

Social and emotional learning for students

In recent years, schools have recognised that many students with an intellectual disability, while learning to express their wants and needs, still struggle to recognise and express their emotional states. Increasing independence for students with an intellectual disability can significantly improve both their ability to reach their potential and quality of life. One key component of developing independence is self-regulation of behaviour.

Teachers in some special schools have begun incorporating elements of emotional self-regulation into lessons, initially as part of PBL programs. Currently these lessons may include use of photos, symbols, and signs to help students learn to recognise and express feelings appropriately, pair feelings with appropriate behaviours, and pair feelings with behavioural choices. Computer programs, such as *The Transporters* (Golan et al., 2006), developed in the UK, and other resources, such as *Mind Reading* (University of Cambridge, 2002, an interactive CD-ROM), resources initially developed to assist students with ASD, are being utilised.

In addition, the review conducted by Dossetor and colleagues (2009) identified five programs that had empirical evidence for effectiveness in schools, and were suitable for addressing the social and emotional learning needs of students with an intellectual disability. Four of these programs are described below, with the addition of a description of a new program developed by The Children's Hospital at Westmead.

Stop, Think, Do social skills training program

The *Stop, Think, Do* program (Petersen, 2002, 2004; Petersen & Adderley, 2002) is an Australian program that focuses on problem solving and resolving conflicts. This program is implemented in groups, and Beck and Horne (1992) reported on its effectiveness in a special school catering primarily for secondary students with mild to moderate intellectual disability and emotional-social problems. Specific applications for this program include anxiety, ADHD and Asperger's syndrome. A parent program is also available.

Promoting Alternative Thinking Strategies (PATHS)

The *Promoting Alternative Thinking Strategies (PATHS)* program (Greenberg & Kusche, 1998), developed in the United States, consists of classroom lessons that teach primary school children how to change behaviours and attitudes that contribute to violence and bullying, how to express and control their emotions, and how to develop effective conflict-resolution strategies. This program has been shown to be effective with a number of special groups, including deaf and hearing-impaired students, behaviour disordered, learning disabled, and gifted students, as well as students from a wide diversity of ethnic, cultural, socioeconomic, and family backgrounds (Kam et al., 2004).

Social Decision Making/Social Problem Solving Program

The Social Decision Making/Social Problem Solving program (Elias & Bruene Butler, 2005), developed in the United States, consists of a series of classroom lessons. The program is designed to help children recognise and use their emotions in solving problems effectively in a wide range of real-life situations inside and outside the classroom. The program focuses on teaching self-control and social awareness skills as important tools for decision-making (Elias, 2004).

Alert Program for self-regulation
The Alert Program (Williams & Shellenberger, 1996) was developed in the United States. It promotes awareness of how to regulate arousal states, and encourages the use of sensorimotor strategies to manage levels of alertness. The program targets students with sensory-processing and/or learning impairments, and can be implemented with individual students or in groups.

Emotion Based Social Skills Training (EBSST)
A more recent program, *Emotion Based Social Skills Training (EBSST)* (Ratcliffe et al., 2010), is a skill-building curriculum for students with autism spectrum disorders (ASD) and a mild intellectual disability. It aims to teach emotional recognition, theory of mind, and problem solving, and therefore skills in relationships. This new program is being implemented in partnership with the Department of Education and Training as a school-based intervention in primary schools in NSW in 2010.

Parenting support and education

In special school settings, schools successfully collaborate with parents and carers for a variety of matters. At a special school in South Western Sydney, for example, such collaboration ranges from sharing information through visual home to school diaries and communication books, to the collaborative development of learning and behavioural programs, and, as needed, collaboration across family, school, and other services. Seminars and workshops are often run collaboratively with disability services and other non-government agencies on topics such as communication, managing behaviour, healthy activities to do with your child, and accessing support services. This valued strategy needs to be expanded and utilised with mental health programs to ensure that the family-based protective factors for positive mental health are developed (see table 26.1).

A Cochrane review by Diggle and McConachie (2002) found that there was some evidence that supported the benefits of parent training with children with ASD and their parents. Schools may be the best place to promote parent training as part of building their alliance with parents and promoting community integration. One mental health promotion program specifically for students with an intellectual disability and their parents is the *Standard Stepping Stones Triple P* program (Sanders et al., 2003). This parenting program can be implemented for individual children with intellectual disability by an accredited practitioner within a school environment. Alternatively, there is *Group Triple P* or *Group Teen Triple P* (Triple P International, n.d.), which provide group-based parent training that could be run within school; however, these are not specific to children with intellectual disability.

The Triple P–Positive Parenting Program 'draws on social learning, cognitive-behavioural and developmental theory, as well as research into risk and protective factors associated with the development of social and behavioural problems in children' (Triple P International, n.d.; The Triple P System section, ¶ 1). The *Standard Stepping Stones* program has been adapted for parents of children and adolescents who have a disability. The approach has been demonstrated to be effective for children with intellectual and physical disabilities who have disruptive behaviour (Roberts et al., 2006).

Early intervention for students experiencing mental health difficulties

Early intervention programs target students who display early signs and symptoms of mental health problems and disorders. Early intervention is essential, as a psychiatric disorder that is left untreated from childhood, or when it first appears, tends to develop into a more serious disorder in adulthood (Hurley, 1996). Indeed, it has been suggested that it is the failure of early detection and early intervention that leads to the long-term psychiatric morbidity, and high costs, particularly in out-of-home residential care. For students with an intellectual disability, the identification and screening of mental health problems and disorders is particularly difficult. This is a result of communication limitations and diagnostic overshadowing, whereby symptoms are attributed to the student's intellectual disability and not to a possible mental health problem or disorder.

Another major barrier to early mental health intervention for students with an intellectual disability is the capacity of professionals working with students to identify early symptoms of mental health problems or disorders. A study from the United Kingdom by Rose and colleagues (2009) surveyed 48 schools to examine the mental health issues of young people with special needs. The study identified that school staff faced problems isolating the features of intellectual disability, challenging behaviour, and mental health indicators, as the boundaries were often unclear, and staff felt ill prepared in dealing with the mental health needs of this group. A major finding of this study was the need to provide professional development on identification of mental health problems or disorders in students with learning disabilities (as intellectual disability is termed in the UK). School staff, such as teachers, require this professional development, as they are often the best placed to detect changes in mood or behaviour in students. In addition, the need to develop curriculum materials that address mental health and well-being issues for students with special needs was highlighted.

Professional development for school staff working with students with an intellectual disability, who may have coexisting mental health problems and disorders, needs to be inclusive of all school staff, not only the school

Advisers
Special education consultant
Special education teachers
Itinerant support teachers
- hearing impairment
- vision impairment
- integration
- transition

School learning support officers (teacher aides)
Support teacher, early intervention
Specialist personnel

Core members
- Parent/carer
- Principal and/or nominee
- Teacher/support teacher
- School counsellor
- Student

Advisers
Physiotherapist
Audiologist
Paediatrician
Psychologist
Community nurse
Speech pathologist
Occupational therapist
Community support worker

Figure 26.1 Supports available to students with disabilities in NSW schools
Source: adapted from NSW Department of Education, 1998

psychologist or counsellor. Professional development also needs to be extended to others who work with or care for children and adolescents with an intellectual disability, to ensure that the presenting problems are treated early, and do not lead to more serious disorders that can have an impact on the quality of life of both child and carer.

Collaboration between professionals

A fundamental element of mental health prevention and promotion programs within a special school setting for students with an intellectual disability is collaboration between professionals. A collaborative framework that includes education, health, disability, and other service areas is essential to ensuring effective prevention and treatment of mental health problems and disorders. Figure 26.1 outlines the array of staff who may be available to students with an intellectual disability in New South Wales (NSW) government schools, and highlights the potential for interagency collaboration, as numerous school and professional staff are recognised and valued as supports within an inclusive framework.

Professional roles

It is important to understand the resources that are available within each school to maximise the effectiveness of collaboration. The core members of a support system for a student with a disability are the parent or carer, principal, classroom and support teachers, and school counsellor (see figure 26.1). The core members and various advisers to the left of the circle are located within the education system, while those advisers listed to the right are located outside education, within the health and disability sectors. The roles of professionals involved in the collaborative process for students with intellectual disability are detailed below.

- *Learning support teams* in schools address the learning needs of students. The team ensures that collaborative planning and programming occur by bringing together key personnel within the school community to address students' many needs (such as curriculum, communication, social skills, personal care, safety, and mobility) (NSW Department of Education (DET), 1998).

- *School counsellors* share the responsibility for student welfare. They are responsible for a variety of assessments, counselling, and working in consultation with other professionals (such as teachers, the school, its management and administrators, parents or caregivers, and other agencies) to improve student learning and behaviour (NSW DET, 1998). In an Australian study, it was found that students were more likely to access a school counselling service than any other mental health service provider (Sawyer et al., 2001). The provision of school counselling differs across government and nongovernment sectors; however, very few school counsellors would have a full time allocation to one school.
- *The school principal* is a key link for interagency collaboration, especially in more specialised settings, when a school counsellor's availability may be limited. The NSW Minister for Education and Training, in a media statement about increased support for principals of specific purpose schools, stated, 'They [school principals] have a unique responsibility to care for some of our most vulnerable children and the challenges they face. They need time to speak with parents and external agencies about each student's learning needs' (Firth, 2008). Furthermore, Rowling (2007) highlighted that the planning and delivery of mental health promotion and prevention approaches within schools require the critical support of the principal and the executive team.
- *Teachers* cater for the diverse range of individual learning needs in classrooms, and are the best placed staff members within a school to detect changes in students' behaviours (Rose et al., 2009). However, in relation to mental health prevention and promotion activities within the classroom, Rowling (2007) argued that teachers need to be convinced of the link between the mental health of students and connectedness to school and academic performance.

Working with students with complex support needs requires close collaboration across the whole school community, including parents and carers. Enhancing communication with parents facilitates consistency in strategies used in both the school and home. Without this collaboration, outcomes for students will decline.

Although figure 26.1 is helpful in conceptualising the array of supports available to students, it does not completely capture the considerable web of professionals available to students with an intellectual disability and mental health problems and disorders. Additional 'advisers' who can be added to create an even more inclusive framework include, but are not limited to, education officers, education specialists, family doctors, developmental paediatricians, paediatric neurologists, geneticists, psychiatrists, family therapists, clinical psychologists, speech pathologists, and social workers. These group of advisers should be consulted and utilised in interagency collaboration for not only the management of a student with a recognised mental health problem or disorder but when developing or implementing promotion, prevention, or early intervention programs.

Baruch (2001) noted that, as special schools usually cater for a smaller number of students, there is greater possibility than in mainstream schools for formal and informal contact between the school psychologist or counsellor and school staff, students, and parents. Therefore opportunities for collaboration between external services and staff in the special school setting may also be improved. This may assist in the implementation of mental health promotion, prevention, and early intervention programs for students with an intellectual disability and complex needs.

A way forward

There are a number of ways of focusing on the mental health of students with an intellectual disability in schools. First, there is a clear need for education on the range of mental health problems that can be identified. Second, there is a need for systematic training in skills that enhance mental health, including the recognition of multidisciplinary subspecialty skills. The need for clear cross-agency pathways to collaboration also needs to be established. Last, more emphasis on mental health promotion, prevention, and early intervention is needed. Dossetor and colleagues (2009) indicated that there were valuable approaches being developed that need further promotion and development. Programs that cater for the complex support needs of students with an intellectual disability in more specialised settings need further developing, as the majority of programs outlined in this chapter are more suitable for students with a mild intellectual disability.

It has been identified that there are opportunities within the special school setting for external professionals to work collaboratively in improving the learning, support, and mental health needs of students with an intellectual disability. Professionals working with this client group need to identify opportunities at various local, regional, state, and even national levels to collaborate with a variety of sectors to best cater for this population. Schools need to remain inclusive in their approach to supporting students, and be recognised for their key role in the partnership with other professionals and agencies that share a responsibility for the optimal mental health of these young people.

A vital element in supporting students with an intellectual disability to realise their full potential is the recognition of the important role of mental heath promotion and prevention strategies as outlined this chapter. Exciting opportunities exist for interagency support and collaboration at the mental health preventative level. If an evidence base is developed for students with an intellectual disability attending special schools, these resources will have a much wider applicability, and include students with an intellectual disability and complex mental health needs in mainstream as well as special school settings.

27

The community clinician and interagency collaboration

Mary Ellen Burke, Meredith A. Martin, and Garry M. Dezilva

Introduction

Adolescents with an intellectual disability and emotional or behavioural difficulties place complex demands on the service system. In order to achieve effective outcomes for and with these clients, best practice includes the expectation that all stakeholders will work collaboratively. Collaboration is best expressed as a process of individuals and groups working together for mutual benefit, with an emphasis on building bridges between people and agencies to bring together the needed clinical skills and resources for the benefit of the patient or client (Darlington et al., 2005; Howarth & Morrison, 2007; Padgett et al., 2004; Sloper 2004).

In practice, the process of working collaboratively is very difficult to establish and maintain. This chapter explores interagency collaboration from the perspective of community clinicians or practitioners. Community clinicians are the individuals or teams who provide a service directly to the client and or his or her family or carer. They could include, for example, the case worker, community nurse, psychologist, psychiatrist, social worker, school counsellor, therapist, special educator, and other care workers, from different agencies or the same agency. Practical information and strategies are provided to assist community clinicians to decide when to choose a collaborative approach to service delivery, and how to participate effectively in collaborative partnerships.

The need for collaboration

The high prevalence of mental health disorders in people with an intellectual disability is a major issue for health and welfare service systems in Australia and elsewhere. Adolescents with an intellectual disability and a possible psychiatric disorder challenge existing service systems. These adolescents present with complex issues to a range of services that are also complex, and include various departments and agencies, each of which is responsible for some aspect of the support service. The clinical challenges have been well documented (see Slevin et al., 2008), and it is generally agreed that to serve this client group there is a need for significant specialised input from a number of sectors, including mental health, health, disability, education, families, and nongovernment agencies. Looking through a single lens is not adequate to meet the needs of these individuals. Effective services need to be based on consideration of the broader social context, individual issues confronting the person and their family or carer, and the characteristics of the agencies involved in providing services.

People with an intellectual disability and emotional or behavioural difficulties require an integrated, holistic approach to assist in and support adequate assessment and effective treatment interventions. What is needed is collaborative engagement of the person, his or her family, and support network with specialists from a range of professional backgrounds. *Collaboration* is a term used extensively when describing ways of providing services to people with complex needs. Reviews of 'good' service models and those that have proven inadequate reinforce the view that *collaboration* is seen as an essential element of good practice in this area. Often it is assumed that the term *collaboration* is understood, and that clinicians are familiar with what constitutes collaborative practice. Clinicians often 'believe' that they function in a collaborative framework. This is not necessarily the case.

Focus on community clinicians

The purpose of this chapter is to provide some practical information and strategies for community clinicians to assist them to (a) decide when it would be appropriate and feasible to establish a collaborative approach to service delivery for clients with complex presentations; and (b) effectively participate in a collaborative process of planning, decision-making, or problem solving.

Collaboration has many faces

Usually the term *collaboration* creates an image of a team of people working together, all focused on the same client. The team meets to determine goals, agree on tasks and processes, and how to measure outcomes. The team works well together, with the assistance of an effective team leader, who provides

Table 27.1 The features of collaborative endeavours

Communication → *Cooperation* → *Coordination* →	*Coalition* → *Integration*
Low-level collaboration	High-level collaboration
Limited or no formal agreements	Formal agreements
Agencies remain autonomous	Agencies sacrifice autonomy
Work towards different targets and goals	Work to shared goals and targets
Agency maintains control of resources and funding	Joint responsibility for resources and funding
Staff managed by individual service	Staff managed by partnership
Focus on individual case	Focus on whole service
Decision-making responsibility of agency	Joint decision-making
Collaboration likely to be voluntary or within guidance	Clear mandate for collaboration at government or state level
Variable practice dependent on individual	Specific focus of activity outlined in strategic plans
Affiliation to own agency and/or discipline	Affiliation to partnership
Accountable to agency	Accountable to partnership
Agency focused	Collaboration focused

Source: reproduced with permission from Howarth & Morrison, 2007, p. 57

clinical leadership to the members. Often this team consists of the client, family, and professionals from different disciplines with different roles in relation to the client. Usually there will be a person identified as the case manager. The membership may change over time as needs or knowledge change; however, everyone in the team has equal standing. In practice, the form of collaboration between agencies often does not look like this ideal, but incorporates key elements of collaborative processes.

The process of collaboration is about building bridges or connections between people rather than breaking down the agency 'silos' that often exist (Darlington & Feeney, 2007; Howarth & Morrison, 2007; Padgett et al., 2004; Sloper, 2004). This process can look different under a variety of conditions, but generally it describes a range of 'working together' arrangements. Howarth and Morrison (2007) have proposed a way of conceptualising the different ways collaborative relationships may look. They describe a possible continuum of collaborative partnerships identifying the features of informal local cooperative partnerships ('low level') to formal whole of agency

Table 27.2 Requirements for collaboration

Collaboration requires:

- inclusion and involvement of the client and significant family or carers throughout the process
- recognising and respecting each person's expertise
- trusting other team members or partners
- sharing knowledge and understanding of the client
- having a shared understanding of how services will be provided
- having a shared understanding of the client's context
- having one plan that sets the direction
- having equal ownership of the plan
- jointly defining needs and priorities
- sharing responsibility for the outcomes
- using a solution-focused problem-solving approach
- being active team members.

It does *not* mean:

- each person having his or her own plan and set of goals
- competition between stakeholders
- individuals doing their own thing and occasionally meeting to tell others what they are doing
- having an expert who directs the process
- ignoring the needs of the person and his or her family or carers
- ignoring the agreed ways of working; attending lots of meetings
- conducting the meeting in such away that contributions are excluded
- everyone doing the same thing.

collaboration ('high level'). Community clinicians need to consider where on the continuum their current arrangement is placed (see table 27.1).

The team or partnership formed around a specific client also needs to be considered. There will be a core team, and possibly secondary support to the core team, whose role may be temporary or intermittent. It is acknowledged that often there are many professionals and agencies involved in the support services. The right people need to be identified to enable collaborative work to be effective. These views of collaboration strongly indicate that community clinicians must consider issues of the team or partnership working as well as specific client-related issues. Membership of teams or partnerships will change over time. Maintaining connections and following agreed ways of working is fundamental to achieving effective outcomes. This means that the two aspects must be addressed, the process involved and the content that must be considered, such as clinical issues. In this chapter, the focus is on the low-level collaborative processes available to all community clinicians (see table 27.1). In practice, it is important that all team members understand that there are specific requirements of successful collaboration. These are outlined in table 27.2.

The experience of collaboration

Community clinicians who have worked in collaborative teams or in a collaborative partnership have different experiences and give varied feedback.

For some, the collaborative experience is a positive one; for example, 'Fabulous! Productive! I learned so much. It was so supportive I felt I could add to the success of the person. I found I did have something useful to contribute' (feedback from a case worker from disability services). For others it is a difficult and frustrating experience; for example, 'Every time we met I got really anxious that they would blame me; they [other agency] think we're hopeless so it was very upsetting; we got nowhere. Everyone tried to blame everyone else; the meeting was a waste of time. We all talked at cross purposes' (feedback from a case manager from mental health services).

Community clinicians are often in the frustrating position of trying to make a group of people function in a collaborative way and not succeeding. This sometimes results in blaming the client or his or her family for being uncooperative, too difficult, or just not engaged, blaming the other agencies for not playing the game properly, or feeling bad because the clinician couldn't get it right. To avoid this negative experience and to address some of the common difficulties, the following strategies are provided for clinicians to consider when establishing effective collaboration or when diagnosing and managing problems. Decisions made are based on the answers to the questions and the results of reflection on personal practice.

Steps in using a collaborative process

Step 1: Determine if collaboration is required

The community clinician needs to determine whether interagency collaboration is useful or necessary for the client and his or her family. There are two main reasons for agencies to collaborate, the needs of the client and the needs of the agencies. These reasons are explained in more detail below.

- *Needs of the client:* the provision of services to most clients with complex needs will require input from a variety of individual professionals within a number of agencies. Involvement can be at different stages of the intervention process—assessment, planning, intervention, and maintenance—and at primary, secondary, or tertiary levels. Often the type, intensity, and level of intervention varies throughout the course of the intervention process. This is particularly the case with people with complex needs where the course of intervention is not clear.
- *Needs of the agencies:* the demands placed upon any one agency to address the varied needs of clients with complex issues usually exceed the capacity of an individual organisation. Sharing of resources across agencies, including expert knowledge, is essential to inform the process of service delivery, creation of new options in response to clients' needs, and achievement of

outcomes. However, all agencies are cost conscious, and therefore it is important to focus on engaging with the minimum number of agencies necessary to meet the needs of the client and family, although discovering which agencies provide a network may be serendipitous.

Answers to the following questions guide decision-making about whether or not to establish a collaborative process.

1 Who needs collaboration? You? Client? Family? Agency?
2 What outcome is required? You? Client? Family? Agency?
3 Which level of the organisation should be engaged in this process—and is it possible?
4 Are there appropriately qualified people who can be involved?
5 What level of collaboration (low or high) is required and is possible? (see table 27.1.)

Step 2: What the community clinician needs to know

If it has been decided that a collaborative process is necessary, what does the community clinician need to know? Based on the literature and the authors' experiences of collaborative processes and teamwork with clients with complex issues, the community clinician will need to consider a number of key elements when attempting to establish effective collaboration partnerships. A checklist of questions to consider is included in appendix 27A (from p. 335). This outlines what community clinicians need to know about the person with complex needs, agencies involved, their own agency, themselves, and the collaborative process.

Step 3: Analysis of information gathered

The *community clinician checklist* (appendix 27A) can be utilised in a number of ways. Depending on the information gathered in response to the questions, it could used: to assist in identifying the skills needed to manage effectively and participate in collaborative processes; to clarify the desirability of engaging multiple agencies in a collaborative process; to determine the level of collaboration that is feasible and will result in effective client outcomes; and to identify significant barriers to the delivery of effective service and subsequent remedial strategies.

Step 4: Finding solutions to collaboration problems

The collaborative process is complex when meeting the needs of adolescents with intellectual disability and emotional and behavioural difficulties. Many issues that may arise when interagency collaboration is occurring may be averted if effective and open communication networks are established between all agencies involved. This is easily done with universal access to email by community clinicians. It is also essential that the client and family are included in the communication network, and that there are agreed criteria for sharing information. This is especially critical in high-risk or emergency situations, where a clear accountability structure within and across agencies is necessary.

Unfortunately, even with the best strategies in place, collaboration with multiple agencies does not always go smoothly. Appendix 27B (from p. 337) provides examples of what may happen or go wrong in the collaborative process, and some indicators for community clinicians that may assist them to identify what may be happening for them and suggestions for how to manage more effectively. A clear accountability structure is also essential when applying a problem-solving approach to the collaborative process.

Community clinicians are beholden to professional standards of conduct and process. They are accountable to management within their organisations. There is also peer group accountability between clinicians, which works on resolving differences and coming to agreements which are properly documented. However, where there are interagency difficulties or tensions in the collaborative team (such as disagreements in action or significant risks to the client), this should be brought to the attention of the managers of the agencies involved. This is where high-level agreement is essential for low-level collaboration to work. The accountability or support structure of each clinician needs to be public knowledge in the collaborative network. A failure to incorporate this knowledge may lead to formal complaints (especially when one agency feels that another is failing to meet their statutory obligations). These complaints can be costly in time and effort and damage future interagency relationships.

Conclusion

Working in a collaborative partnership to address the complex needs of adolescents with an intellectual disability and emotional or behavioural difficulties is not an easy task. The decision to move toward a collaborative endeavour should be made deliberately, following consideration of the ability of the partners to work and problem-solve together effectively. The responsibility of community clinicians is to develop skills in collaborative work, as well as in their specialist or professional area. All agreements or disagreements and outcomes of the collaborative process should be properly documented and circulated within the communication network. Documentation not only provides a formal and legal record, but it is also a measure of professional and clinical standards, and ensures the quality of the collaborative work.

The skill in managing the collaborative partnership is being comprehensive in framework and strategic planning, decision-making, and recommendations. The results of collaborative work can be judged from evaluation of outcomes for the clients and the development of networks of specialists prepared to jointly create new options and solutions for people with complex needs.

Acknowledgment

The authors would like to acknowledge the assistance of Janice Carroll from the New South Wales Department of Community Services in the development of this chapter. Her insights and experiences are incorporated into the chapter.

Appendix 27A

Community clinician checklist: key elements in establishing effective collaboration

What you need to know about the person with complex needs	*What you need to know about the other agencies involved*
• The reason the person is considered to be complex. Is this because there is not enough knowledge or information about the person's issues? Is the context difficult or complex? • Has anyone identified the needs holistically, or is everyone only looking at his or her part of the picture about the person? • Is the problem about diagnosis or treatment? • Which agencies agree on the analysis of what the 'clients problem' is and/or what is needed now? • Does the person and family have a relationship with the clinician or agency, and how does he or she experience it? • What are the outcomes expected by the client and his or her family and carer from a joint intervention?	• What agencies are actually involved? • What they are responsible for? • What is their involvement? Is it current? Is it within their usual client or service framework? • The personnel involved and their role in their agency: are they representing a service or themselves? • How does the agency usually provide a service? • What is the culture of the service? (including practices of sharing of information, process of decision-making, types of intervention, and length of involvement) • What is the language used to describe the agencies' service, and/or what is meant by terms usually involved in service delivery (such as assessment, individual plan)? • If a formal management plan exists, does it incorporate collaborative work with other agencies or identify them as being 'needed'? • What response does the agency provide in high-risk or emergency situations?
What you need to know about your own agency	*What you need to know about yourself*
• The reason your agency is involved • Whether the client falls within your agency's usual client group • Whether there is another reason for this client's high profile • If your agency supports interagency work, does a *memorandum of understanding* (MOU) between agencies or specific policies exist?	• Your role with this case • Limitations to your involvement • Your role in the process of collaboration • Whether you have the skills required to manage this case, i.e. substantive knowledge as a professional • Whether you have the experience and procedural knowledge of the agencies involved in the collaborative team

What you need to know about your own agency (Continued)	*What you need to know about yourself (Continued)*
• Identify who has decision-making responsibility • Whether your view of what should be implemented is supported by your agency • The philosophy of service delivery • Terminology that may need to be interpreted for other agency clinicians • The history of collaboration between agencies or individual clinicians (effective or ineffective?)	• Whether you have case management responsibility • The support you have from your manager or agency to participate in the collaborative process • Where you fit in terms of power and/or authority in the collaborative team
What you need to know about the collaborative process	
• Has the actual process of partnership been agreed? • Have goals been set for the client and stakeholders, and agreed upon by all agencies? • Has agreement been reached about accountability and commitment by all parties? • Has a process for communication been agreed for the primary team and for higher-level communication by all agencies? • Is there commitment by both senior and direct staff to the process? • Is there strong leadership or a multiagency steering group for this process? • Does an agreement exist about implementation time frames?	

Source: adapted from Carnaby, 2007; Darlington & Feeney, 2007; Howarth & Morrison, 2007; Kvarnstrom, 2008; Mohr et al., 2002; NSW Department of Ageing Disability and Home Care, 2004; Sloper, 2004; Simpson, 2007; Xyrichis & Lowton, 2008

Appendix 27B

Common experiences of collaboration

What's happening	*Indicators*	*Where do I go?*
Pseudo-collaboration	• Agencies are either unable or unwilling to share information. There may be different understandings and policies related to privacy and confidentiality • Statements by team members such as: 'We have our own plans'; 'It's really your problem'; 'You will need to sort out your management problems if you want us to help'; or inability to move beyond repeated descriptions or declarations of 'the problem' • A feeling that an agency is showing 'all care but no responsibility' • No time being spent establishing common ground for all those involved	• Focus on establishing or reestablishing the collaborative process, including agreements and common ground about goals, processes, roles and expectations • Clarify privacy provisions • If necessary, engage the hierarchy of both (all) agencies involved to address systemic issues, such as sharing of information • Understand the limitations and strengths of each agency or service, then look at ways to be more innovative and creative to achieve the desired outcomes
Just sort it out!	• Interagency collaboration is often seen as a 'fix-it' solution to a 'crisis'. Higher levels of management can direct this to happen, particularly when there is a crisis or there is some political pressure to solve the problem quickly	• Pressure to solve problems does not always create an environment of cooperation and collaboration between agencies and clinicians. While the identification of a team to address problems may be seen as an answer, it is really the first step only • The team needs to develop a joint understanding and agreement of what is actually required • Examine and prioritise short-term, medium-term, and long-term options • Raise the strategies and analysis with senior people in each organisation

What's happening	*Indicators*	*Where do I go?*
Who's in charge of this team?	• A person or agency appears to have greater authority than others, which does not match agreed roles and responsibilities. Often this is an informal arrangement that can undermine collaborative casework	• The team leader's role needs to be clarified and assigned • Decision-making processes to be agreed, including an escalation process for issues of concern • Joint training and supervision to maintain agreed focus and roles
Contact is not collaboration	• Team members have no contact of any kind between meetings • Partners may feel that 'we meet because we have to' • Little or no progress is made on agreed tasks from meeting to meeting	• Team leader to assess lines of functional communication and monitor compliance • Team leader to actively manage the interaction, focused on attaining goals and agreed actions
Agency ambush!	• Disagreements or concerns within an agency may result in additional people attending the team meeting or bringing internal issues to this forum • Raising issues unrelated to the intervention and support plan	• Establish who attends the meetings and what role they fulfil • New attendees need to be introduced with a purpose that relates to implementing the agreed plan or to inform the understanding of the client's needs and issues • Shared understanding of how meetings will be conducted • Identify team leader to manage the meetings
Blame the others	• The unstated views of some team members or partners are that others are not working competently with the client. Individuals or agencies presume that they have the 'right view' and/or attempt to direct others to 'do their jobs properly' • There is an assumption that one agency is better or more professional than another	• Participants need to take time to listen and learn about each service or agency and the context in which the clinicians operate. Also see section above on pseudo-collaboration • Acknowledge the specialised knowledge and contribution of others • Focus on a strengths-based approach
Passing the hot potato	• Despite attempts to address issues, no progress has been made • Comments such as: – 'What more can we do? This client is beyond our resources.' – 'Lucky you're here—we have done all we can so now it's up to you!'	• There may be a sense of the client being dumped • Work through the requirements for collaboration • Stick with the agreed process of how you will operate and escalate issues of concern • Apply the escalation process to more senior levels in agencies to assist in resolving areas of concern (see table 27.1)

Conclusion

David Dossetor

Developmental framework for neuropsychiatric conditions

There is no doubt that children and adolescents with intellectual disability and mental health problems are challenging for families and the practitioners who support them. There may be no easy answers or solutions, but there are some valuable lessons to help make a difference. This includes the application of holistic professional practice that combines a bio-developmental-psycho-social-cultural framework, evidence-based medicine, values-based practice, and collaboration.

The developmental component of the framework is the area of importance for this population. The term *developmental* has traditionally been used to imply that certain aspects of behaviour change over time. In those with intellectual disability the emphasis is on the need to consider development as a sequence of acquiring skills, understanding, and, indeed, conscious mindfulness. In the absence of adequate scientific knowledge of the complexity of development and of deviancy from these processes, developmental theory provides a guiding framework for understanding disability and intervention.

Considering symptoms from several theoretical frameworks at the same time is not new for child mental health practitioners. Similarly, models of the development of emotional recognition, theory of mind, an internal voice, intersubjectivity, and social reciprocity may do more to help us understand and treat autistic spectrum disorders (ASD) than tracking genetic or biochemical markers. There is little doubt that the problems that children and adolescents with intellectual disability present with are frequently a result of biological difference, and are often among the most challenging that professionals working in mental health encounter.

Service differentiation of mental health disorders

One experience of the training events for the educational program was that some of the ideas and information presented were commonplace for some practitioners, but novel for others. This variation was dependent on the practitioners' professional backgrounds, previous training, experiences, and work settings (such as disability services, mental health services, and educational settings). Approaches to understanding difficult behaviour are dichotomised into *challenging behaviour* and *mental disorder.* The former (externalising and disruptive disorders) are based on a linear model of behaviour (antecedent, behaviours, and consequences), the latter on the recognition of syndromes or patterns of behaviour that go together in meaningful associations. One is derived from behavioural and social psychology, and the other from the medical model. However, both these models have come to rely on both environmental and biological causal factors, such as neurochemical systems and physical ill-health.

All practitioners have to be aware of these models, albeit to different degrees. However, in practice, many mental health services do not provide significant treatment services for externalising and disruptive disorders, with a few exceptions. Additionally, it is suggested that there is a third group of developmental psychiatric conditions that are now not seen as core mental health. This group includes young people with autism and ADHD, for whom paediatricians provide the mainstream of service. This is not to malign mental health services, but illustrates that as understanding grows about mental health needs, resources do not, so are devolved to general paediatrics and community health.

Furthermore, the *Diagnostic and Statistical Manual of Mental Disorders* (DSM) and *International Classification of Diseases* (ICD) have grown from a process of categorising members of the community who present with severe mental health impairment requiring treatment services. With the expansion of psychology and epidemiology, there is growing acceptance that most troubled emotion and behaviour can be better understood in a dimensional frame of more healthy and competent to less healthy and impaired (Hudziak et al., 2007). However, when working with children and adolescents with intellectual disability and mental health problems, the developmental context has to be taken into account. That is, their mental health should be considered in relation to the norms for developmental competence or mental developmental age before taking account of other dimensional or categorical models of understanding mental ill-health, whether this is due to environmental vulnerability (as occurs in conduct disorder) or genetic vulnerability (as occurs in ADHD).

Validity of the developmental framework

A developmental model is difficult to validate. A number of child psychiatric disorders have moved from a categorical to a dimensional concept with epidemiological-based research, notably in the diagnosis of ASD and ADHD. This reflects moving from a research hypothesis of single gene or brain defect as an explanation of these disorders to a multifactorial model of growing complexity. Psychometric studies don't help us either. The measures of autism, in terms of social intelligence, compared with a normal population, are two to three standard deviations outside of the norm. With this level of difference, it isn't possible to determine whether this might be a developmental or dimensional disorder. As observed in chapter 20, there are significant questions about the reliability and validity of mainstream psychiatric disorders in those with moderate and severe intellectual disability. Particularly in those with intellectual disability, there is room for constructive questioning of mental health orthodoxy. The implicit risk and harm of a categorical or deconstructive model is that it medicalises a disorder, such as autism, and assumes there will be a specific medical intervention. Such assumptions contribute to the stigma of difference and families feeling powerless to help such a child.

Developmental models, such as those of Piaget and Kohlberg, have had powerful influences in child psychology. Attachment theory, in addition to cognitive development, emphasises the importance of the environment and relationships to development. In practice, many specialist clinicians of different disciplines working with children and adolescents with intellectual disability work from an underlying developmental framework. It has not, however, been promoted as a coherent crossdisciplinary model. A developmental framework makes such disorders understandable by comparison with other children of equivalent mental or social developmental age. This is humanising for the child and family, and creates a common language and goal to promote development rather than cure.

There remains a tension between basic research, which uses deconstructive hypotheses, versus child- and family-centred clinical approaches, which work from the face validity of a developmental framework. This tension is helpful in terms of enhancing knowledge of the efficacy of different interventions. However, the best evidence supports family- and environment-based interventions for parenting skills and behaviour management. Neuroscience and psychopharmacology also have a role, but this is the language of subspecialty disciplines with limited demonstrated validity. In the absence of a scientific leap creating a paradigm shift, the dominant framework should be developmental. Science will continue to make incremental advances, but it is probable that the development of the brain and the mind is sufficiently complex that a paradigm shift is not likely. It is more likely that small shifts will add to the understanding of developmental processes and sequences. Although child psychiatry teaches clinicians to consider competing explanatory models of disorder, in the mental health of children and adolescents with intellectual disability, the developmental model of emotions and behaviour is central.

Collaboration and the modern multidisciplinary team (MDT)

A developmental framework enables a common language across different members of the multidisciplinary team. In practice in Australia, where there is no specialist mental health service for people with intellectual disability, these models help guide where first to seek help. For example, challenging behaviour is first dealt with by disability services, developmental psychiatric conditions by paediatricians, and other psychiatric syndromes by mainstream mental health services. The more complex, severely disabling, and co-occurring conditions require close collaboration between these three service systems and special education services.

Families are the cornerstone, not just of the care of these children and adolescents, but the best source of management and treatment of their most troubling problems. Families have not been sufficiently engaged in the partnership with practitioners in the process of understanding what they can do for their children and what service providers need to do to enable them. This partnership still needs to advocate for significantly greater recognition and greater provision of services in communities.

The establishment of a common language and knowledge base through the educational program has begun the process of defining what distinct specialist skills and training are required for expert clinical practice in meeting the mental health problems in intellectual disability (see table C1). Working at the coal face of tertiary clinical cases with clinical research questioning is likely to be the most fruitful source of innovation in intervention (Kealey, 2008).

Skills development in the clinical areas highlighted in table C1 would assist clinicians in the provision of specific interventions for addressing the needs of this complex group of young people with autism and intellectual disability. Recently, the importance of treatment approaches focused on skill building was emphasised by a parent presenter at a seminar for parents and carers. The parent spoke with the clarity of experience when she advised, 'Don't waste your time looking for a cure for autism; there is no cure for autism. What matters is working on building skills for your child in both their strengths and their weaknesses' (Wilson, 2009).

Table C1 Areas of clinical expertise and innovation in mental health and intellectual disability

	Clinical expertise and innovation
1	Specialist evidence-based parent training skills e.g., *Stepping Stones Triple P* (Sanders et al., 2003)
2	General health promotion and prevention, especially with a focus on other chronic disabilities
3	School-based prevention and early interventions e.g.: • a Positive behaviour learning • b Inclusion approaches and practices • c Inclusive communication strategies • d Focus on developing mindfulness of self and others • e Focus on emotion-based social skills learning
4	The role of exercise and coordination for self-esteem, motor–sensory modulation, and attention
5	Sensory profiling and sensory diet interventions for management of arousal levels and motor calmness, relaxation, and playfulness e.g., floortime (Greenspan & Wieder, 1998)
6	Augmentative and alternate communication, especially capitalising on using new electronic devices for socially acceptable forms of visual communication
7	Problem-solving and self-monitoring skills
8	Emotion-based social skills training
9	Modification of cognitive behaviour skills therapy
10	Neurobiological research e.g., based on behavioural phenotypes, new metric and imaging techniques, and the effects of medication

The need for an action plan of service development and function

The need to have access to the skills of a *multidisciplinary team (MDT)* (as outlined in table C1) for complex cases necessitates collaboration (at minimum) between doctors, dentists, psychiatrists, psychologists, speech pathologists, occupational therapists, family therapists, physiotherapists, nurses, teachers, and school counsellors. There is evidence to indicate that equity of access requires availability to each of these disciplines. However, these clinicians also need to have specialist experience and expertise in intellectual disability, and be supporting of and engaged with their non-specialist colleagues in the same discipline. Multidisciplinary collaboration is required between practitioners in the different agencies of health, mental health, disability, and education. The family needs also require the engagement of a whole-of-government approach, including social services and welfare, housing, police, criminal justice, advocacy, legal services, and, of course, the growing non-government sector.

The collaborative process is difficult in terms of practitioner skills and organisational rationing of services, but essential for complex cases. Complex cases therefore need a charter of collaboration for adequate service provision. Limited resources require a tier structure of services, whereby higher tiers provide case-centred management advice and educational support for lower tiers. Distance need not be an excuse, with modern video consultations between tiers of service. The quality of collaboration has to be measured across agency to provide an external measure of efficacy. Services need to be designed to be 'forever learning'. The services, the tiers, the charter of collaboration, and measures of outcomes and collaboration need to be made open to public access and scrutiny.

Holland (2009) described some of the components for and complexity of assessment and formulation for adults with intellectual disability, components that can also be applied to children and adolescents with intellectual disability. They include:

- consideration of individuals' different trajectories of development because of biological, temperamental, and environmental qualities
- assessment of the nature and extent of impairments and associated disabilities
- the contribution of developmental disorders, sensory issues, physical health, and psychiatric illnesses
- the influence of life circumstances
- skills to cope with the demands of their environment
- system factors, including the quality of attachment and relationships with family, community, and services.

Such assessments lead to a formulation and a hypothesis of what may be causing the current predicament, which is then tested by the process of intervention. However, formulation requires the MDT to be able to weight the different components of the evaluation and apply clinical judgments. Optimal clinical judgment is only possible with experience, mutual professional trust, and flexibility, as not all team members will be equal in understanding a clinical predicament. Thus many, various intervention approaches may be taken by the MDT. Some examples of different clinical formulations include:

- nothing further can be done without a shift in family relationships and attitudes, treating parental mental health problems or responding to parental burnout, including respite care
- medication is a first necessity for bringing about change for other approaches to be helpful
- a combination of approaches is needed, such as a functional analysis, enhancing communication skills, a sensory assessment, family and cultural assessment, and neuropsychiatric testing

- a systems theory review of individual, family, and service provider relationships is required.

There are also clinical ethical considerations associated with engagement, assessment, and intervention; for example, that of identifying disability in the absence of adequate services for the juvenile offender with impaired communication and moral insight, who prefers to be identified as 'bad' rather than 'disabled'.

The need for multidisciplinary subspecialty mental health teams

It is evident that, for the more intellectually disabled and those with more serious disturbance and disorder, it is important to have psychiatrists and clinicians from other allied health disciplines who identify as having special expertise in intellectual disability. Not only is such expertise needed for optimal service provision for different subgroups of those with intellectual disability in terms of quality of life, morbidity, and mortality, but it is likely to save significant costs for the broader community through enhancing autonomy and reducing dependency on long-term government welfare and care. Recognising the need for subspecialty skills also challenges professional organisations to recognise their value and to support workforce development in such subspecialty skills. This is a huge challenge, as professional bodies all too readily marginalise subspecialty expertise, under similar political and social pressures faced by people with an intellectual disability of any age.

Advocacy: families that care, and acceptance by the community

The breakdown of extended family networks and loss of community connection is slowly generating a catastrophe of care, particularly for children and adolescents with intellectual disability. More needs to be done to help break down the prejudice, stigma, and social isolation that these families experience. The frequency with which practitioners encounter parents with murder–suicide ideation reflects the lack of community recognition of need and inadequate community-based support services. Murder–suicide is such a publicly horrific event when it occurs. Every clinician, friend, and neighbour should be alert to this alarm bell of coping breakdown, and recognise their duty to make a difference. The level of distress and potential for adverse events should be a wake-up call for the need for comprehensive mental health services for children and adolescents with intellectual disability.

Studying the development of the mind: is it a prerequisite to understanding losing one's mind?

Development of the mind involves developing capacities of:

- identification of self and non-self
- motor regulation and coordination
- arousal modulation and selective attention
- communication skills and an internal voice
- mood regulation
- self-concept
- reciprocal social interaction
- reality testing and perspective taking.

The external validation of this process is the capacity for developing good-quality peer attachment relationships as the best measure of youth mental health and future mental health as an adult.

Nonetheless, the closer professionals get to understanding the neurobiology of the basis of mental illness, it is suspected that it will be found that there are a range of commonalities between the processes of development of the mind and losing one's mind (Starling & Dossetor, 2009). Indeed, genetic research suggests that biology of mental processes involves considerable commonality of processes between the two (Mouridsen & Hauschild, 2008). Mainstream psychiatry and mental health services should pay greater heed to understanding the developmental processes witnessed in those with intellectual disability and autism, even if it is only to further understand the processes of mental illness of the mainstream adult population. Mainstream mental health clinicians may also be drawn to the fascination of better understanding the developing mind, and as a result show greater interest in the plight of those with intellectual disability and mental health problems, and add their voice to advocate for this needy population.

References

Aarts, M. (2008). *Marte Meo: Basic Manual* (rev. 2nd edn). Eindhoven, Netherlands: Aarts Productions.

Abbeduto, L. & Hesketh, L. J. (1997). Pragmatic development in individuals with mental retardation: Learning to use language in social situations. *Mental Retardation and Developmental Disabilities Research Reviews, 3*, 323–3.

Abbeduto, L., Warren, S. F., & Conners, F. A. (2007). Language development in Down syndrome: From the prelinguistic period to the acquisition of literacy. *Mental Retardation and Developmental Disabilities Research Reviews, 13*, 247–61.

Abrams, E. Z. & Goodman, J. F. (1998). Diagnosing developmental problems in children: Parents and professionals negotiate bad news. *Journal of Paediatric Psychology, 23*(2), 87–98.

Abu-Akel, A. (2003). The neurochemical hypothesis of 'theory of mind'. *Medical Hypotheses, 60*(3), 382–6.

Access Economics (2005). *The Economic Value of Informal Care: Report by Access Economics Pty Limited for Carers Australia.* Retrieved 24 November 2009 from <http://www.communities.wa.gov.au/serviceareas/seniorscard/Documents/The_Economic_value_of_informal_care_2005.pdf>.

Achenbach, T. M. (1991). *Manual for the Child Behavior Checklist/4–18 and 1991 Profile.* Burlington, VT: Department of Psychiatry, University of Vermont.

Adamson, W. C. (1972). Helping parents of children with learning disabilities. *Journal of Learning Disabilities, 5*, 326–30.

Adnams, C. (2008). *Poverty and Intellectual Disabilities: A View from Africa.* Cape Town: Plenary Presentation at the 13th IASSID World Congress. Abstract: *Journal of Intellectual Disability Research, 52*(8–9), 639.

Ægisdóttir, S., White, M. J., Spengler, P. M., Maugherman, A. S., Anderson, L. A., Cook, R. S., Nichols, C. N., Lampropoulous, G. K., Walker, B. S., Cohen, G., & Rush, J. D.. (2006). The meta-analysis of clinical judgment project: Fifty-six years of accumulated research on clinical versus statistical prediction. *Counseling Psychologist, 34*(3), 341–82.

Ahn, R. R., Miller, L. J., Milberger, S., & McIntosh, D. N. (2004). Prevalence of parents' perceptions of sensory processing disorders among kindergarten children. *American Journal of Occupational Therapy, 58*(3), 287–93.

Alborz, A. (2003). Transitions: Placing a son or daughter with intellectual disability and challenging behaviour in alternative residential provision. *Journal of Applied Research in Intellectual Disabilities, 16*, 75–88.

Aldwin, C. M. (1994). *Stress, Coping, and Development: An Integrative Perspective.* New York: Guildford Press.

Alexander, F. & Selesnick, S. (1966). *The History of Psychiatry: An Evaluation of Psychiatric Thought and Practice from Prehistoric Times to the Present.* New York: Harper & Row.

Allen, D. & Davies, D. (2007). Challenging behaviour and psychiatric disorder in intellectual disability. *Current Opinion in Psychiatry, 20*(5), 450–5.

Allen, G., Buxton, R. B., Wong, E. C., & Courchesne, E. (1997). Attentional activation of the cerebellum independent of motor involvement. *Science, 275*(5308), 1940–3.

Allet, L., Burge, E., & Monnin, D. (2008). ICF: Clinical relevance for physiotherapy? A critical review. *Advances in Physiotherapy, 10*(3), 127–37.

Allington-Smith, P. (2006). Mental health of children with learning disabilities. *Advances in Psychiatric Treatment, 12,* 130–40.

Aman, M. G. (1991a). *Assessing Psychopathology and Behavior Problems in Persons with Mental Retardation: A Review of Available Instruments.* Rockville, MD: US Department of Health and Human Services.

Aman, M. G. (1991b). Review and evaluation of instruments for assessing emotional and behavioural disorders. *Australia and New Zealand Journal of Developmental Disabilities, 17,* 127–45.

Aman, M. G. (1993). Efficacy of psychotropic drugs for reducing self-injurious behaviour in the developmental disabilities. *Annals of Clinical Psychiatry, 5,* 171-88.

Aman, M. G. & Singh, N. N. (1986). *Aberrant Behavior Checklist Manual.* East Aurora, NY: Slosson Educational Publications.

Aman, M. G. & Singh, N. N. (1994). *Supplement to the Aberrant Behavior Checklist Manual.* East Aurora, NY: Slosson Educational Publications.

Aman, M. G., Tassé, M. J., Rojahn, J., & Hammer, D. (1996). The Nisonger CBRF: A child behavior rating form for children with developmental disabilities. *Research in Developmental Disabilities, 17,* 41–57.

American Academy of Child and Adolescent Psychiatry (AACAP, 2007). Practice parameters for the assessment and treatment of children and adolescents with attention deficit hyperactivity disorder. *Journal of the American Academy of Child and Adolescent Psychiatry, 46*(7), 894–920.

American Association of Intellectual and Developmental Disability (AAIDD, 2002a). *Family Support Position Statement.* Retrieved 17 December 2008 from <http://www.aaidd.org/content_149.cfm?navID=31>.

American Association of Intellectual and Developmental Disability (AAIDD, 2002b). *Inclusion Position Statement.* Retrieved 17 December 2008 from <http://www.aaidd.org/content_161.cfm?navID=31>.

American Association of Intellectual and Developmental Disability (AAIDD, 2009). *Frequently Asked Questions: What Is the Official AAIDD Definition of Intellectual Disability?* Retrieved 13 November 2009 from <http://www.aaidd.org/IntellectualDisabilityBook/content_2678.cfm?navID=282>.

American Psychiatric Association (APA, 1994). *Diagnostic and Statistical Manual of Mental Disorders* (4th edn). Washington, DC: American Psychiatric Association.

American Psychiatric Association (APA, 2000). Diagnostic and statistical manual of mental disorders (4th ed., text revision). Washington, DC: Author.

Anderson, H., Angelo, F., Stewart, R., & Taylor, J. (2007). Special boys' business. Victoria, Australia: Secret Girls' Business.

Angelo, F., Pritchard, H., Stewart, R., & Davey, J. (2005). *Special Girls' Business.* Melbourne: Secret Girls' Business.

Anger, N. (1999). Communication disorders in child and adolescent mental health. *Australian Communication Quarterly*, February 1999, 5–13.

Antshel, K., Phillips, M., Gordon, M., Barkley, R., & Faraone, S. (2006). Is ADHD a valid disorder in children with intellectual delays? *Clinical Psychology Review, 26*(5), 555–72.

Attfield, E. (2009). Blue sky thinking? I don't think so. *Advances in Mental Health and Learning Disabilities, 3*(2), 36–9.

Attwood, T. (2004). *Exploring Feelings: Cognitive Behaviour Therapy to Manage Anger.* Slacks Creek, QLD: Future Horizons.

Audet, L. R. & Hummel, L. J. (1990). A framework for assessment and treatment of language-learning disabled children with psychiatric disorders. *Topics in Language Disorders, 10*(4), 57–74.

Australian Bureau of Statistics (ABS, 2005). *Australian Social Trends 2005* (ABS Document cat. no. 4102.0). Available from <http://www.abs.gov.au/AUSSTATS/abs@.nsf/DetailsPage/4102.02005?OpenDocument>.

Australian Bureau of Statistics (ABS, 2006). *Australia's Population. Census Data 2006.* Retrieved 8 December 2009 from <http://www.abs.gov.au/>.

Australian Institute of Health and Welfare (AIHW, 2004). *Carers in Australia: Assisting Frail Older People and People with a Disability.* AIHW Cat. No AGE 41. Canberra: AIHW (Aged Care Series No 8). Retrieved 13 November 2009 from <http://www.aihw.gov.au/publications/index.cfm/title/10064>.

Australian Medical Workforce Advisory Committee (AMWAC, 1999). *The Specialist Psychiatry Workforce in Australia: Supply, Requirements and Projections 1999–2010.* AMWAC Report 1999.7. Retrieved 10 December 2009 from <http://www.nhwt.gov.au/documents/Publications/1999/The%20specialist%20psychiatry%20workforce%20in%20Australia.pdf>.

Bagenholm, A. & Gillberg, C. (1991). Psychosocial effects on siblings of children with autism and mental retardation: A population based study. *Journal of Mental Deficiency Research, 35*, 291–307.

Bagner, D. M. & Eyberg, S. M. (2007). Parent–child interaction therapy for disruptive behaviour in children with mental retardation: A randomized controlled trial. *Journal of Clinical Child and Adolescent Psychology, 36*, 418–29.

Bailey Jr, D. B., Armstrong, F. D., Kemper, A. R., Skinner, D., & Warren, S. F. (2009). Supporting family adaptation to presymptomatic and 'untreatable' conditions in an era of expanded newborn screening (Electronic version). *Journal of Pediatric Psychology, 34*(6), 648–61.

Baker, B. L., & Feinfield, K.A. (2007). Early intervention and parent education. In Carr, A. (ed.). *The Handbook of Intellectual Disability and Clinical Psychology Practice* (pp. 336–64). New York: Routledge, Taylor, & Francis.

Baker, B. L., McIntyre, L. L., Blachner, J., Crnic, K., Edelbrock, C., & Low, C. (2003). Pre-school children with and without developmental delay: Behaviour problems and parenting stress over time. *Journal of Intellectual Disability Research, 47*(4/5), 217–30.

Baker, J. E. (2003). Social skills training, for children and adolescents with Asperger syndrome and social-communication problems. Shawnee Mission, KS: Autism Asperger Publishing Company.

Balogh, R., Bretherton, K., Whibley, S. Berney, T., Graham, S. Richold, P., Worsley, C., & Firth, H. (2001). Sexual abuse in children and adolescents with intellectual disability. *Journal of Intellectual Disability Research, 45*(3), 194–201.

Baranek, G. T., Boyd, B. A., David, F. J., Poe, M. D., & Watson, L. R. (2007). Hyperresopnsive sensory patterns in young children with autism, developmental delay, and typical development. *American Journal on Mental Retardations, 112*(4), 233–45.

Baranek, G. T., Foster, L. G., & Berkson, G. (1997). Tactile defensiveness and stereotyped behaviors. *American Journal of Occupational Therapy, 51*(2), 91–5.

Barkley, R. A. (1997). *ADHD and the Nature of Self-control*. New York: Guilford Press.

Barlow, D. H., Raffa, S. D., & Cohen, E. M. (2002). Psychosocial treatments for panic disorders, phobias, and generalized anxiety disorder. In Nathan, P. E. & Gordon, J. M. (eds). *A Guide to Treatments that Work* (2nd edn) (pp. 301–36). New York: Oxford University Press.

Barlow, D. H., & Rapee, R. M. (1997). *Mastering Stress: A Lifestyle Approach*. Sydney: Lifestyle Press.

Barnhill, G. P. (2002). Designing social skills intervention for students with Asperger syndrome (electronic version). *NASP Communique*, 31(3). Retrieved 2 October 2006 from <www.nasponline.org/publications/cq313asperger_ss.html>.

Barrett, P. M. (2000).Treatment of childhood anxiety: Developmental aspects. *Clinical Psychology Review, 20*(4), 479–94.

Barrett, P. M. (2004). *Friends for Life! For Children: Participant Workbook And Leaders Manual*. Brisbane: Australian Academic Press.

Barrett, P. M. (2005). *Friends for Life! For Youth: Participant Workbook and Leader Manual*. Brisbane: Australian Academic Press.

Barrett, P. M. (2007a). *Fun Friends. Family Learning Adventure: Resilience Building Activities for 4, 5, and 6 Year Old Children*. Brisbane: Fun Friends Publishing.

Barrett, P. M. (2007b). *Fun Friends. The Teaching and Training Manual for Group Leaders*. Brisbane: Fun Friends Publishing.

Barrett, R. P., Feinstein, C., & Hole, W.T. (1989). Effects of naloxone and naltrexone on self-injury: A double-blind, placebo controlled analysis. *American Journal on Mental Retardation, 93*, 644–51.

Bartolo, P. A. (2002). Communicating a diagnosis of developmental disability to parents: Multiprofessional negotiation frameworks (electronic version). *Child: Care, Health and Development, 28*(1), 65–71.

Baruch, G. (2001). Mental health services in schools. *Journal of Adolescence, 24*(4), 549–70.

Bates, P., Priest, H., & Gibbs, M. (2004). The education and training needs of learning disability staff in relation to mental health issues. *Nurse Education in Practice, 4*, 30–8.

Baum, S. (2006). The use of the systemic approach to adults with intellectual disabilities and their families: Historical overview and current research. In Baum, S. & Lynggaard, H. (eds). *Intellectual Disabilities: A Systemic Approach* (pp. 21–41). London: Karnac Books.

Baumgart, D., Johnson, J., & Helmsletter, E. (1990). *Augmentative and Alternative Communication for Persons with Moderate and Severe Disabilities*. Baltimore: Paul H. Brookes.

Baxter, C., Cummins, R., & Polak, S. (1995). A longitudinal study of parental stress and support: From diagnosis of disability to leaving school. *International Journal of Disability, Development and Education, 42*(2), 125–36.

Beange, H. & Lennox, N. (1998). Physical aspects of health in the learning disabled. *Current Opinion in Psychiatry, 11*(5), 531–4.

Beange, H., McElduff, A., & Baker, W. (1995). Medical disorders of adults with mental retardation: A population study. *American Journal of Mental Retardation, 99*, 595–604.

Beck, A., Hastings, R. P., Daley, D., & Stevenson, J. (2004). Pro-social behaviour and behaviour problems independently predict maternal stress. *Journal of Intellectual and Developmental Disability, 29*(4), 339–49.

Beck, J., & Horne, D. (1992). A whole school implementation of the Stop, Think Do! social skills training program at Minerva Special School. In Willis, B. & Izard, J. (eds). *Student Behaviour Problems: Directions, Perspectives and Expectations*. Hawthorn, VIC: Australian Council for Educational Research.

Becker-Wiedman, A. (2006). Treatment for children with trauma-attachment disorders: Dyadic Developmental Psychology. *Child and Adolescent Social Work Journal, 23*, 147–171.

Begun, A. L. (1989). Sibling relationships involving developmentally disabled people. *American Journal of Mental Retardation, 93*, 566–74.

Bell, K., Kinder, T., & Huby, G. (2008). What comes around goes around: On the language and practice of 'integration' in health and social care in Scotland. *Journal of Integrated Care, 16*(4), 40–8.

Bellini, S. C. (2003). *Anxiety in Individuals with Autism Spectrum Disorders: The Role of Social Skill Deficits*. Bellini, Indiana: Scott Curtis.

Benderix, Y. & Sivberg, B. (2007). Siblings' experiences of having a brother or sister with autism and mental retardation: A case study of 14 siblings from 5 families. *Journal of Pediatric Nursing*, 22, 410–18.

Benson, H. (2000). *The Relaxation Response*. New York: HarperCollins.

Bernard, S., & Turk, J. (2009). *Developing Mental Health Services for Children and Adolescents with Learning Difficulty: A Toolkit for Clinicians*. London: Royal College of Psychiatrists Publications.

Bernard-Opitz, V., Ross, K., & Tuttas, M. L. (1990). Computer asssisted instruction for autistic children. *Annals of the Academy of Medicine*, *19*(5), 611–16.

Bernard-Opitz, V., Sriram, N., & Nakhoda-Sapuan, S. (2001), Enhancing social problem solving in children with autism and normal children through computer-assisted instruction, *Journal of Autism Developmental Disorders*, *31*, 377–84.

Berument, S. K., Rutter, M., Lord, C., Pickles, A., & Bailey, A. (1999). Autism screening questionnaire: Diagnostic validity. *British Journal of Psychiatry*, *175*, 444–51.

Beukelman, D. R. & Mirenda, P. (2005). *Augmentative and Alternative Communication: Supporting Children and Adults with Complex Communication Needs* (3rd edn). Baltimore: Paul H. Brookes.

Bhatara, V., Loudenberg, R., & Ellis, R. (2006). Association of attention deficit hyperactivity disorder and gestational alcohol exposure: An exploratory study. *Journal of Attention Disorders*, *9*(3), 515–22.

Bhaumik, S. & Branford, D. (2008). *The Frith Prescribing Guidelines for Adults with Intellectual Disability* (2nd edn). London: HealthComm UK Ltd.

Bigby, C. (2000). *Moving On without Parents: Planning, Transitions and Sources of Support for Middle-Aged and Older Adults with Intellectual Disability*. Sydney: MacLennan & Petty.

Billstedt, E., Gillberg, C., & Gillberg, C. (2005). Autism after adolescence: Population-based 13 to 22 year follow-up study of 120 individuals with Autism diagnosed in childhood. *Journal of Autism and Developmental Disorders*, *35*(3), 351–60.

Birch, J. (1986). Enchantment as a cybernetic metaphor: Problems some families encounter with intellectual disability. *Dulwich Centre Review*, Winter, 40–6.

Bjorklund, D. F. (2005). *Children's Thinking: Cognitive Development and Individual Differences* (4th edn). Belmont, CA: Thomson-Wadsworth.

Blacher, J. & Baker, B. L. (2007). Positive impact of intellectual disability on families. *American Journal on Mental Retardation*, *112*(5), 330–48.

Blacher, J. & McIntyre, L. L. (2006). Syndrome specificity and behavioural disorders in young adults with intellectual disability: Cultural differences in family impact. *Journal of Intellectual Disability Research*, *50*(3), 184–98.

Black, L. A. & Devine, M. (n.d.). *Head Start. Promoting Positive Mental Health for Children and Young People with a Learning Disability: A Guide for Parents, Carer, Educators and Health and Social Care Staff.* Belfast: South Eastern Health and Social Care Trust. Retrieved 5 March 2010 from <http://www.wellnet-ni.com/publications/1Head_Start.pdf>.

Blanchett, W. J. & Wolfe, P. S. (2002). A review of sexuality education curricula: Meeting the sexuality education needs of individuals with moderate and severe intellectual disabilities. *Research and Practice for Persons with Severe Disabilities, 27*(1), 43–57.

Bloom, Y. & Bhargava, D. (2004). *Using AAC to Develop Emotions and Problem Solving Skills.* Sydney: Innovative Programming. Available from <www.innovativeprogramming.net.au>.

Bloomberg, K., West, D., & Johnson, H. (2004). *InterAACtion: Strategies for Intentional and Unintentional Communicators.* Melbourne: Scope.

Bloomquist, M. L. (2006). *Skills training for Children with Behaviour Problems: A Parent and Practitioner Guidebook.* New York: Guilford Press.

Blum, R. W. M., Garell, D., Hodgman, C. H., Jorissen, T. W., Okinow, N. A., Orr, D. P., et al. (1993). Transition from child-centred to adult health-care systems for adolescents with chronic conditions: A position paper of the Society for Adolescent Medicine. *Journal of Adolescent Health, 14*(7), 570–6.

Boardman, E. (2003). *An Investigation into International Best Practice in Facilitating the Transition of Tertiary Education Students with Disabilities into their Post-Graduate Careers.* Rockhampton: National, Regional Disability Liaison Officer Initiative, Central Queensland University.

Boldizsar, C., Simon, M., Schmelting, B., Heimke, C., & Fuchs, E. (2006). Astroglial plasticity in the hippocampus is affected by chronic psychosocial stress and concomitant fluoxetine treatment. *Neuropsychopharmacology, 31,* 1616–26.

Bolte, S. & Poustka, F. (2002). The relation between general cognitive level and adaptive behavior domains in individuals with autism with and without co-morbid mental retardation. *Child Psychiatry and Human Development, 33*(2), 165–72.

Bopp, K., Brown, K., & Mirenda, P. (2004). Speech-language pathologists' roles in the delivery of positive behavior support for individuals with developmental disabilities. *American Journal of Speech-Language Pathology, 13,* 5–19.

Bor, W., Sanders, M., & Markie-Dadds, C. (2002). The effects of the Triple P-Positive Parenting Program on preschool children with co-occurring disruptive behavior and attentional/hyperactive difficulties. *Journal of Abnormal Child Psychology, 30*(6), 571–87.

Bosch, J., Mraz, R., Masbruch, J., Tabor, A., Van Dyke, D., & McBrien, D. (2002). Constipation in young children with developmental disabilities. *Infants and Young Children, 15*(2), 66–77.

Bowlby, J. (1969). *Attachment and loss: Attachment, Vol. 1.* New York: Basic Books.

Bowlby, J. (1982). *Attachment and loss: Attachment, Vol. 1* (2nd edn). New York: Basic Books.

Bowlby, J. (1988). *A Secure Base*. London: Routledge.

Boyd, A. (2001). Process for delivering bad news: Supporting families when a child is diagnosed. *Journal of Neuroscience Nursing, 33*(1), 14–20.

Bradley, E. A. & Isaacs, B. J. (2006). Inattention, hyperactivity, and impulsivity in teenagers with intellectual disabilities, with and without autism. *Canadian Journal of Psychiatry, 51*(9), 598–606.

Bradley, E., Summers, J. A., Wood, H. L., & Bryson, S. E. (2004). Comparing rates of psychiatric and behaviour disorders in adolescents and young adults with severe intellectual disability with and without Autism. *Journal of Autism and Developmental Disorders, 34*(2), 151–61.

Bratel, J., Baldry, E., Dunsel, M., & Durrant, M. (2002). Keeping families safely together: A report on quantitative and qualitative investigation of program elements that help to keep children with disabilities safely within their homes (on-line). Available: <http://www.thespasticcentre.org.au/ifso/papers/keepingfamsafe.pdf>.

Brereton, A. V., Tonge, B. J., & Einfeld, S. L. (2006). Psychopathology in children and adolescents with autism compared to young people with intellectual disability. *Journal of Autism and Developmental Disorders, 36*(7), 863–70.

Bretherton, I. (1992). The origins of attachment theory: John Bowlby and Mary Ainsworth. *Developmental Psychology, 28*, 759–75.

Brewster, S. J. (2004). Putting words into their mouths? Interviewing people with learning disabilities and little/no speech. *British Journal of Learning Disabilities, 32*, 166–9.

Bridges, W. (2004). *Transitions: Making Sense of Life's Changes*. Cambridge, MA: Da Capo Press.

Brigance, A. (2004). *Brigance Inventory of Early Development (IED-II)* (2nd edn). North Billerica, MA: Curriculum Associates Inc.

Bright, T., Bittick, K., & Fleeman, B. (1981). Reduction of self-injurious behavior using sensory integrative techniques. *American Journal of Occupational Therapy, 35*(3), 167–72.

Brofenbrenner, U. (1979). *The Ecology of Human Development*. Cambridge, MA: Harvard University Press.

Brown, E. C., Aman, M. G., & Havercamp, S. M. (2002). Factor analysis and norms on parent ratings with the Aberrant Behavior Checklist community for young people in special education. *Research in Developmental Disabilities, 23*, 45–60.

Brown, R. & Brown, I. (2005). The application of quality of life. *Journal of Intellectual Disability Research, 49*(10), 718–27.

Brown, C. & Dunn, W. (2002). *Adolescent/adult Sensory Profile*. San Antonio: Psychological Corporation.

Brugha, T. S. (1988). *Reliability Study of Diagnosis of Schizophrenia with PSE* (abstract). Dublin: 8th World Congress of the International Association for the Scientific Study of Mental Deficiency.

Bruno, J. & Trembath, D. (2006). Use of aided language stimulation to improve syntactic performance during weeklong intervention program. *Augmentative and Alternative Communication, 22*(4), 300–13.

Buccafusco, J. J. (1992). Neuropharmacologic and behavioural actions of clonidine: Interactions with central neurotransmitters. *International Review of Neurobiology, 33*, 55–107.

Bullis, M., Walker, H. M., & Sprague, J. R. (2001). A promise unfulfilled: Social skills training with at risk and antisocial children and youth. *Exceptionality, 9*(1–2), 67–90.

Bunce, M. & Rickards, A. (2004). *Working with Bereaved Children: A Guide*. Colchester: University of Essex: Children's Legal Centre.

Burack, J. (2008). From dawn to dusk: Developing developmental frameworks in understanding persons with ID across the life span. Cape Town: plenary presentation at the 13th IASSID World Congress. (Abstract: *Journal of Intellectual Disability Research, 52*(8–9), 640).

Burge, P., Oulettette-Kuntz, H., McCreary, B., Bradley, E., & Leichner, P. (2002). Senior residents in psychiatry: Views on training in developmental disabilities. *Canadian Journal of Psychiatry, 47*(6), 568–71.

Burgess, A. & Gutstein, S. (2007). Quality of life for people with autism: Raising the standard for evaluating successful outcomes. *Child and Adolescent Mental Health, 12*(2), 80–6.

Burkhart, L. J. (2008). Key concepts for using augmentative communication with children who have complex communication needs (handout). Retrieved 4 March 2010 from <http://www.lburkhart.com/hand_AAC_OSU_6_08.pdf>.

Burris, K. D., Molski, T. F., Xu, C., Ryan, E., Tottori, K., Kikuchi, T., Yocca, F. D., & Molinoff, P. B. (2002). Aripiprazole, a novel antipsychotic, is a high-affinity partial agonist at human dopamine D2 receptors. *Journal of Pharmacology and Experimental Therapies, 302*(1), 381–9.

Busch, C., De Maret, P. S., Flynn, T., Kellum, R., Le, S., Meyers, B., Sanders, M., White, P., & Palmquist, M. (2005). *Writing Guides: Content Analysis*. Retrieved 16 June 2008 from Fort Collins: Writing@CSU, Colorado State University Department of English: <http://writing.colostate.edu/guides/research/content/>.

Butler, J., Leighton, D., & Galea, J. (2003). *The Assessment of Sexual Knowledge*. Melbourne: Centre for Developmental Disability Health Victoria.

Byrne, E., Cunningham, C., & Sloper, P. (1988). *Families and their Children with Down's Syndrome: One Feature in Common*. London: Routledge.

Calabrese, J. R., Fatemi, S. H., & Woyshville, M. J. (1996). Antidepressant effects of lamotrigine in rapid cycling bipolar disorder (letter). *American Journal of Psychiatry, 153*, 1236.

Cameron, L. & Murphy, J. (2002). Enabling young people with a learning disability to make choices at a time of transition. *British Journal of Learning Disabilities, 30*, 105–12.

Campbell, D., Coldicott, T., & Kinsella, K. (1994). *Systemic Work with Organizations*. London: Karnac Books.

Candler, C. (2003). Sensory integration and therapeutic riding at summer camp: Occupational performance outcomes. *Physical and Occupational Therapy in Pediatrics, 23*, 51–64.

Cardinali, D. P., & Pandi-Perumal, S. R. (Eds.) (2005). Neuroendocrine correlates of sleep/wakefulness (pp. 264-6). New York, Springer-Verlag.

Carley, K. (1993). Coding choices for textual analysis: A comparison of content analysis and map analysis. *Sociological Methodology, 23*, 75–126.

Carnaby, S. (2007). Developing good practice in the clinical assessment of people with profound disabilities and multiple impairment. *Journal of Policy and Practice in Intellectual Disabilities, 4*(2), 88–96.

Carr A. (2004). *Family Therapy: Concepts, Process and Practice*. London: John Wiley.

Carr, A., O'Reilly, G., Walsh, P., & McEvoy, J. (2007). *The Handbook of Intellectual Disability and Clinical Psychology Practice*. London: Routledge.

Carr, E. G., Dunlap, G., Horner, R. H., Koegel, R. L., Turnbull, A. P., Sailor, W., Anderson, J., Albin, R. W., Koegel, L. K., & Fox, L. (2002). Positive Behaviour Support: Evolution of an applied science. *Journal of Positive Behaviour Interventions, 4*, 4–16, 20.

Carter, M. A. & Santomauro, J. (2004). *Space Travellers: An Interactive Program for Developing Social Understanding, Social Competence and Social Skills for Students with AS, Autism and Other Social Cognitive Challenges*. Shawnee Mission, KS: Autism Asperger Publishing Company.

Carter, M. A., & Santomauro, J. (2007). *Pirates: An Early Years Group Program for Developing Social Understanding and Social Competence for Children with Autism Spectrum Disorders and Related Challenges*. Shawnee Mission, KS: Autism Asperger Publishing Company.

Carvill, S. (2001). Sensory impairments, intellectual disability and psychiatry. *Journal of Intellectual Disability Research, 45*(6), 467–83.

Case-Smith, J. & Bryan, T. (1999). The effects of occupational therapy with sensory integration emphasis on preschool age children with autism. *American Journal of Occupational Therapy, 53*, 489–97.

Caspi, A. & Moffitt, T. (2006): Gene-environment interactions in psychiatry: joining forces with neuroscience. *Nature Reviews Neuroscience, 7*, 583–90.

Cass, H., Sekaran, D., & Baird, G. (2006). Medical investigation of children with autistic spectrum disorders. *Child: Care, Health and Development, 32*(5), 521–33.

Cermak, S. A. & Daunhauer, L. A. (1997). Sensory processing in the post-institutionalised child. *American Journal of Occupational Therapy, 51*, 500–7.

Chadwick, P., Trower, P., & Dagnan, D. (1999). Measuring negative person evaluations: The evaluative beliefs scale. *Cognitive Therapy and Research, 23*, 549–59.

Chapparo, C. & Mora, L. (2008). The impact of the sensory protocol on functional and behavioural performance of children with severe sensory defensiveness, behavioural disturbance and intellectual disability. Melbourne: paper presented at Federal Congress of the Australian Occupational Therapy Association.

Chappell, P. B., Scahill, L., & Leckman, J. F. (1997). Future therapies of Tourette syndrome. *Neurologic Clinics, 15*, 429–50.

Chivers, J. & Mathieson, S. (2000). Training in sexuality and disability: An Australian model. *Sexuality and Disability, 18*(1), 73–80.

Cho, S. J., Singer, G. H. S., & Brenner, B. M. (2003). A comparison of adaptation to childhood disability in Korean immigrant and Korean mothers. *Focus on Autism and Other Developmental Disabilities, 18*(1), 9–19.

Christie, D. & Wilson, C. (2005). CBT in paediatric and adolescent health settings: A review of practice-based evidence. *Pediatric Rehabilitation, 8*(4), 241–7.

Cicirelli, V. G. (1995). *Sibling Relationships across the Lifespan*. New York: Plenum.

Clarke, M., McConachie, H., Price, K., & Wood, P. (2001). Views of young people using augmentative and alternative communication systems. *International Journal of Communication Disorders, 36*(1), 107–15.

Clegg, J., Hollis, C., Mawhood, L., & Rutter, M. (2005). Developmental language disorders: A follow-up in later adult life: Cognitive, language and psychosocial outcomes. *Journal of Child Psychology and Psychiatry, 46*(2), 128–49.

Clegg, J. & Sheard, C. (2002). Challenging behaviour and insecure attachment. *Journal of Intellectual Disability Research, 46*, 503–6.

Clendon, S. & Erickson, K. (2009). Literacy instruction for individuals with complex communication needs. *ACQuiring Knowledge in Speech, Language and Hearing, 11*(2), 77–80.

Cliffe, S., Black, D., Bryant, J., & Sullivan, E. (2008). Maternal deaths in New South Wales, Australia: A data linkage project. *Australian and New Zealand Journal of Obstetrics and Gynaecology, 48*(3), 255–60.

Cockram, J. (2005). *Equal Justice? The Experiences and Needs of Repeat Offenders with Intellectual Disabilities in Western Australia*. Perth: Activ Foundation Inc.

Coe, D. A., Matson, J. L., Russell, D. W., Slifer, K. J., Capone, G. T., Baglio, C., & Stallings, S.. (1999). Behaviour problems of children with Down syndrome and life events. *Journal of Autism and Developmental Disorders, 29*(2), 149–56.

Cohen, I. L., Tsiouris, J. A., Flory, M. J., Kim, S. Y., Freedland, R., Heaney, G., Pettinger, J., & Brown, W. T. (2009). A large scale study of the psychometric characteristics of the IBR Modified Overt Aggression Scale: Findings and evidence for increased self-destructive behaviors in adult females with Autism Spectrum Disorder (online version). *Journal of Autism and Developmental Disorders*.

Cohn, E. S. (2001). Parent perspectives of occupational therapy using a sensory integrative approach. *American Journal of Occupational Therapy, 55,* 285–94.

Cohn, E., Miller, L. J., & Tickle-Degnen, L. (2000). Parental hopes for therapy outcomes: Children with sensory modulation disorders. *American Journal of Occupational Therapy, 54,* 36–43.

Cole, P., Michel, M., & Teti, L. (1994). The development of emotion regulation and dysregulation: A clinical perspective. *Monographs of the Society for Research in Child Development, 59*(2–3), 73–100.

Coles, D. (2001). The challenge of disability: Being solution focussed with families. *Australia and New Zealand Journal of Family Therapy, 22*(2), 98–107.

Commonwealth Department of Health and Aged Care (CDHAC, 2000). *Promotion, Prevention and Early Intervention for Mental Health: A Monograph.* Canberra: Mental Health and Special Programs Branch, CDHAC. Available from <http://www.health.gov.au/internet/main/publishing.nsf/Content/mental-pubs-p-prommon>.

Commonwealth Department of Health and Ageing (CDHA, n.d.). *KidsMatter-Primary: Australian Primary Schools Mental Health Initiative.* Retrieved 15 September 2009 from <http://www.kidsmatter.edu.au>.

Connor, D. F. & Meltzer B. M. (2006). *Paediatric Psychopharmacology: Fast Facts.* New York: W.W. Norton.

Constantino, J. N. (2002). *The Social Responsiveness Scale.* Los Angeles: Western Psychological Services.

Constantino, J., Przybeck, T., Friensen, D., & Todd, R. (2000). Reciprocal social behaviour in children with and without pervasive developmental disorders. *Journal of Behavioral Pediatrics, 21,* 2–11.

Constantino, J. & Todd, R. (2000). The genetic structure of reciprocal social behaviour. *American Journal of Psychiatry, 157,* 2043–5.

Cook, A., Spinazzola, J., Ford, J., Lanktree, C., Blaustein, M., Sprague, C., Cloitre, M., DeRosa, R., Hubbard, R., Kagan, R., Liautard, J., Mallah, K., Olafson, E., & van der Kolk, B. (2005). Complex trauma in children and adolescents. *Psychiatric Annals, 35,* 390–8.

Cooley, C. (2004). Providing a primary medical home for children and young people with cerebral palsy. *Pediatrics, 114*(4), 1106–13.

Cooper, J., Goodfellow, H., Muhlheim, E., Paske, K., & Pearson, L. (2007). *PALS Social Skills Program: Playing and Learning to Socialise* (3rd edn). Exeter, NSW: Inscript Publishing.

Cooper, S. & Bailey, N. (2001). Psychiatric disorders amongst adults with learning difficulties: Prevalence and relationship to ability levels. *Irish Journal of Psychological Medicine, 18*(2), 45–53.

Cooper, S., Morrison, J., Melville, C., Finlayson, J., Allan, L., Martin, G. & Robinson, E. H. (2006). Improving the health of people with intellectual disabilities: Outcomes of a health screening programme after 1 year. *Journal of Intellectual Disability Research, 50*(9), 667–77.

Cooper, S., Smiley, E., Morrison, J., Williamson, A., & Allan, L. (2007). Mental ill-health in adults with intellectual disabilities: Prevalence and associated factors. *British Journal of Psychiatry,* 190, 27-35.

Copeland, M. E. (1993). *The Depression Workbook.* Oakland, CA: New Harbinger Publications.

Corfield, D. & Brearley, K. (2009). Transition: More than an event. In White, D., Dossetor, D., & Whatson, L. (eds). A framework for professional practice: A seminar for disability, health, and education professionals. Paper presented in Pilot Educational Program. Sydney: The Children's Hospital at Westmead and Statewide Behaviour Intervention Service, NSW Department of Ageing, Disability and Home Care.

Cormack, K. F. M., Brown, A. C., & Hastings, R. P (2000). Behavioural and emotional difficulties in students attending schools for children and adolescents with severe intellectual disability. *Journal of Intellectual Disability Research, 44*(2), 124–9.

Cornell, T. & Hamrin, V. (2008). Clinical interventions for children with attachment problems. *Journal of Child and Adolescent Psychiatric Nursing, 21,* 35–47.

Cornish, U. & Ross, F. (2003). *Social Skills Training for Adolescents with General Moderate Learning Difficulties.* London: Jessica Kingsley Publishers.

Costello, H. & Bouras, N. (2006). Assessment of mental health problems in people with intellectual disabilities. *Israel Journal of Psychiatry and Related Sciences, 43*(4), 241–51.

Costello, H., Bouras, N., & Davis, H. (2007). The role of training in improving community care staff awareness of mental health problems in people with intellectual disabilities. *Journal of Applied Research in Intellectual Disabilities, 20,* 228–35.

Costello, H., Holt, G., Cain, N., Bradley, E., Torr, J., Davis, R., Edwards, N., Lennox, N., & Weber, G. (2007). Professional training for those working with people with intellectual disabilities and mental health problems. In Bouras, N. & Holt, G. (eds). *Psychiatric and Behavioural Disorders in Intellectual and Developmental Disabilities* (2nd edn) (pp. 400–11). Cambridge: Cambridge University Press.

Costello, H., Moss, S. C, Prosser, H., & Hatton, C. (1997). Reliability of the ICD10 version of the Psychiatric Assessment Schedule of Adults with Developmental Disability (PAS-ADD). *Social Psychiatry and Psychiatric Epidemiology, 32,* 339–43.

Cotton, S. & Richdale, A. (2006). Brief report: Parental descriptions of sleep problems in children with autism, Down syndrome, and Prader-Willi syndrome. Research in Developmental Disabilities, 27, 151-161.

Coyle, J. T. & Puttfarcken, P. (1993). Oxidative stress, glutamate and neurodegenerative disorders. *Science, 262,* 689–95.

Crabtree, S. A. (2007). Maternal perceptions of care-giving of children with developmental disabilities in the United Arab Emirates. *Journal of Applied Research in Intellectual Disabilities, 20*(3), 247–55.

Craighead, W. E., Hart, A. B., Craighead, L. W., & Ilardi, S. S. (2002). Psychosocial treatments for major depressive disorder. In Nathan, P. E. & Gordon, J. M. (eds). *A Guide to Treatments That Work* (2nd edn) (pp. 245–62). New York: Oxford University Press.
Cress, C. J., & Marvin, C. A. (2003). Common questions about AAC services in early intervention. *Augmentative and Alternative Communication, 19*(4), 254–72.
Crittenden, P. M. (1999). Atypical attachment in infancy and early childhood among children at developmental risk. VII. Danger and development: The organization of self-protective strategies. *Monographs of the Society for Research in Child Development, 64*, 145–71.
Crittenden, P. M. (2000a). Introduction. In Crittenden, P. M. & Claussen, A. H. (eds). *The Organization of Attachment Relationships: Maturation, Culture and Context*. Cambridge: Cambridge University Press.
Crittenden, P. M. (2000b). Dynamic maturational exploration of the meaning of security and adaptation. In Crittenden, P. M. & Claussen, A. H. (eds). *The Organization of Attachment Relationships: Maturation, Culture and Context*. Cambridge: Cambridge University Press.
Crittenden, P. M. (2008). *Raising Parents: Attachment, Parenting and Child Safety*. Cullompton, Devon: Willan Publishing.
Cross, M. (1999). Lost for words. *Child and Family Social Work, 4*, 249–57.
Cross, M. (2004). *Children with Emotional and Behavioural Difficulties and Communication Problems: There Is Always a Reason*. London: Jessica Kingsley Publishers.
Cross, M., Blake, P., Tunbridge, N., & Gill, T. (2001). Collaborative working to promote the communication skills of a 14-year-old student with emotional, behavioural, learning and language difficulties. *Child Language, Teaching and Therapy, 17*(3), 227–46.
Crozier, S. & Tincani, M. (2007). Effects of social stories on prosocial behavior of preschool children with autism spectrum disorders. *Journal of Autism and Developmental Disorders, 37*, 1803–14.
Cummins, R. A. (2005). Issues in the systematic assessment of quality of life. In Hogg, J. & Langa, A. (eds). *Assessing Adults with Intellectual Disabilities: A Service Provider's Guide* (pp. 9–21). London: British Psychological Society and Blackwell Publishing Ltd.
Cummins, R., Hughes, J., Tomyn, A., Gibson, A., Woerner, J., & Lai, L. (2007). *The Wellbeing of Australians: Carer Health and Wellbeing*. Australian Unity Wellbeing Index, Survey 17.1, Special Report. Geelong: Deakin University, Australian Unity and Carers Australia.
Cunningham, C. C., Morgan, P. A., & McGucken, R. V. (1984). Down's syndrome: Is dissatisfaction with disclosure of diagnosis inevitable? *Developmental Medicine and Child Neurology, 26*, 33–9.
Cunningham, C. E., Siegel, L. S., & Offord, D. R. (1991). A dose-response analysis of the effects of methyphenidate on the peer interactions and

simulated classroom performance of ADD children with and without conduct problems. *Journal of Child Psychology and Psychiatry and Allied Disciplines, 32*, 439–52.

Curran, J. & Kyrkou, M. (2008). Diversity is the SPICE of life: Working to improve the emotional and mental health assessment of people with developmental disabilities and mental health problems. Paper presented at 43rd ASSID Conference, Melbourne. Retrieved 10 December 2009 from <http://www.assid.org.au/ConferencePapers/tabid/59/Default.aspx>.

Cuskelly, M. & Gunn, P. (2006). Adjustment of children who have a sibling with Down Syndrome: Perspectives of mothers, fathers and children. *Journal of Intellectual Disability Research, 50*, 917–25.

Czobor, P., Volavka, J., & Meibach, R. C. (1995). Effect of risperidone on hostility in schizophrenia. *Journal of Clinical Psychopharmacology, 15*, 243–9.

Dada, S. & Alant, E. (2009). The effect of aided language stimulation on vocabulary acquisition in children with little or no functional speech. *American Journal of Speech-Language Pathology, 18*, 50–64.

Dagnan, D. (2007). Psychosocial interventions for people with intellectual disabilities and mental ill-health. *Current Opinion in Psychiatry, 20*, 456–60.

Dagnan, D., Chadwick, P., & Proudlove, J. (2000). Toward an assessment of suitability of people with mental retardation for cognitive therapy. *Cognitive Therapy and Research, 24*(6), 627–36.

Dagnan, D., Jahoda, A., & Kroese, B. (2007). Cognitive behaviour therapy. In Carr, A., O'Reilly, G., Walsh, P., & McEvoy, J. (eds). *Handbook of Intellectual Disability and Clinical Psychology Practice*. New York: Routledge.

Dagnan, D. & Lindsay, W. R. (2004). Cognitive therapy with people with learning disabilities. In Emerson, E., Hatton, C., Thompson, T., & Parmenter, T. (eds). *International Handbook of Research and Evaluation in Intellectual Disabilities* (pp. 517–30). Chichester, UK: Wiley.

Dagnan, D. & Proudlove, J. (1997). Using Makaton drawing to assess the ability to recognize facial expressions of emotion in people with learning disabilities. *Clinical Psychology Forum, 105*, 3–5.

D'Arcy, F., Flynn, J., McCarthy, Y., O'Connor, C., & Tierney, E. (2005). Sibshops: An evaluation of an interagency model. *Journal of Intellectual Disabilities, 9*, 43–57.

Darlington, Y., Feeney, J., & Rixon, K. (2005). Interagency collaboration between child protection and mental health services: Practices, attitudes and barriers. *Child Abuse and Neglect, 29*, 1085–98.

Darlington, Y. & Feeney, J. (2007). Collaboration between mental health and child protection services: Professionals' perceptions of best practice. *Children and Youth Services Review, 30*, 187–98.

Datta, S. S., Russell, P. S. S., & Gopalakrishna, S. C. (2002). Burden among the caregivers of children with intellectual disability: Associations and risk factors. *Journal of Learning Disabilities* (London), *6*(4), 337–50.

Davies, P. L., & Gavin, W. J. (2007). Validating the diagnosis of sensory processing disorders using EEG technology. *American Journal of Occupational Therapy, 61*(2), 176–89.

Davis, E., Barnhill, L. J., & Saeed, S. A. (2008). Treatment models for treating patients with combined mental illness and developmental disability. *Psychiatric Quarterly, 79*, 205–23.

Davis, M., Eshelman, E. R., & McKay, M. (2000). *The Relaxation and Stress Reduction Workbook* (5th edn). Oakland, CA: New Harbinger.

Dawes, R. M., Faust, D., & Meehl, P. E. (1989). Clinical versus actuarial judgment. *Science, 243*, 1668–1774.

Dawkins, R. (2009). *The Genius of Charles Darwin*. Retrieved 24 February 2010 from <www.youtube.com/view_play_list?p=6B2A3E5FE91D59CF>.

Deb, S. & Unwin, G. L. (2007). Psychotropic medication for behaviour problems in people with intellectual disability: A review of the current literature. *Current Opinion in Psychiatry, 20*, 461–6.

Dekker, M. C., Koot, H. M., van der Ende, J., & Verhulst, F. C. (2002). Emotional and behavioural problems in children and adolescents with and without intellectual disability. *Journal of Child Psychology and Psychiatry, 43*(8), 1087–98.

De Leersnyder, H., Claustrat, B., Munnich, A., & Verloes, A. (2006). Circadian Rhythm in a rare disease: Smith-Magenis syndrome. *Molecular and Cellular Endocrinology, 252*(1–2), 88–91.

De Leersnyder, H., de Blois, M. C., Vekemans, M., Sidi, D., Villain, E., Kindermans, C., & Munnich, A. (2001). β1-adrenergic antagonists improve sleep and behavioural disturbances in a circadian disorder, Smith–Magenis syndrome. *Journal of Medical Genetics, 38*, 586–90.

Department for Children, Schools and Families/Department of Health (2008). *Transition: Moving On Well*. Retrieved 3 April 2008, from <http://www.dh.gov.uk/en/Publicationsandstatistics/Publications/PublicationsPolicyAndGuidance/DH_083592>.

Department of Ageing, Disability and Home Care (DADHC, 2004). *Supporting Children and Young People with a Disability* (New South Wales Government policy document). Retrieved 30 September 2009 from <http://www.dadhc.nsw.gov.au/NR/rdonlyres/67F2202C-243C-48EB-B8C5-5378872383F1/1440/Supportingchildrenandyoungpeoplewithadisability-and.pdf>.

Department of Education (2008). *My Future Let's Plan*. Retrieved 18 April 2008 from <http://www.education.tas.gov.au/school/health/disabilities/transitionplanning>.

Department of Families, Housing, Community Services and Indigenous Affairs (FaHCSIA, 2008). Carer Payment (Child): *A New Approach: Report of the Carer Payment (Child) Review Taskforce*. Canberra: Commonwealth of Australia. Retrieved 17 December 2008 from <http://www.facsia.gov.au/carers/carer_payment_review_report/ch4.htm>.

Department of Health (2007). *Services for People with Learning Disabilities and Challenging Behaviour or Mental Health Needs: Report of a Project Group* (Chairman: Prof. J. L. Mansell) (rev. edn). Retrieved 7 February 2010 from <http://www.kent.ac.uk/tizard/staff/documents/dh2007mansell-report%20_revised.pdf>.

Department of Health/Department for Education and Skills (2006). *Getting It Right for Young People.* Retrieved 19 February 2008, from <http://www.dh.gov.uk/en/Publicationsandstatistics/Publications/PublicationsPolicyAndGuidance/DH_4132145>.

De Schipper, J. C., Stolk, J., & Schuengel, C. (2006). Professional caretakers as attachment figures in day care centres for children with intellectual disability and behaviour problems. *Research in Developmental Disabilities, 27,* 203–16.

de Shazer, S. (1982). *Patterns of Brief Family Therapy: An Ecosystemic Approach.* New York: Guilford Press.

Dhikav, V. & Anand, K. S. (2007). Is hippocampal atrophy a future drug target? *Medical Hypotheses, 68*(6), 1300–6.

Diana, M. (1998). Drugs of abuse and dopamine cell activity. *Advances in Pharmacology, 42,* 998–1001.

DiClemente, C. C. & Velasquez, S. K. (2002). Motivational interviewing and the stages of change. In Miller, W. R. & Rollnick, S. (eds). *Motivational Interviewing: Preparing People for Change* (2nd edn). New York: Guilford Press.

Diggle, T., & McConachie, H. H. R. (2002). Parent-mediated early intervention for young children with autism spectrum disorder. *Cochrane Database of Systematic Reviews,* Issue 2, CD003496.

Diken, I. H. (2006). Turkish mothers' interpretation of the disability of their children with mental retardation. *International Journal of Special Education, 21,* 8–27.

Di Marco, M. & Iacono, T. (2007). Mental health assessment and intervention for people with complex communication needs associated with developmental disabilities. *Journal of Policy and Practice in Intellectual Disabilities, 4*(1), 40–59.

Dingledine, R., McBain, C. J., & McNamara, J. O. (1990). Excitatory amino acid receptors in epilepsy. *Trends in Pharmacological Sciences, 11,* 334–8.

Dodd, P., Dowling, S., & Hollins, S. (2005). A review of the emotional, psychiatric and behavioural responses. *Journal of Clinical Child and Adolescent Psychology, 34,* 260–71.

Donnellan, A. M., Mirenda, P. L., Mesaros, R. A., & Fassbender, L. L. (1984). Analysing the communicative functions of aberrant behaviour. *Journal of the Association for Persons with Severe Handicaps, 9*(3), 201–12.

Dorner, S. (1975). The relationship of physical handicap to stress in families with an adolescent with spina bifida. *Developmental Medicine and Child Neurology, 17,* 765–76.

Dosen, A. (2005a). Applying the developmental perspective in the psychiatric assessment and diagnosis of persons with intellectual disability: Part I. Assessment. *Journal of Intellectual Disability Research*, *49*(1), 1–8.

Dosen, A. (2005b). Applying the developmental perspective in the psychiatric assessment and diagnosis of persons with intellectual disability: Part II. Diagnosis. *Journal of Intellectual Disability Research*, *49*(1), 9–15.

Dossetor, D. (2001). Parenting a disabled child: The chosen and those that choose. *The Clinician: Hope & Anxiety*, *1*(1), 61–3.

Dossetor, D. (2003). Intellectual disability. In Nunn, K. & Dey, C. (eds). *Psychotropic Prescribing in Children and Adolescents* (pp. 248–61). Sydney: Department of Psychological Medicine, The Children's Hospital at Westmead; available at <www.CHWSchoollink.edu.au>.

Dossetor, D. (2004). The evolution of the 'photon catcher': Implications for social development and autism. *Clinical Child Psychology and Psychiatry*, *9*(3), 443–51.

Dossetor, D. (2007). 'All that glitters is not gold': Misdiagnosis of psychosis in pervasive developmental disorders: A case series. *Clinical Child Psychology and Psychiatry*, *12*(3), 437–48.

Dossetor, D. R. (1991). A study of the dependency needs of adolescents with developmental retardation: An evaluation of short-term care usage, expressed emotion in the primary carer, and the contribution of community services. Unpublished dissertation for Doctorate of Medicine, University of Cambridge, UK.

Dossetor, D. R., Caruana, J. A, Goltzoff, H., & Saleh, H. (2009). Leading the way in mental health and intellectual disability: A focus on the needs of children and adolescents in schools for specific purposes in NSW (unpublished manuscript). Sydney: The Children's Hospital at Westmead.

Dossetor, D. R., Nicol, A. R., & Stretch, D. D. (1993). Hostel-based respite care for adolescents with developmental retardation: The need for normalised resources. *Journal of Child Psychology and Psychiatry*, *34*(3), 391–412.

Dossetor, D. R., Santhanam, R., Rhodes, P., Holland, T. J., & Nunn, K. P. (2005). Developmental neuropsychiatry: A new model of psychiatry for young people with and without and intellectual disability? *Clinical Child Psychology and Psychiatry*, *10*(3), 277–304.

Douglas, V. I., Barr, R. G., Desiletes, J., & Sherman, E. (1995). Do high doses of stimulants impair flexible thinking in attention-deficit hyperactivity disorder? *Journal of the American Academy of Child and Adolescent Psychiatry*, *34*(7), 877–85.

Douglas, V. I., Barr, R. G., O'Neill, M. E., & Britton, B. G. (1988). Dosage effects and individual responsivity to methylphenidate in attention deficit disorder. *Journal of Child Psychology and Psychiatry*, *29*(4), 453–75.

Douma, J. C. H., Dekker, M. C., & Koot, H. M. (2006). Supporting parents of youths with intellectual disabilities and psychopathology. *Journal of Intellectual Disability Research*, *50*(8), 570–81.

Downing, J. E. (2005). Inclusive education for high school students with severe intellectual disabilities: Supporting communication. *Augmentative and Alternative Communication, 21*(2), 132–48.

Drinkwater, J. A. & Stewart, A. B. (2002). Cognitive behaviour therapy for young people. *Current Opinion in Psychiatry, 15*(4), 377–81.

Dugmore, O. & Hurcombe, R. (2007). *Quality Improvement Network for Multi-Agency CAMHS (QINMAC): Learning Disability Standards.* London: Royal College of Psychiatrists. Retrieved 10 December 2009 from <http://www.rcpsych.ac.uk/clinicalservicestandards/centreforqualityimprovement/servicestandards.aspx>.

Dunn, L., Whetton, C., & Burley, J. (1997). *The British Picture Vocabulary Scale* (2nd edn). Slough, UK: NFER-Nelson.

Dunn, W. (1999). *Sensory Profile.* San Antonio: Psychological Corporation.

Durlak, J. A., Fuhrman, T., & Lampron, C. (1991). Effectiveness of cognitive-behavioral therapy for maladapting children: A meta-analysis. *Psychological Bulletin, 110*(2), 204–14.

Dutar, P. & Nicoll, R. A. (1988). A physiological role for GABAB receptors in the central nervous system. *Nature, 332,* 156–8.

Dykens, E. M. (2000). Annotation: Psychopathology in children with intellectual disability. *Journal of Child Psychology and Psychiatry, 41*(4), 407–17.

Dykens, E. M. & Hodapp, R. M. (2001). Research in mental retardation: Toward an etiologic approach. *Journal of Child Psychology and Psychiatry and Allied Disciplines, 42*(1), 49–71.

Echemendia, R. J. & Westerveld, M. (2006). Cultural perspectives in paediatric rehabilitation. In Farmer, J. E., Donders, J., & Warschausky, S. (eds). *Treating Neurodevelopmental Disabilities: Clinical Research and Practice* (chapter 16). New York: Guildford Press.

Edelson, S. M., Edelson, M. G., Kerr, D., & Grandin, T. (1999). Behavioural and physiological effects of deep pressure on children with autism: A pilot study evaluating the efficacy of Grandin's hug machine. *American Journal of Occupational Therapy, 53,* 145–52.

Ehninger, D., de Vries, P. J., & Silva, A. J. (2009). From mTOR to cognition: Molecular and cellular mechanisms of cognitive impairments in tuberous sclerosis. *Journal of Intellectual Disability Research, 53*(10), 838–51.

Einfeld, S. & Emerson, E. (2008). Intellectual disability. In Rutter, M., Bishop, D., Pine, D., Scott, S., Stevenson, J. S., Taylor, E. A., Thapar, A. (eds). *Rutter's Child and Adolescent Psychiatry* (5th edn) (pp. 820–40). Oxford: Blackwell Publishing Ltd.

Einfeld, S. L., Piccinin, A. M., Mackinnon, A., Hofer, S. M., Taffe, J., Gray, K. M., Bontempo, D. E., Hoffman, L. R., Parmenter, T., & Tongue, B. J. (2006). Psychopathology in young people with intellectual disability. *Journal of the American Medical Association, 296*(16), 1981–9.

Einfeld, S. L. & Tonge, B. J. (1992). *Manual for the Developmental Behaviour Checklist*. Clayton: Monash University for Developmental Psychiatry, and Sydney: School of Psychiatry, University of New South Wales.

Einfeld, S. L. & Tonge, B. J. (1995) The Developmental Behavior Checklist: The development and validation of an instrument to assess behavioral and emotional disturbance in children and adolescents with mental retardation. *Journal of Autism and Developmental Disorders, 25*(2), 81–104.

Einfeld, S. L. & Tonge, B. J. (1996a). Population prevalence of psychopathology in children and adolescents with intellectual disability: I. Rationale and methods. *Journal of Intellectual Disability Research, 40*(2), 91–8.

Einfeld, S. L. & Tonge, B. J. (1996b). Population prevalence of psychopathology in children and adolescents with intellectual disability: II. Epidemiological findings. *Journal of Intellectual Disability Research, 40*(2), 99–109.

Einfeld, S. L. & Tonge, B. T. (2002). *Manual for the Developmental Behaviour Checklist* (2nd edn): *Primary Carer Version (DBC-P)* and *Teacher Version (DBC-T)*. Clayton: Monash University Centre for Developmental Psychiatry, and Sydney: Psychology and School of Psychiatry, University of New South Wales.

Einfeld, S., Tonge, B., Chapman, L., Mohr, C., Taffe, J., & Horstead, S. (2007). Inter-rater reliability of the diagnosis of psychosis and depression in individuals with intellectual disabilities. *Journal of Applied Research in Intellectual Disabilities, 20*(5), 384–90.

Eisenberg, N., Fabes, R., Murphy, B., Maszk, P., Smith, M., & Karbon, M. (1995). The role of emotionality and regulation in children's social functioning: A longitudinal study. *Child Development, 66*, 1360–84.

Eisenhower, A. S., Baker, B. L., & Blacher, J. (2005). Preschool children with intellectual disability: Syndrome specificity, behaviour problems, and maternal well being. *Journal of Intellectual Disability Research, 49*(9), 657–71.

Elias, M. J. & Bruene Butler, L. (2005). *Social Decision Making/Social Problem Solving for Middle School Students: Skills and Activities for Academic, Social and Emotional Success*. Champaign, IL: Research Press.

Elias, M. J. (2004). The connection between social-emotional learning and learning disabilities: Implications for intervention. *Learning Disability Quarterly, 27*, 53–63.

Elliott, C. D. (1990). *Differential Ability Scales (DAS)*. San Antonio, TX: Psychological Corporation.

Ello, L. M., & Donovan, S. J. (2005). Assessment of relationship between parenting stress and a child's ability to functionally communicate. *Research on Social Work Practice, 15*(6), 531–44.

El Naggar Gaad, E. (2001). Educating children with Down syndrome in the United Arab Emirates. *British Journal of Special Education, 28*(4), 195–203.

Elsea, S. H. & Girirajan, S. (2008). Smith-Magenis syndrome. *European Journal of Human Genetics, 16*, 412–21.

Emerson, E. (2000). Behaviour analysis. In Gillberg, C. & O'Brien, G. (eds). *Developmental Disability and Behaviour* (pp. 77–88). London: Mac Keith Press.

Emerson, E. (2001). *Challenging Behaviour: Analysis and Intervention in People with Severe Intellectual Disabilities* (2nd edn). Cambridge: Cambridge University Press.

Emerson, E. (2003a). Prevalence of psychiatric disorders in children and adolescents with and without intellectual disability. *Journal of Intellectual Disability Research, 47*(1), 51–8.

Emerson, E. (2003b). Mothers of children and adolescents with intellectual disability: Social, and economic situation, mental health status, and the self-assessed social and psychological impact of the child's difficulties. *Journal of Intellectual Disability Research, 47*(4–5), 385–99.

Emerson, E. (2004). Poverty and children with intellectual disabilities in the world's richer countries. *Journal of Intellectual and Developmental Disability, 29*(4), 319–87.

Emerson, E., Cummings, R., Barrett, S., Hughes, H., McCool, C., & Toogood, A. (1988). Challenging behaviour and community services. Who are the people who challenge services? *Mental Handicap, 16*, 16–19.

Emerson, E. & Hatton, C. (2007). Mental health of children and adolescents with intellectual disabilities in Britain. *British Journal of Psychiatry, 191*, 493–9.

Emerson, E., Robertson, J., & Wood, J. (2005). Emotional and behavioural needs of children and adolescents with intellectual disabilities in an urban conurbation. *Journal of Intellectual Disability Research, 49*(1), 16–24.

Esbensen, A. J. & Benson, B. A. (2006). A prospective analysis of life events, problem behaviours and depression in adults with intellectual disability. *Journal of Intellectual Disability Research, 50*(4), 258–58.

Esbensen, A. J., Rojahn, J., Aman, M. G., & Ruedrich, S. (2003). Reliability and validity of an assessment instrument for anxiety, depression, and mood among individuals with mental retardation. *Journal of Autism and Developmental Disorders, 33*, 617–29.

Evans, E., Taffe, J., Einfeld, S., Tonge, B., & Grey, K. (2003). *Manual for the DBC Score for Windows Version C: Scoring Checklist for the DBC*. Clayton: Monash University Centre for Developmental Psychiatry and Psychology, and Sydney: School of Psychiatry, University of New South Wales.

Family Planning NSW (2004). *Sex Safe and Fun. Reader's Guide: A Guide for Supporting the Learning of Positive Safer Sex Messages*. Sydney: FPA Health.

Family Planning NSW (2007). *Love and Kisses: The DVD*. Sydney: Family Planning NSW.

Family Planning Queensland (2002). *Feel safe: CD ROM*. Brisbane: Family Planning Queensland.

Family Planning Victoria (1997). *Human Relations and Sexuality: Knowledge and Awareness Assessment for People with an Intellectual Disability*. Melbourne: Family Planning Victoria.

Fannon, D. (2008). E-interview: Bill Fulford. *Psychiatric Bulletin, 32*(1), ibc.

Farber, N. B., Newcomer, J. W., & Olney, J. W. (1999). Glycine agonists: What can they teach us about schizophrenia? *Archives of General Psychiatry, 56*, 13–17.

Fertel-Daly, D., Bedell, G., & Hinojsa, J. (2001). Effects of a weighted vest on attention to task and self-stimulatory behaviors in preschoolers with pervasive developmental disorders. *American Journal of Occupational Therapy, 55*, 829–40.

Fiddell, B. (2000). Exploring the use of family therapy with adults with a learning disability. *Journal of Family Therapy, 22*, 308–23.

Fidler, D. J., Barret, K. C., & Most, D. E. (2005). Age-related differences in smiling and personality in Down syndrome. *Journal of Developmental and Physical Disabilities, 17*, 263–80.

Firth, V. (2008). New support for principals of 'Specific Purpose Schools'. (Media Statement from NSW Minister for Education and Training, 23 September.). Retrieved 15 November 2009 from <https://www.det.nsw.edu.au/media/downloads/aboutus/ministerial/mr080923_principals_ssp.pdf>.

Fisman, S., Wolf, L., Ellison, D., Gillis, B., Freeman, T., & Szatmari, P. (1996). Risk and protective factors affecting the adjustment of siblings of children with chronic disabilities. *Journal of the American Academy of Child and Adolescent Academy, 35*(11), 1532–41.

Fleming, B. (2010). Positive behaviour for learning statistics 2008–09. Unpublished raw data.

Fletcher, R., Loschen, E., Stavrakaki, C., & First, M. (eds) (2007). *Diagnostic Manual: Intellectual Disability (DM-ID): A Textbook of Diagnosis of Mental Disorders in Persons with Intellectual Disability*. Kingston, NY: NADD Press.

Flores, G. (2000). Culture and the patient–physician relationship: Achieving cultural competency in health care. *Journal of Pediatrics, 136*, 14–23.

Flores, G., Abreu, M., Schwatz, I., & Hill, M. (2000). The importance of language and culture in pediatric care: case studies from the Latino community. *Journal of Pediatrics, 137*, 842–8.

Folgelson, D. L. & Sternbach, H. (1997). Lamotrigine treatment of refractory bipolar disorder. *Journal of Clinical Psychiatry, 58*, 271–3.

Fombonne, E. (2003). Epidemiological surveys of autism and other pervasive developmental disorders: An update. *Journal of Autism and Developmental Disorders, 33*, 365–82.

Forrester-Jones, R., Cambridge, P., Carpenter, J., Tate, A., Beecham, J., Hallam, A., Knapp, M., Coolen-Schrijner, P., & Wopolff, D. (2006). The social networks of people with intellectual disability living in the community 12 years after resettlement from long-stay hospitals. *Journal of Applied Research in Intellectual Disabilities, 19*, 285–95.

Foss, A., Swinth, Y., McGruder, J., & Tomlin, G. (2003). *Sensory Modulation Dysfunction and the Wilbarger Protocol: An Evidence Review*. OT Practice, CE 1–7.

Frances, A., First, M. B., & Pincus, H. A. (1995). *DSM-IV Guidebook*. Washington, DC: American Psychiatric Press.

Freedman, R., Adler, L. E., & Waldo, M. (1987). Gating of the auditory evoked potential in children and adults. *Psychophysiology, 24*, 223–7.

Frey, K. S., Greenberg, M. T., & Frewell, R. R. (1989). Stress and coping among parents of handicapped children: A multidimensional approach. *American Journal on Mental Retardation, 94*, 240–9.

Fung, C. W. & Wong, V. (2005). Program for Chinese children with developmental disabilities: The Hong Kong model. *Brain and Development, 27*(2), 141–7.

Gallimore, R., Weisner, T. S., Bernheimer L. P., Guthrie D., & Nihira, K. (1993). Family responses to young children with developmental delays: Accommodation activity in ecological and cultural context. *American Journal of Mental Retardation, 98*(2), 185–206.

Garb, H. N. (1994). Toward a second generation of statistical prediction rules in psychodiagnosis and personality assessment. *Computers in Human Behavior, 10*, 377–94.

Garber, J. & Robinson, N. S. (2007). Cognitive vulnerability in children at risk for depression. *Cognition and Emotion, 11*, 619–35.

Gardner, W. I. (2002). *Aggression and Other Disruptive Behavioural Challenges: Biomedical and Psychosocial Assessment and Treatment*. New York: NADD Press.

Garmezy, N. (1984). Children vulnerable to major mental disorders: Risk and protective factors. In Greenspoon, L. (ed.). *Psychiatry Update*, Vol. 3 (pp. 91–104), Washington DC: American Psychiatric Press.

Garwood, M. & McCabe, M. P. (2000). Impact of sex education programs on sexual knowledge and feelings of men with a mild intellectual disability. *Education and Training in Mental Retardation and Developmental Disabilities, 35*(3), 269–83.

Gavidia-Payne, S. & Hudson, A. (2002). Behavioural supports for parents of children with an intellectual disability and problem behaviours: An overview of the literature. *Journal of Intellectual and Developmental Disability, 27*, 31–55.

Geula, C. (1998). Abnormalities of neural circuitry in Alzheimer's disease: Hippocampus and cortical cholinergic innervations. *Neurology, 51*, S18–29.

Ghaziuddin, M., Ghaziuddin, N., & Greden, J. (2002). Depression in persons with autism: Implications for research and clinical care. *Journal of Autism and Developmental Disorders, 32*(4), 299–306.

Giacobini, E. (1998). Cholinergic foundations of Alzheimer's disease therapy. *Journal of Physiology, 92*, 283–7.

Giallo, R. & Gavidia-Payne, S. (2006). Child, parent and family factors as predictors of adjustment for siblings of children with disability. *Journal of Intellectual Disability Research, 50*, 937–48.

Giarratano, L. (2004). *Managing Psychological Trauma: Clinician and Client Resources for the Clinical Skills Series*. Mascot, NSW: Talomin Books.

Gibbs, M. & Priest, H. M. (1999). Designing and implementing a 'dual diagnosis' module: A review of the literature and some preliminary findings. *Nurse Education Today, 19*(5), 357–63.

Giddan, J. J., Bade, K. M., Rickenberg, D., & Ryley, A. T. (1995). Teaching the language of feelings to students with severe emotional and behavioural handicaps. *Language, Speech and Hearing Services in the Schools, 26*, 3–10.

Giddan, J. J. & Milling, L. (1999). Comorbidity of psychiatric and communication disorders in children. *Child and Adolescent Psychiatric Clinics of North America, 8*(1), 19–36.

Gillberg, C. & Billstedt, E. (2000). Autism and Asperger syndrome: Coexistence with other clinical disorders. *Acta Psychiatrica Scandinavica, 102*(5), 321–30.

Gillett, Y. & DePompei, R. (2004). The potential of electronic organizers as a tool in the cognitive rehabilitation of young people. *NeuroRehabilitation, 19*, 233–43.

Glazer, W. M. & Dickson, R. A. (1998). Clozapine reduces violence and persistent aggression in schizophrenia. *Journal of Clinical Psychiatry, 59*(S3), 8–14.

Goddard, J., Lehr, R., & Lapadat, J. (2000). Parents of children with disabilities: Telling a different story. *Canadian Journal of Counseling, 34*(4), 273–89.

Golan, O., Humphrey, A., Chapman, E., Gómez de la Cuesta, G., Peabody, K., Weiner, B., Lever, N., Harcup, C., & Baron-Cohen, S. (2006). *The Transporters: Teaching Emotion Recognition to Preschoolers with Autism* (animation DVD). Cambridge, UK: Autism Research Centre, University of Cambridge.

Goldberg, D., Magrill, L., Hale J., Damaskinidou, K., & Tham, S. (1995). Protection and loss: Working with learning-disabled adults and their families. *Journal of Family Therapy, 17*, 263–80.

Goldman-Rakic, P. S. (1998). The cortical dopamine system: Role in memory and cognition. *Advances in Pharmacology, 42*, 707–11.

Goldstein, S. & Schwebach, A. J. (2004). The comorbidity of pervasive developmental disorder and attention deficit hyperactivity disorder: Results of a retrospective chart review. *Journal of Autism and Developmental Disorders, 34*(3), 329–39.

Goodfellow, J. & Camilleri, M. (2003). *Beyond Belief, Beyond Justice: Final Report of Stage 1 of the Disability Discrimination Legal Services Sexual Offences Project*. Melbourne: Disability Discrimination Legal Services.

Goossens, C., Crain, S., & Elder, P. (1992). *Engineering the Preschool Environment for Interactive, Symbolic Communication: 18 Months to 5 Years*. Birmingham, AL: Southeast Augmentative Communication Conference Publications Clinician Series.

Graham, I. D., Logan, J., Harrison, M., Straus, S. E., Tetroe, J., Caswell, W., & Robinson, N. (2006). Lost in knowledge translation: Time for a map? *Journal of Continuing Education in the Health Professions, 26*, 13–24.

Grant, G., Nolan, M., & Keady, J. (2003). Supporting families over the life course: Mapping temporality. *Journal of Intellectual Disability Research, 47*(4–5), 342–51.

Gray, A. (2001). Accommodation, resistance and transcendence: Three narratives of autism. *Social Science and Medicine, 53*, 1247–57.

Gray, C. A. (1994). *Comic Strip Conversations: Colorful, Illustrated Interactions with Students with Autism and Related Disorders*. Jenison, MI: Jenison High School.

Gray, C. A. (1995). Teaching children with autism to 'read' social situations. In Quill, K. (ed.). *Teaching Children with Autism: Strategies to Enhance Communication and Socialization* (pp. 219–41). Albany, NY: Delmar.

Greaves, D. (1997). The effect of rational-emotive parent education on the stress of mothers of young children with Down syndrome. *Journal of Rational-Emotive and Cognitive Behaviour Therapy, 15*, 249–67.

Greenberg, J. S., Seltzer, M. M., Orsmond, G. I., & Krauss, M. W. (1999). Siblings of adults with mental illness or mental retardation: Current involvement and expectation of future caregiving. *Psychiatric Services, 50*, 1214–19.

Greenberg, M. T. & Kusche, C. A. (1998). Preventive intervention for school-age deaf children: The PATHS curriculum. *Journal of Deaf Studies Deaf Education, 3*(1), 49–63.

Greenberg, M. T., Kusche, C. A., Cook, E.T., & Quamma, J.P. (1995). Promoting emotional competence in school-aged deaf children: The effects of the PATHS curriculum. *Development and Psychopathology, 7*, 117–36.

Greenberger, D. & Padesky, C. A. (1995). *Mind Over Mood: Change The Way You Feel by Changing The Way You Think*. New York: Guildford Press.

Greenspan, S. I. & Wieder, S. (1998). *The Child with Special Needs: Intellectual and Emotional Growth*. Reading, MA: Addison Wesley Longman.

Greenspan, S. I. & Wieder, S. (2008). The interdisciplinary council on developmental and learning disorders diagnostic manual for infants and young children: An overview. *Journal of the Canadian Academy of Child and Adolescent Psychiatry, 17*(2), 76–89.

Grey, I. M., & Hastings, R. P. (2005). Evidence-based practices in intellectual disability and behaviour disorders. *Current Opinion in Psychiatry, 18*(5), 469–75.

Griffiths, R. (1970). *The Abilities of Young Children: A Comprehensive Assessment of Mental Measurement of the First 8 Years of Life*. High Wycombe, UK: The Test Agency.

Grizenko, N. & Vida, S. (1988). Propranolol treatment of episodic dyscontrol and aggressive behaviour in children (letter). *Canadian Journal of Psychiatry, 33*, 776–8.

Grobin, A. C., Matthews, D. B., Devaud, L. L., & Morrow, A. L. (1998). The role of GABA(A) receptors in the acute and chronic effects of ethanol. *Psychopharmacology, 139*, 2–19.

Grotstein, J. S. (1987). The borderline as a disorder of self-regulation. In Grotstein, J. S., Solomon, M. F., & Lang, J. A. (eds). *The Borderline Patient: Emerging Concepts in Diagnosis, Psychodynamics, and Treatment*, Vol. 1 (pp. 347–83). Hillsdale, NJ: Analytic Press.

Grove, W. M., Zald, D. H., Lebow, B. S., Snitz, B. E., & Nelson, C. (2000). Clinical vs. mechanical prediction: A meta-analysis. *Psychological Assessment, 12*(1), 19–30.

Gualtieri, C. T. (2002). *Brain Injury and Mental Retardation: Psychopharmacology and Neuropsychiatry*. Hagerstown, MD: Lippincott Williams & Wilkins.

Haddock, K. & Jones, R. S. P. (2006). Practitioner consensus in the use of cognitive behaviour therapy for individuals with a learning disability. *Journal of Intellectual Disabilities, 10*(3), 221–30.

Hagerman, R., Berry-Kravis, E., Hessl, D., Coffey, S., Schneider, A., Nguyen, D., Hervey, C., Hutchinson, L., & Snape, M. (2008). Trial of fenobam, a mGluR5 antagonist, in adults with Fragile X syndrome. *Journal of Intellectual Disability Research, 52*(10), 814.

Hall, I. (2000). Young offenders with a learning disability. *Advances in Psychiatric Treatment, 6*, 278–86.

Hames, A. (1998). Do the younger siblings of learning-disabled children see them as similar or different? *Child: Care, Health and Development, 24*, 157–68.

Handen, B. L. (2007). Intellectual disability (mental retardation). In Mash E. J. & Barkley, R. A. (eds). *Assessment of Childhood Disorders* (4th edn) (pp. 551–97). NY: Guilford Press.

Hanft, B. E., Miller, L. J., & Lane, S. J. (2000). Toward a consensus in terminology in sensory integration theory and practice: Part 3: Observable behaviors: Sensory integration dysfunction. *Sensory Integration Special Interest Section Quarterly, 23*(3), 1–4.

Hanline, M. F. (1991). Transitions and critical events in the family life cycle: Implications for providing support to families of children with disabilities. *Psychology in Schools, 28*, 53–9.

Hardan, A. & Sahl, R. (1997). Psychopathology in children and adolescents with developmental disorders. *Research in Developmental Disabilities, 18*, 369–82.

Harris, J. C. (2006). *Intellectual Disability: Understanding Its Development, Causes, Classification, Evaluation and Treatment*. New York: Oxford University Press.

Harris, J. C. (2008). Neuromodulatory treatment for dystonia and self injurious behaviour in Lesch-Nyhan disease. *Journal of Intellectual Disability Research, 52*(8–9), 656.

Harris, S. (1982). The family systems approach to behavioural training with parents of intellectually disabled children. *Child and Family Behaviour Therapy, 4*(1), 21–40.

Harris, M. & Reichle, J. (2004). The impact of aided language stimulation on symbol comprehension and production in nonverbal children with moderate cognitive disabilities. *American Journal of Speech-Language Pathology, 13,* 155–67.

Harrison, P. L. & Oakland, T. (2003). *Adaptive Behaviour Assessment System* (2nd edn) (ABAS-II). San Antonio, TX: Psychological Corporation.

Hartley, S. L., Sikora, D. M., & McCoy, R. (2008). Prevalence and risk factors of maladaptive behaviour in young children with autistic disorder. *Journal of Intellectual Disability Research, 52*(10), 819–29.

Harty, M., Alant, E., & Uys, C. J. E. (2007). Maternal self-efficacy and maternal perception of child language competence in pre-school children with a communication disability. *Child: Care, Health and Development, 33*(2), 144–54.

Harvey, S. T., Boer, D., Meyer, L. H. & Evans, I. M. (2009). Updating a meta-analysis of intervention research with challenging behaviour: Treatment validity and standards of practice. *Journal of Intellectual and Developmental Disability, 34*(1), 67–80.

Hassall, R., Rose, J., & McDonald, J. (2005). Parenting stress in mothers of children with an intellectual disability: The effects of parental cognitions in relation to child characteristics and family support. *Journal of Intellectual Disability Research, 49*(6), 405–18.

Hassiotis, A., Barron, D. A., & Hall, I. (eds) (2009). *Intellectual Disability Psychiatry: A Practical Handbook.* Chichester: Wiley-Blackwell.

Hassiotis, A. A. & Hall, I. (2008). Behavioural and cognitive-behavioural interventions for outwardly-directed aggressive behaviour in people with learning disabilities. *Cochrane Database of Systematic Reviews,* Issue 3, CD003406.

Hastings, R. P. (2002). Parental stress and behaviour problems of children with developmental disability. *Journal of intellectual and Developmental Disability, 27,* 149–60.

Hastings, R. P. & Beck, A. (2004). Practitioner review: Stress intervention for parents of children with intellectual disabilities. *Journal of Child Psychology & Psychiatry, 45*(8), 1338–49.

Hastings, R. P., Hatton, C., Taylor, J. L., & Maddison, C. (2004). Life events and psychiatric symptoms in adults with intellectual disabilities. *Journal of Intellectual Disability Research, 48*(1), 42–6.

Hastings, R. P. & Mount, R. H. (2001). Early correlates of behavioural and emotional problems in children and adolescents with severe intellectual disabilities: A preliminary study. *Journal of Applied Research in Intellectual Disabilities, 14,* 381–91.

Hatton, C. & Emerson, E. (2004). The relationship between life events and psychopathology amongst children with intellectual disabilities. *Journal of Applied Research in Intellectual Disabilities, 17,* 109–17.

Hauser-Cram P., Warfield, M., Shonkoff, J., Krauss, M., Sayer, A., & Upshur, C. C. (2001). Children with disabilities: A longitudinal study of child development and parent well-being. *Monographs of the Society for Research in*

Child Development, 66(3), i–viii, 1–114, discussion 115–26. Retrieved from MEDLINE with Full Text database.

Haveman, M., Van Berkum, G., Hölscher, P., & Van Wallegam, M. (2000). Needs for services expressed by parents with young intellectually disabled children: A comparison of results in Germany, the Netherlands and Belgium (Abstract no 471). *Journal of Intellectual Disability Research, 44*(4–5), 310–11.

Havighurst, S. S. & Downey, L. (2009). Clinical reasoning for child and adolescent mental health practitioners: The mindful formulation. *Clinical Child Psychology and Psychiatry, 14*(2), 251–71.

Hawkins, N. E. & Singer, G. H. S. (1989). A skills training approach for assisting parents to cope with stress. In Singer, G. H. S. & Irvin, L. K. (eds). *Support for Caregiving Families: Enabling Positive Adaptation to Disability* (pp. 71–102). Baltimore: Paul H. Brookes.

Hebert, J. R., Brandt, H. M., Armstead, C. A., Adams, S. A., & Steck, S. E. (2009). Interdisciplinary, translational, and community-based participatory research: Finding a common language to improve cancer research. *Cancer Epidemiology, Biomarkers and Prevention, 18*(4), 1213–17.

Heckers, S. & Konradi, C. (2000). Anatomic and molecular principles of psychopharmacology: A primer for psychiatrists. *Child and Adolescent Psychiatric Clinics of North America: Psychopharmacology, 9*(1), 1–22.

Helen, M. & Francey, S. (1991). *Friendly Kids: Friendly Classrooms.* Melbourne: Pearson Education.

Hemmings, C. P. (2007). The relationship between challenging behaviours and psychiatric disorders in people with severe intellectual disabilities. In Bouras, N. & Holt, G. (eds). *Psychiatric and Behavioural Disorders in Intellectual and Developmental Disabilities* (2nd edn) (pp. 62–75). Cambridge: Cambridge University Press.

Hendren, R., Birrell Weisen, R., & Orley, J. (1994). *Mental Health Programs in Schools.* Geneva: Division of Mental Health, World Health Organization; available from <http://whqlibdoc.who.int/hq/1993/WHO_MNH_PSF_93.3_REV.1.pdf>.

Henry, B., Caspi, A., Moffitt, T. E., & Silva, P. A. (1996). Temperamental and familial predictors of violent and nonviolent criminal convictions: Age 3 to age 18. *Developmental Psychology, 32*, 614–23.

Hérault, J., Petit, E., Martineau, J., Cherpi, C., Perrot, A., Barthélémy, C., Lelord, G., & Müh, J. P. (1996). Serotonin and autism: Biochemical and molecular biology features. *Psychiatry Research, 65*(1), 33–43.

Herring, S., Gray, K., Taffe, B., Sweeney, D., & Einfeld, S. (2006). Behaviour and emotional problems in toddlers with pervasive developmental disorders and developmental delay: Associations with parental mental health and family functioning. *Journal of Intellectual Disability Research, 50*(12), 874–82.

Heslop, P., Mallett, R., Simons, K., & Ward, L. (2002). *Bridging the Divide at Transition: What Happens for Young People with Learning Difficulties and their Families.* Kidderminster: British Institute of Learning Disabilities.

Hetzroni, O. E. (2003). A positive behaviour support: A preliminary evaluation of a school-wide plan for implementing AAC in school for students with intellectual disabilities. *Journal of Intellectual and Developmental Disability, 28*(3), 283–96.

Hill, J. W. & Coufal, K. L. (2005). Emotional/behavioral disorders: A retrospective examination of social skills, linguistics, and student outcomes. *Communication Disorders Quarterly, 27*(1), 33–46.

Hirsch, E. (2005). Childhood epilepsy syndromes with both focal and generalized seizures. *Acta Neurologica Scandinavica, 112*(Suppl. 181), 52–6.

Hodapp, R. M. (1995). Parenting children with Down syndrome and other types of mental retardation. In Bornstein, M. H. (ed.). *Handbook of Parenting. Vol. 1: Children and Parenting* (pp. 233–53). Mahwah, NJ: Lawrence Erlbaum Associates.

Hodapp, R. M. (1997). Direct and indirect behavioural effects of different genetic disorders of mental retardation. *American Journal on Mental Retardation, 102*(1), 67–79.

Hodapp, R. & Barack, J. (2006). Developmental approaches to children with mental retardation: A second generation? In Cicchetti, D. & Cohen, D. (eds). *Developmental Psychopathology: Vol. 3. Risk, Disorder and Adaptation* (2nd ed.) (pp. 235–67). London: John Wiley.

Hodapp, R. M., & Urbano, R. C. (2007). Adult siblings of individuals with Down Syndrome versus with autism: Findings from a large-scale US survey. *Journal of Intellectual Disability Research, 51*, 1018–29.

Hoffman, L., Marquis, J., Poston, D., Summers, J. A., & Turnbull, A. (2006). Assessing family outcomes: Psychometric evaluation of the beach center family quality of life scale. *Journal of Marriage and Family, 68*(4), 1069–83.

Holden, M. J. (with Mooney, A. J., Holden, J. C., Kuhn, I. F., Morgan, C. S., Taylor, R., Bidleman, D., et al.) (2001). *Therapeutic Crisis Intervention* (5th edn): *Student Workbook.* Ithaca, NY: Family Life Development Center, Cornell University.

Holland, A. (2009). What is special in psychiatry for people with intellectual disability? Mental health and challenging behaviour: Understanding the complexity of the relationship. Amsterdam: keynote lecture presented at 7th European Congress of Mental Health in Intellectual Disability, September.

Hollis, C. (2008). Schizophrenia and allied disorders. In Rutter, M., Bishop, D., Pine, D., Scott, S., Stevenson, J. S., Taylor, E. A., Thapar, A. (eds). *Rutter's Child And Adolescent Psychiatry* (5th edn) (pp. 737–58). Oxford: Blackwell.

Horner, R. H. & Carr, E. G. (1997). Behavioral support for students with severe disabilities: Functional assessment and comprehensive intervention. *Journal of Special Education, 31*, 84–104.

Horrigan, J. P. & Barnhill, L. J. (1997). Risperidone and explosive aggressive autism. *Journal of Autism and Developmental Disorders, 27*, 313–23.

Horwitz, A., Tessler, R., Fisher, G., & Gamache, G. M. (1992). The role of adult siblings in providing social support to the severely mentally ill. *Journal of Marriage and the Family, 54*(1), 233–41.

Horwitz, N., & Ellis, J. (2007). Paediatric SpRs' experiences of breaking bad news. *Child: Care, Health and Development, 33*(5), 625–30.

Howarth, J. & Morrison, T. (2007). Collaboration, integration and change in children's services: Critical issues and key ingredients. *Child Abuse and Neglect, 31*, 55–69.

Howlin, P., Baron-Cohen, S., & Hadwin, J. (1999). *Teaching Children with Autism to Mind-Read: A Practical Guide*. Chichester: Wiley.

Hsieh, S. F. & Shannon, S. E. (2005). Three approaches to qualitative content analysis. *Qualitative Health Research, 15*, 1277–88.

Huang, W., O'Brien, H. R., Kalinowski, C. M., Vreeland, R. G., Keinbub, L., & Hall, G. A. (2007). Multidisciplinary approach to optimizing pharmacological and behavioural interventions for persons with developmental disabilities who are on psychotropic medications. *Journal of Developmental and Physical Disabilities, 19*, 237–50.

Hudson, B. (2003). From adolescence to young adulthood: The partnership challenge for learning disability services in England. *Disability and Society, 18*(3), 259–76.

Hudson, B. (2006). Making and missing connections: Learning disability services and the transition from adolescence to adulthood. *Disability and Society, 21*(1), 47–60.

Hudson, A., Cameron, C., & Matthews, J. (2008). The wide-scale implementation of a support program for parents of children with an intellectual disability and difficult behaviour. *Journal of Intellectual and Developmental Disability, 33*, 117–26.

Hudson, A. M., Matthews, J. M., Gavidia-Payne, S. T., Cameron, C. A., Mildon, R. L., & Radler, G. A.(2003). Evaluation of an intervention system for parents of children with intellectual disability and challenging behaviour. *Journal of Intellectual Disability Research, 47*(4–5), 238–49.

Hudziak, J. (ed.) (2008). *Developmental Psychopathology and Wellness: Genetic and Environmental Influences*. Washington DC: American Psychiatric Publishing Inc.

Hudziak, J., Achenback, T., Althoff, R., & Pine, D. (2007). A dimensional approach to developmental psychopathology. *International Journal of Methods in Psychiatric Research, 16*(Suppl. 1), S16–23.

Hulbert-Williams, L., & Hastings, R. P. (2008). Life events as a risk factor for psychological problems in individuals with intellectual disabilities: A critical review. *Journal of Intellectual Disability Research, 52*(11), 883–95.

Hurley, A. (1989). Individual psychotherapy with mentally retarded individuals: A review and call for research. *Research in Developmental Disabilities, 10,* 261–75.

Hurley, A. (2008). Depression in adults with intellectual disability: Symptoms and challenging behaviour. *Journal of Intellectual Disability Research, 52*(11), 905–16.

Hurley, A. D. (1996). Psychiatric disorders in children and adolescents with mental retardation and developmental disabilities. *Current Opinion in Pediatrics, 8*(4), 361–5.

Hustard, K. C. & Shapley, K. L. (2003). AAC and natural speech in individuals with developmental disabilities. In Light, J. C., Beukelman, D. R., & Reichle, J. (eds). *Communicative Competence for Individuals Who Use AAC: From Research to Effective Practice* (pp. 41–62). Baltimore: Paul H. Brookes.

Hutchings, J. & Lane, E. (2006) Reaching those who need it most. *Psychologist, 19*(8), 480–3.

Imber-Black, E. (1987). *The Mentally Handicapped In Context.* Family Systems Medicine, 5428–45.

Imms, C. (2006). The international classification of functioning, disability and health: They talking our language. *Australian Occupational Therapy Journal, 53*(2), 65–6.

International Association for the Scientific Study of Intellectual Disabilities (IASSID, 2001). *Mental Health and Intellectual Disabilities: Addressing the Mental Health Needs of People with Intellectual Disabilities. Report of the Mental Health Special Interest Research Group of the IASSID to the World Health Organization.* Geneva: World Health Organization.

Ireland, M. (2007). 007 Licence to communicate. Opening address at Melbourne: AGOSCI 8th Biennial National Conference, March.

Jackson; J. H. (1931). *Selected Writings of John Hughlings Jackson,* Vols 1–2. London: Hodder & Stoughton.

Jacobson, S. A. & Wilhite, B.C. (1999). Residential transitions in the lives of older adults with developmental disabilities: An ecological perspective. *Therapeutic Recreation Journal, 33*(3), 195–208.

Jaffe, A. V., & Gardner, L. (2006). *My Book Full of Feelings: How to Control and React to the Size of Your Emotions.* Shawnee Mission, KS: Autism Asperger Publishing Co.

Jahromi, L. B., Gulsrud, A., & Kasari, C. (2008). Emotional competence in children with Down syndrome: Negativity and regulation. *American Journal of Mental Retardation, 113*(1), 32–43.

Janssen, C. G. C., Schuengel, C., & Stolk, J. (2002). Understanding challenging behaviour in people with severe and profound intellectual disability: A stress-attachment model. *Journal of Intellectual Disability, 46,* 445–53.

Janus, M., Kopechanski, L., Cameron, R., & Hughes, D. (2008). In transition: Experiences of parents of children with special needs at school entry. *Early Childhood Education Journal, 35,* 479–85.

Jess, G., Torr, J., Cooper, S. A., Lennox, N., Edwards, N., Galea, J., & O'Brien, G. (2008). Specialist versus generic models of psychiatry training and service provision for people with intellectual disabilities. *Journal of Applied Research in Intellectual Disabilities, 21*, 183–93.

Jette, A. M. (2006). Toward a common language for function, disability and health. *Physical Therapy, 86*(5), 726–34.

Johnson, B. A., Rosenthal, N., Capece J. A., Wiegand, F., Mao, L., Beyers, K., McKay, A., Ait-Daoud, N., Anton, R. F., Ciraulo, D.A., Kranzler, H. R., Mann, K., O'Malley, S. S., & Swift, R. M. (2007). Topiramate for treating alcohol dependence: a randomized controlled trial. *Journal of the American Medical Association, 298*(14), 1641–51.

Johnson, B. S. (2000). Mothers' perceptions of parenting children with disabilities. *American Journal Maternal Child Nursing, 25*(3), 127–32.

Jordan, R. (2001). *Autism with Severe Learning Difficulties: A Guide for Parents and Professionals*. London: Souvenir Press.

Kalat, J. W. (2009). *Biological Psychology* (10th edn). Belmont, CA: Wadsworth, Cengage Learning.

Kam, C. M., Greenberg, M. T., & Kusché, C. A. (2004). Sustained effects of the PATHS curriculum on the social and psychological adjustment of children in special education. *Journal of Emotional and Behavioral Disorders, 12*, 66–78.

Kaminski, J. W., Valle, L. A., Filence, J. H., & Boyle, C. L. (2008). A meta-analytic review of components associated with parent training program effectiveness. *Journal of Abnormal Child Psychology, 36*, 567–89.

Kandel, E. R., Schwartz, J. H., & Jessell, T. M. (2000). *Principles of Neural Science* (4th edn). New York: McGraw-Hill.

Kauffman, J. M. (1997). *Characteristics of Emotional and Behavioural Disorders of Children and Youth* (6th edn). Columbus, OH: Charles E. Merrill.

Kealey, T. (2008). *Sex, Science and Profits: How People Evolved to Make Money*. London: William Heinemann.

Kelly, A. (1996). *Talkabout: A Social Communication Skills Package*. Milton Keynes, UK: Speechmark Publishing Ltd.

Kendall, P. C. (1993). Cognitive-behavioural therapies with youth: Guiding theory, current status and emerging developments. *Journal of Consulting and Clinical Psychology, 61*, 235–47.

Kenny, K. & McGilloway, S. (2007). Caring for children with learning disabilities: An exploratory study of parental strain and coping. *British Journal of Learning Disabilities, 35*(4), 221–8.

Kevan, F. (2003). Challenging behaviour and communication difficulties. *British Journal of Learning Disabilities, 31*, 75–80.

Kim, K. & Turnbull, A. (2004). Transition to adulthood for students with severe intellectual disabilities: Shifting toward person-family interdependent planning. *Research and Practice for Persons with Severe Disabilities, 29*(1), 53–7.

Kimball, J. G. (1999). Sensory integration frame of reference: Theoretical base, function/dysfunction continua and guide to evaluation. In Kramer, P. & Hinojosa, J. (eds). *Frames of Reference for Pediatric Occupational Therapy* (2nd edn) (pp. 119–68). Philadelphia: Lippincott Williams & Wilkins.

King, G. A., Baldwin, P. J., Currie, M., & Evans, J. (2005). Planning successful transitions from school to adult roles for youth with disabilities. *Children's Health Care, 34*(3), 195–216.

King, M. & Anderson, N. (2002). *Managing Innovation and Change.* Sydney: Thompson Learning.

Kingsley, E. P. (1987). *Welcome to Holland.* Retrieved 12 November 2009 from <http://www.our-kids.org/Archives/Holland.html>.

Kinnealey, M. (1998). Princess or tyrant: A case report of a child with sensory defensiveness. *Occupational Therapy International, 5,* 293–303.

Kiresuk, T. J. & Sherman, R. E. (1968). Goal attainment scaling: A general method for evaluating comprehensive community mental health programs. *Community Mental Health Journal, 4*(6), 443–53.

Kluft, R. P. (1985). The treatment of multiple personality disorder (MPD): Current concepts. In Flach, F. F. (ed.). *Directions in Psychiatry.* New York: Hatherleigh.

Koegel, L., Koegel, R., & Dunlap, G. (eds) (1996). *Positive Behavioural Support: Including People with Difficult Behaviour in the Community.* Baltimore: Paul H. Brookes.

Kohler, P. D. (1996). *Taxonomy for Transition Programming: Linking Research and Practice.* Urbana-Champaign: Transition Research Institute, University of Illinois.

Koob, G. F. (1998). Circuits, drugs and drug addiction. *Advances in Pharmacology, 42,* 978–82.

Koskentausta, T., Iivanainen, M., & Almqvist, F. (2007). Risk factors for psychiatric disturbance in children with intellectual disability. *Journal of Intellectual Disability Research, 51*(1), 43–53.

Kostelnik, M., Whiren, A., Soderman, A., Stein, L., & Gregory, K. (2006). *Guiding Children's Social Development* (5th edn). Florence, KY: Delmar Cengage Learning.

Kotler, M. & Matar, M. A. (1998). Lamotrigine in the treatment of resistant bipolar disorder. *Clinical Neuropharmacology, 21,* 65–7.

Kozlowska, K. & Hanney, L. (2002). The network perspective: An integration of attachment and family system theories. *Family Process, 41,* 285–312.

Kraijer, D. (2000). Review of adaptive behavior studies in mentally retarded persons with autism/pervasive developmental disorder. *Journal of Autism and Developmental Disorders, 30*(1), 39–47.

Kralik, D., Visentin, K., & van Loon, A. (2006). Transition: A literature review. *Journal of Advanced Nursing, 55*(3), 320–9.

Krippendorff, K. (2004). *Content Analysis: An Introduction to its Methodology* (2nd edn). Thousand Oaks, CA: Sage.

Kuperman, S. & Stewart, M. A. (1987). Use of propranolol to decrease aggressive outbursts in younger patients. *Psychosomatics, 28,* 315–19.

Kvarnstrom, S. (2008). Difficulties in collaboration: A critical incident of interprofessional healthcare teamwork. *Journal of Interprofessional Care, 22*(2), 191–203.

Kwok, H. & Cheung, P. W. H. (2007). Co-morbidity of psychiatric disorder and medical illness in people with intellectual disabilities. *Current Opinion in Psychiatry, 20,* 443–9.

LaCava, P. G. (2005). Facilitate transitions. *Intervention in School and Clinic, 41*(1), 46–8.

Lachman, H. M., Nolan, K. A., Mohr, P., Saito, T., & Volavka, J. (1998). Association between catechol-O-methyltransferase genotype and violence in schizophrenia and schizoaffective disorder. *American Journal of Psychiatry, 155*(6), 835–7.

Lambert, N., Nihira, K., & Leland, H. (1993). *AAMR Adaptive Behavior Scale: School and Community* (2nd edn). Austin, TX: Pro-Ed.

Landa, R. (2007). Early communication development and intervention for children with autism. *Mental Retardation and Developmental Disabilities Research Reviews, 13,* 16–25.

Larson, E. (1998). Reframing the meaning of disability to families: The embrace of paradox. *Social Science and Medicine, 47*(7), 865–75.

Lask, B., Taylor, S., & Nunn, K. P. (2003). *Practical Child Psychiatry: The Clinician's Guide.* London: BMJ Books.

LaVigna, G. W. & Willis, T. J. (1995). Challenging behaviour: A model for breaking the barriers to social and community integration. *Positive Practices, 1*(1), 1, 8–15.

LaVigna, G. W., Willis, T. J., & Donnelan, A. M. (1989). The role of positive programming in behavioral treatment. In Cipani, E. (ed.). *The Treatment of Severe Behavior Disorders: Behavior Analysis Approaches* (pp. 59–83). Washington, DC: American Association on Mental Retardation.

Leahy, R. L. (2003). *Cognitive Therapy Techniques: A Practitioner's Guide.* New York: Guildford Press.

Lecavalier, L. & Aman, M. G. (2005). Rating instruments. In Matson, J. L., Laud, R. B., & Matson, M. L. (eds). *Behavior Modification for Persons with Developmental Disabilities: Empirically Supported Treatments,* Vol. 1 (pp. 160–89). Kingston, NY: National Association for the Dually Diagnosed.

Leckman, J. F., Ort, S., Caruso, K. A., Anderson, G. M., Riddle, M. A., & Cohen D. J. (1986). Rebound phenomena in Tourette's syndrome after abrupt withdrawal of clonidine. *Archives of General Psychiatry, 43,* 1168–76.

Lee, D. O. & Ousley, O. Y. (2006). Attention-deficit hyperactivity disorder symptoms in a clinic sample of children and adolescents with pervasive developmental disorders. *Journal of Child and Adolescent Psychopharmacology, 16*(6), 737–46.

Lee, P., Moss, S., Friedlander, R., Donnelly, T., & Honer, W. (2003). Early-onset schizophrenia in children with mental retardation: Diagnostic reliability and stability of clinical features. *Journal of American Academy of Child and Adolescent Psychiatry, 42*(2), 162–9.

Lennox, N., Rey-Conde, T., & Cooling, N. (2006). Comprehensive health assessments during de-institutionalization: an observational study. *Journal of Intellectual Disability Research, 50*(10), 719–24.

Leonard, B. J., Johnson, A. L., & Brust, J. D. (1993). Preventing mental health problems in children with chronic illness or disability. *Children's Health Care, 20*(3), 150–61.

Levy, F., Hay, D. A., McStephen, M., Wood, C., & Waldman, I. (1997). Attention-deficit hyperactivity disorder: A category or a continuum? Genetic analysis of a large-scale twin study. *Journal of the American Academy of Child and Adolescent Psychiatry, 36*(6), 737–44.

Lewis, A. (1995). *Children's Understanding of Disability.* London: Routledge.

Lewis, P., Abbeduto, L., Murphy, M., Richmond, E., Giles, N., Bruno, L., Schroeder, S., Anderson, J. A., & Orsmond, G. (2006). Psychological well being of mothers of youth with Fragile X syndrome: Syndrome specificity and within syndrome variability. *Journal of Intellectual Disability Research, 50*(12), 894–904.

Leyfer, O. T., Folstein, S. E., Bacalman, S., Davis, N. O., Dinh, E., Morgan, J., Tager-Flusberg, H., & Lainhart, J. E. (2006). Comorbid psychiatric disorders in children with Autism: Interview development and rates of disorders. *Journal of Autism and Developmental Disorders, 36*(7), 849–61.

Life Support Productions (2002a). *Jason's Private World* (DVD). London: Life Support Productions.

Life Support Productions (2002b). *Kylie's Private World* (DVD). London: Life Support Productions.

Light, J. C. (2003). Shattering the silence: Development of communicative competence by individuals who use AAC. In Light, J. C., Beukelman, D. R., & Reichle, J. (eds). *Communicative Competence for Individuals Who Use AAC: From Research to Effective Practice* (pp. 3–38). Baltimore: Paul H. Brookes.

Light, J. & Drager, K. (2007). AAC technologies for young children with complex communication needs: State of the science and future research directions. *Augmentative and Alternative Communication, 23,* 204–16.

Linderman, T. & Stewart, D. (1999). Sensory integrative-based occupational therapy and functional outcomes in young children with pervasive developmental disorders: A single subject study. *American Journal of Occupational Therapy, 53,* 145–52.

Lindsay, W. R. (2005). Model underpinning treatment for sex offenders with mild intellectual disability: Current theories of sex offending. *Mental Retardation, 43*(6), 428–41.

Lipinski, J. F., Sallee, F. R., Jackson, C., & Sethuraman, C. (1997). Dopamine agonist treatment of Tourette disorder in children: Results of an open-label trial of pergolide. *Movement Disorders, 12*, 402–7.

Llewellyn, G., Dunn, P., Fante, M., Turnbull, L., & Grace, R. (1999). Family factors influencing out-of-home placement decisions. *Journal of Intellectual Disability Research, 43*(3), 219–41.

Lobato, D. (1993). Issues and interventions for young siblings of children with medical and developmental problems. In Stoneman, Z. & Berman, P. (eds). *The Effects of Mental Retardation, Disability and Illness on Sibling Relationships: Research Issues and Challenges* (pp. 85–98). Baltimore, MD: Paul H Brookes.

Lobato, D. L. & Kao, B. T. (2005). Brief report: Family-based group intervention for young siblings of children with chronic illness and developmental disability. *Journal of Pediatric Psychology, 30*, 678–82.

Lobato, D., Kao, B. T., Engel, R., & Plante, W. (2000). Sibling parent communication about a child's illness or disability. Poster presented at Cleveland, OH: meeting of the Biannual Great Lakes Regional Conference of the Society for Pediatric Psychology.

Lochman, J. E., White, K. J., & Wayland, K. K. (1991). Cognitive-behavioural assessment and treatment with aggressive children. In Kendall, P. C. (ed.). *Child and Adolescent Therapy: Cognitive Behavioural Procedures* (pp. 25–65). New York: Guilford Press.

Löfgren-Mårtenson, L. (2004). 'May I?' About sexuality and love in the new generation with intellectual disabilities. *Sexuality and Disability, 22*(3), 197–207.

Lord, C., Rutter, M., DiLavore P.C., & Risi, S. (1999). *Autism Diagnostic Observation Schedule (ADOS)*. Los Angeles, CA: Western Psychological Services.

Lord, C., Rutter, M., & Le Couteur, A. (1994). Autism Diagnostic Interview-Revised: A revised version of a diagnostic interview for caregivers of individuals with possible pervasive developmental disorders. *Journal of Autism and Developmental Disorders, 24*(5), 659–85.

Loscher, W. (1998). Pharmacology of glutamate receptor antagonists in the kindling model of epilepsy. *Progress in Neurobiology, 54*, 721–41.

Loveland, K. A. & Tunali-Kotoski, B. (1997). The school age child with autism. In Cohen, D. J. & Volkmar, F. R. (eds). *Handbook of Autism and Pervasive Developmental Disorders* (2nd edn) (pp. 283–308). New York: John Wiley.

Lovibond, S. H. & Lovibond, P. F. (1995). *Manual for the Depression, Anxiety, Stress Scales*. Sydney: Psychology Foundation.

Lumley, V. A. & Scotti, J. R. (2001). Supporting the sexuality of adults with mental retardation: Current status and future directions. *Journal of Positive Behaviour Interventions, 3*(1), 109–19.

McCathren, R. B., Warren, S. F., & Yoder, P. J. (1996). Prelinguistic predictors of later language development. In Cole, K. N., Dale, P. S., & Thal, D. J. (eds).

Communication and Language Intervention Series: Vol. 6. Advances in Assessment of Communication and Language (pp. 57–75). Baltimore: Paul H. Brookes.

McCarthy, J. (2007). Children with autism spectrum disorders and intellectual disability. *Current Opinion in Psychiatry, 20*, 472–6.

McConkey, R. (2009). Social inclusion. Paper presented at Amsterdam: 7th European Congress of Mental Health in Intellectual Disability, September.

McConkey, R. & Ryan, D. (2001). Short report: Experiences of staff in dealing with client sexuality in services for teenagers and adults with intellectual disability. *Journal of Intellectual Disability Research, 45*(1), 83–7.

McConnell, S. R. (2002). Interventions to facilitate social interaction for young children with Autism: Review of available research and recommendations for educational intervention and future research. *Journal of Autism and Developmental Disabilities, 32*, 351–72.

McDonagh, A., Barrett, J., & Ryan, L. (2000). *Design and Deliver: Developing Training Programs in Sexuality, Sexual Health and Intellectual Disability.* Sydney: FPA Health.

McDougle, C. J., Kresch, L. E., Goodman, W. K., Naylor, S. T., Volkmar, F. R., Cohen, D. J., & Price, L. H. (1995). A case-controlled study of repetitive thoughts and behavior in adults with autistic disorder and obsessive-compulsive disorder. *American Journal of Psychiatry, 152*(5), 772–7.

McElroy, S. L., Hudson, J. I., Capece, J. A., Beyers, K., Fisher, A. C., & Rosenthal, N. R. (2007). Topiramate for the treatment of binge eating disorder associated with obesity: a placebo-controlled study. *Biological Psychiatry, 61*(9), 1039–48.

McGoldrick, M. & Gerson, R. (1986). *Genograms in Family Assessment.* New York: Norton.

McGrath, H. & Francey, S. (1991). *Friendly Kids: Friendly Classrooms.* Melbourne: Pearson Education.

MacHale, R. & Carey, S. (2002). An investigation of the effects of bereavement on mental health and challenging behaviour in adults with learning disability. *British Journal of Learning Disabilities, 30*, 113–17.

McIntosh, D. N., Miller, L. J., Shyu, V., & Dunn, W. (1999). The Short Sensory Profile (SSP). In Dunn, W. (ed.). *The Sensory Profile: Examiner's Manual* (pp. 59–83). San Antonio, TX: Psychological Corporation.

McIntyre, L. L., Blacher, J., & Baker, B. L. (2002). Behaviour/mental health problems in young adults with intellectual disability: The impact on families. *Journal of Intellectual Disability Research, 46*(3), 239–49.

McIntyre, L. L., Blacher, J., & Baker, B. L. (2006). The transition to school: Adaptation in young children with and without intellectual disability. *Journal of Intellectual Disability Research, 50*(5), 349–61.

McLeod, S. & McKinnon, D. H. (2007). The prevalence of communication disorders compared with other learning needs in 14,500 primary and secondary school students. *International Journal of Language and Communication Disorders, 42*(S1), 37–59.

McNaughton, D. & Bryen, D. N. (2007). AAC technologies to enhance participation and access to meaningful societal roles for adolescents and adults with developmental disabilities who require AAC. *Augmentative and Alternative Communication, 23*, 217–29.

McVilly, K. R. (2002). *Positive Behaviour Support for People with Intellectual Disability: Evidence-based Practice, Promoting Quality of Life*. Putney, NSW: Australian Society for the Study of Intellectual Disability.

Maes, B., Broekman, T. G., Dosen, A., & Nauts, J. (2003). Caregiving burden of families looking after persons with intellectual disability and behavioural or psychiatric problems. *Journal of Intellectual Disability Research, 47*(6), 447–55.

Main, M. & Solomon, J. (1990). Procedures for identifying infants as disorganized-disoriented during the Ainsworth Strange Situation. In Greenberg, M., Cicchetti, D., & Cummings, E. M. (eds). *Attachment in the Preschool Years: Theory, Research, and Intervention* (pp. 121–60). Chicago: University of Chicago Press.

Malhotra, S. & Santosh, P. J. (1998). An open clinical trial of buspirone in children with attention deficit/hyperactivity disorder. *Journal of the American Academy of Child and Adolescent Psychiatry, 37*, 364–71.

Malone, R. P., Cater, J., Sheikh, R. M., Choudhury, M. S., & Delaney, M. A. (2001). Olanzapine versus haloperidol in children with autistic disorder: An open pilot study. *Journal of the American Academy of Child and Adolescent Psychiatry, 40*(8), 887–94.

Manasco, H. (2006). *The Way to A: Empowering Children with Autism Spectrum and Other Neurological Disorders to Monitor and Replace Aggression and Tantrum Behaviour*. Shawnee Mission, KS: Autism Asperger Publishing Company.

Manchester, D. (2007). *Motivational Interviewing: For All Clinicians in Mental Health, Forensic, and Brain Injury Services*. Sydney: training course provided by MLR Consulting Psychology, May.

Mangeot, S. D., Miller, L. J., McIntosh, D. N., McGrath-Clarke, J., Simon, J., Hagerman, R.J. & Goldson, E. (2001). Sensory modulation dysfunction in children with attention-deficit-hyperactivity disorder. *Developmental Medicine and Child Neurology, 43*(6), 399–406.

Mannix, D. (1993). *Social Skills Activities for Special Children*. San Franciso, CA: Jossey-Bass.

March, J. S. & Benton, C. M. (2007). *Talking Back to OCD: The Program that Helps Kids and Teens Say 'No Way' and Parents Say 'Way To Go'*. London: Guilford Press.

March, J. S. & Mulle, K. (1998). *OCD in Children And Adolescents: A Cognitive-Behavioural Treatment Manual*. New York: Guilford Press.

Marks, I. (2005). Common language for psychotherapy procedures. *Behaviour Therapist, 28*(4), 81–3.

Marshall, P. J., Bar-Haim, Y., & Fox, N. A. (2004). The development of P50 suppression in the auditory event-related potential. *International Journal of Psychophysiology, 51*, 135–41.

Martin, N. C., Piek, J. P., & Hay, D. (2006). DCD and ADHD: A genetic study of their shared aetiology. *Human Movement Science, 25*(1), 110–24.

Maslow, A. H. (1954, 1970). *Hierarchy of Needs*. Retrieved 21 February 2010 from <www.businessballs.com/maslow>.

Matson, J. L., Anderson, S. J., & Bamburg, J.W. (2000). The relationship of social skills to psychopathology for individuals with mild and moderate mental retardation. *British Journal of Developmental Disabilities, 46*(1), 15–22.

Matson, J. L., Matson, M. L., & Rivet, T. T. (2007). Social-skills treatments for children with autism spectrum disorders: An overview. *Behavior Modification, 31*(5), 682–707.

Matson, J. L. & Shoemaker, M. (2009). Intellectual disability and its relationship to autism spectrum disorders. *Research in Developmental Disabilities, 30*(6), 1107–14.

Matson, J. L. & Wilkins, J. (2007). A critical review of assessment targets and methods for social skills excesses and deficits for children with autism spectrum disorders. *Research in Autism Spectrum Disorders, 1*(1), 28–37.

Mayer, J. D., Salovey, P., & Caruso, D. (2000). Models of emotional intelligence. In Sternberg, R. J. (ed.). *The Handbook of Intelligence* (pp. 396–420). New York: Cambridge University Press.

Maynard, D. W. (1991). The Perspective-Display Series and the delivery and receipt of diagnostic news. In Boden, D. & Zimmerman, D. H. (eds). *Talk and Social Structure: Studies in Ethnomethodolgy and Conversation Analysis* (pp. 164–92). Los Angeles: University of California Press.

Maynard, D. W. (1995). On 'labelling' in actual interaction: Delivering and receiving diagnoses of developmental disabilities. *Social Problems, 42*(1), 11–37.

Meehl, P. E. (1954). *Clinical versus Statistical Prediction: A Theoretical Analysis and a Review of the Evidence*. Northvale, NJ: Jason Aronson.

Meehl, P. E. (1957). When shall we use our heads instead of the formula? *Journal of Counseling Psychology, 4*, 268–73.

Meehl, P. E. (1959). A comparison of clinicians with five statistical methods of identifying psychotic MMPI profiles. *Journal of counseling Psychology, 6*(2), 102–9.

Meert, K. L., Eggly, S., Pollack, M., Anand, K. J. S., Zimmerman, J., & Carcillo, J. (2008). Parents' perspectives on physician-parent communication near the time of a child's death in the pediatric intensive care unit. *Pediatric Critical Care Medicine, 9*(1), 2–7.

Mental Health Act (1983). Retrieved 22 December 2009 from Department of Health, UK, at <http://www.dh.gov.uk/en/PublicationsAndStatistics/Legislation/ActsAndBills/DH_4002034>.

Mental Health Act (2007). Retrieved 2 February 2010 from *New South Wales Consolidated Acts* at <http://www.austlii.edu.au/au/legis/nsw/consol_act/mha2007128/>.

Mento, G., Suppiej, A., & Bisiacchi, P. (2009). *When does Right Functional Hemispheric Lateralization Arise? Evidence from Preterm Infants.* Retrieved 21 February 2010 from <Nature Preceedings at http://hdl.handle.net/10101/npre.2009.3204.1>.

Mesulam, M. M. (1998). From sensation to cognition. *Brain, 121,* 1013–52.

Michaels, C. A. & Ferrara, D. L. (2005). Promoting post-school success for all: The role of collaboration in person-centered transition planning. *Journal of Educational and Psychological Consultation, 16*(4), 287-313.

Miller, L. J., Reisman, J. E., McIntosh, D. N., & Simon, J. (2001). An ecological model of sensory modulation: Performance of children with fragile X syndrome, autistic disorder, attention-deficit/hyperactivity disorder, and sensory modulation dysfunction. In Smith-Roley, S., Blanche, E. I., & Schaaf, R. C. (eds). *Understanding the Nature Of Sensory Integration with Diverse Populations* (pp. 57–88). San Antonio, TX: Therapy Skill Builders.

Miller, P. R., Dasher, R., Collins, R., Griffiths, P., & Brown, F. (2001). Inpatient diagnostic assessments: 1. Accuracy of structured vs. unstructured interviews. *Psychiatry Research, 105*(3), 255–64.

Miller, W.R. & Rollnick, S. (eds) (2002). *Motivational Interviewing: Preparing People for Change.* New York: Guilford Press.

Minichiello, V., Aroni, R., Timewell, E., & Alexander, L. (1995). *In-depth Interviewing: Principles, Techniques, Analysis* (2nd edn). Sydney: Longman.

Minnes, P. (1988). Family resources and stress associated with having a mentally retarded child. *American Journal on Mental Retardation, 93,* 184–92.

Minnes, P. (1998). Mental retardation: The impact upon the family. In Burack, J. A., Hodapp, R. M., & Zigler, E. (eds). *Handbook of Mental Retardation and Development* (pp. 693–712). New York: Cambridge University Press.

Minuchin, S. (1974). *Families and Family Therapy.* Cambridge, MA: Harvard University Press.

Mirenda, P. (2008). A back door approach to autism and AAC. *Augmentative and Alternative Communication, 24,* 219–33.

Moeschler, J. B. (2008). Genetic evaluation of intellectual disabilities. *Seminars in Pediateric Neurology, 15*(1), 2–9.

Mohr, C., Curran, J., Coutts, A., & Dennis, S. (2002). Collaboration: Together we can find the way in dual diagnosis. *Issues in Mental Health Nursing, 23*(2), 171–80.

Mohr, C., Phillips, A., Curran, J., & Rymill, A. (2002). Interagency training in dual disability. *Australasian Psychiatry, 10*(4), 356–64.

Molteno, G., Molteno, C., Finchilescu, G., & Dawes, A. (2001) Behavioural and emotional problems in children with intellectual disability attending special schools in Cape Town, South Africa. *Journal of Intellectual Disability Research, 45*(6), 515–20.

Mooney, M., Dobia, B., Yeung, A. S., Barker, K., Power, A., & Watson, K. (2008). *Positive Behaviour for Learning: Investigating the Transfer of a United States System into the New South Wales Department of Education and Training Western Sydney Region Schools* (report). Penrith, NSW: University of Western Sydney. Retrieved 25 February 2010 from <http://arrow.uws.edu.au:8080/vital/access/manager/Repository/uws:132/SOURCE2>.

Moore, K. M., & Henry, A. D. (2002). Treatment of adult psychiatric patients using the Wilbarger protocol. *Occupational Therapy in Mental Health, 18*(1), 43–63.

Moreno, J. (1934). *Who Shall Survive?* Roanoke, VA: Royal Publishing Company.

Moss, S. (2000). *The Mini PAS-ADD Handbook. Psychiatric Assessments Schedules for Adults with Developmental Disabilities.* Brighton, UK: Pavilion Publishing.

Moss, S. C., Patel, P., Prosser, H., Goldberg, D. P., Simpson, N., Rowe, S. & Lucchino, R. (1993). Psychiatric morbidity in older people with moderate and severe learning disability: 1. Development and reliability of the patient interview (PAS-ADD). *British Journal of Psychiatry, 163*, 471–80.

Moss, S. C., Prosser, H., Costello, H., Simpson, N., Patel, P., Rowe, S., Turner, S., & Hatton, C. (1998). Reliability and validity of the PAS-ADD Checklist for detecting psychiatric disorders in adults with intellectual disability. *Journal of Intellectual Disability Research, 42*(2), 173–83.

Mouridsen, S. & Hauschild, K. (2008). A longitudinal study of schizophrenia—and affective spectrum in individuals diagnosed with a developmental language disorder as children. *Journal of Neural Transmission, 115*(11), 1591–7.

Mulligan, S. (2003). Examination of the evidence for occupational therapy using a sensory integration framework with children: Part 2. *Sensory Integration Special Interest Section Quarterly, 26*(2), 1–5.

Mulroy, S., Robertson, L., Aiberti, K., Leonard, H., & Bower, C. (2008). The impact of having a sibling with an intellectual disability: Parental perspectives in two disorders. *Journal Intellectual Disability Research, 52*(3), 216–29.

Murphy, J. & Cameron, L. (2008). The effectiveness of talking mats for people with intellectual disability. *British Journal of Learning Disability, 36*(4), 232–41.

Murphy, O., Healy. O., &. Leader, G (2009). Risk factors for challenging behaviors among 157 children with autism spectrum disorders in Ireland. *Research in Autism Spectrum Disorders, 3*, 474–82.

Murray-Slutsky, C. & Paris, B. A. (2005). *Is It Sensory or Is It Behaviour? Behaviour Problem Identification, Assessment and Intervention*. San Antonio, TX: PsychCorp.

Myrbakk, E. & von Tetzcher, S. (2008). Psychiatric disorders and behaviour problems in people with intellectual disability. *Research in Developmental Disabilities, 29*, 316–32.

Nada Raja, S., McGee, R., & Stanton, W. A. (1992). Perceived attachments to parents and peers and psychological well-being in adolescence. *Journal of Youth and Adolescence, 21*(4), 471–85.

Nankervis, K., Rosewarne, A., & Vassos, M. (2009). *Review of the Causal Factors Resulting in Unavailable Respite Beds: Final Report*. Melbourne: Division of Disability Studies: RMIT University.

National Federation of Voluntary Bodies (2007). *Informing Families of their Child's Disability: National Best Practice Guidelines*. Retrieved 20 May 2009 from Oranmore, Co. Galway, Ireland: National Federation of Voluntary Bodies Providing Services to People with Intellectual Disability at <http://www.fedvol.ie/National_Federation_Publications/Default.757.html>.

Nicholson, D., Artz, S., Armtiage, A., & Fagan, J. (2000). Working relationships and outcomes in multidisciplinary collaborative practice settings. *Child and Youth Care Forum, 29*(1), 39–73.

Nicoll, N., Dowling, C., & Thomas, B. (eds) (2004). *Lessons from My Child: Parent's Experiences of Life with a Disabled Child*. Sydney: Finch Publishing.

Nihira, K., Leland, H., & Lambert, N. (1993). *Adaptive Behavior Scales: Residential and Community Edition* (2nd edn): *Examiner's Manual*. Austin, TX: Pro-Ed.

Nijenhuis, E. R. S., Van der Hart, O., & Steele, K. (2004). *Trauma-related Structural Dissociation of the Personality*. Retrieved 27 September 2009 from <http:www.trauma-pages.com/a/nijenhuis-2004.php>.

Noh, S., Dumas, J. E., Wolf, L. C., & Frisman, S. N. (1989). Delineating sources of stress in parents of exceptional children. *Family Relations, 38*(4), 456–61.

Nota, L., Ferrari, L., Soresi, S., & Wehmeyer, M. (2007). Self-determination, social abilities and the quality of life of people with intellectual disability. *Journal of Intellectual Disability Research, 51*(11), 850–65.

Nott, M. & Chapparo, C. (2008). Measuring information processing in a client with extreme agitation following traumatic brain injury using the Perceive, Recall, Plan and Perform System of Task Analysis. *Australian Occupational Therapy Journal, 55*(3), 188–98.

Noyes-Grosser, D. M. (2007). Children and youth with disabilities and public health: A model syllabus for health professionals. *Infants and Young Children, 20*(3), 202–21.

NSW Commission for Children and Young People (2002). *Report of an Inquiry into the Best Means of Assisting Children and Young People with No-One to Turn To*. Sydney: NSW Commission for Children and Young People.

NSW Department of Ageing Disability and Home Care (2004). *Working Together: Collaborative Planning for Children and Young People with Disabilities* (*Workshop Curriculum, Training Manual Teaching Aids,* and *Facilitators Guide*). Sydney: NSW Department of Ageing Disability and Home Care.

NSW Department of Education (DET) (1998). *Special Education Handbook for Schools.* Sydney: NSW Department of Education Student Services Directorate. Available at <https://www.det.nsw.edu.au/policies/general_man/general/spec_ed/handbook.pdf>.

Nuehring, M. I. & Sitlington, P. L. (2003). Transition as a vehicle: Moving from high school to an adult vocational service provider. *Journal of Disability Policy Studies, 14*(1), 23–35.

Nugent, J. A. (2005). *A Handbook on Dual Diagnosis: Supporting People with a Developmental Disability and a Mental Health Problem* (3rd edn). Mississauga, Ontario: Nugent Training and Consulting Services Publishing.

Nurcombe, B., Anger, N., & Hoyland, M. (2001). *The Role of Speech and Language Pathology in Child and Youth Mental Health Services.* Brisbane: Institute for Child and Youth Mental health Royal Children's Hospital and Health Services and University of Queensland.

Oliver, C. (2008). Environmental responses to genetic disorders: Getting beyond dialogue and toward transaction. Paper presented at Cape Town: 13th IASSID World Congress. (Abstract: *Journal of Intellectual Disability Research, 52*(8–9), 639).

Oliver, C., Arron, K., Sloneem, J., & Hall, S. (2008). Behavioural phenotype of Cornelia de Lange syndrome: Case-control study. *British Journal of Psychiatry, 193,* 466–70.

Oliver, C., Moss, J., Petty, J., Arron, K., Sloneem, J., & Hall, S. (2003). *Self-injurious Behaviour in Cornelia De Lange Syndrome: A Guide for Parents and Carers.* Coventry, UK: Trident Communications Ltd.

Olsen, R. W. & Tobin, A. J. (1990). Molecular biology of GABAA receptors. *Federation of American Societies for Experimental Biology (FASEB) Journal, 4,* 1469–80.

Olson, L .J. & Moulton, H. J. (2004). Occupational therapists' reported experiences using weighted vests with children with specific developmental disorders. *Occupational Therapy International, 11,* 52–66.

O'Neill, R. E., Horner, R. H., Albin, R. W., Storey, K., & Sprague, J. R. (1990). *Functional Analysis of Problem Behavior: A Practical Assessment Guide.* Sycamore, IL: Sycamore Publishing Company.

Orsmond, G. I. & Seltzer, M. M. (2007a). Siblings of individuals with autism or Down syndrome: Effects on adult lives. *Journal of Intellectual Disability Research, 51*(9), 682–96.

Orsmond, G. I. & Seltzer, M. M. (2007b). Siblings of individuals with autism spectrum disorders across the life course. *Mental Retardation and Developmental Disabilities Research Reviews, 13,* 313–20.

Osgood, A. (2004). *Doing It for Attention: Non-Physical Reactive Strategies* (electronic). Retrieved 5 January 2009, from NHS Evidence—Learning Disabilities at <http://www.library.nhs.uk/learningdisabilities/viewresource.aspx?resid=250450>.

Owen, D. M., Hasting, R. P., Noone, S. J., Chinn, J., Harman, K., Roberts, J., et al. (2004). Life events as correlates of problem behaviour and mental health in a residential population of adults with developmental disabilities. *Research in Developmental Disabilities, 25,* 209–320.

Padgett, S. M., Bekemeier, B., & Berkowitz, B. (2004). Collaborative partnerships at the state level: Promoting systems changes in public health infrastructure. *Journal of Public Health Management Practice, 10*(3), 251–7.

Parette Jr., H. P., Brotherson, M. J., & Huer, M. B. (2000). Giving families a voice in augmentative and alternative communication decision-making. *Education and Training in Mental Retardation and Developmental Disabilities, 35*(2), 177–90.

Parkes, C. M. (1993). Bereavement as a psychosocial transition: Processes of adaptation to change. In Stroebe, M. S., Stroebe, W., & O'Hansson, R. (eds). *Handbook of Bereavement.* Cambridge, UK: Press Syndicate of the University of Cambridge.

Patterson, G. R. (1982). *Coercive Family Process.* Eugene, OR: Castalia Publishing.

Patterson, G. R. & Chamberlain, P. (1994). A functional analysis of resistance during parent training therapy. *Clinical Psychology and Scientific Practice, 1,* 53–70.

Patterson, G. R., DeBaryshe, B., & Ramsey, E. (1990). A developmental perspective on antisocial behaviour. *American Psychologist, 44,* 329–35. Reprinted in: Gauvain, M. & Cole, M. (eds) (1993). *Readings on the Development of Children* (2nd edn) (pp. 263–72). New York: Freeman.

Paul, S., Sinen, P., Johnson, J., Latshaw, C., Newton , J., Nelson, A., & Powers, R. (2003). The effects of a sensory motor activities protocol based on the theory of sensory integration on children with preprimary impairments. *Occupational Therapy in Health Care, 17,* 19–34.

Paykel, E. S. (2001). The evolution of life events research in psychiatry. *Journal of Affective Disorders, 62,* 141–9.

PBIS TA Center (n.d.). *National Technical Assistance Center on Positive Behavioral Interventions and Supports.* US Department of Education, Office of Special Education Programs. Retrieved 30 October 2009 from <www.pbis.org>.

Pegram, M. H. (1989). A logotherapeutic support group for mothers of special children. *International Forum for Logotherapy, 12,* 23–7.

Perkins, J. J. & Sanson-Fisher, R. W. (1996). Increased focus on the teaching of interactional skills to medical practitioners. *Advances in Health Sciences Education, 1*(1), 17–28.

Perry, A., Reilly, S., Cotton, S., Bloomberg, K., & Johnson, H. (2004). A demographic survey of people who have a disability and complex communication needs in Victoria, Australia. *Asia Pacific Journal of Speech, Language and Hearing, 9*(3), 259–71.

Perry, B. D. & Szalavitz, M. (2006). *The Boy who Was Raised as a Dog: And Other Stories From a Child Psychiatrist's Notebook. What Traumatized Children Can Teach Us about Loss, Love and Healing.* New York: Basic Books.

Petersen, L. (1995). *Stop and Think Learning. A Teacher's Guide for Motivating Children to Learn: Including Those with Special Needs.* Melbourne: ACER Press.

Petersen, L. (with Adderly, A.) (2002). *Stop, Think, Do! Social Skills Training: Early Years of Schooling Ages 4–8.* Melbourne: ACER Press.

Petersen, L. (with Lewis, P.) (2004). *Stop, Think, Do! Social Skills Training: Supplement for Middle Years of Schooling Ages 12–15.* Melbourne: ACER Press.

Petersen, L. & Adderley, A. (2002). *Stop, Think, Do! Social Skills Training: Primary Years of Schooling Ages 8–12.* Melbourne: ACER Press.

Phillips, A., Morrison, J., & Davies, R. W. (2004). General practitioners' educational needs in intellectual disability health. *Journal of Intellectual Disability Research, 48*(2), 142–9.

Phillips, W., Gomezt, J. C., Baron-Cohen, S., Laat, V., & Rivieret, A. (1995). Treating people as objects, agents, or 'subjects': How young children with and without autism make requests. *Journal of Child Psychology and Psychiatry, 36*(8), 1383–98.

Piaget, J. (1972). *The Psychology of the Child.* New York: Basic Books.

Pickover, S. (2002). Breaking the cycle: A clinical example of disrupting an insecure attachment system. *Journal of Mental Health Counseling, 24,* 358–66.

Pilowsky, T., Yirmiya, N., Gross-Tsur, V., & Shalev, R. S. (2007). Neuropsychological functioning of siblings of children with autism, siblings of children with developmental language delay and siblings of children with mental retardation of unknown genetic aetiology. *Journal of Autism and Developmental Disorders, 37,* 537–52.

Plant, K. M. & Sanders, M. R. (2007). Reducing problem behavior during caregiving in families of preschool-aged children with developmental disorders. *Research in Developmental Disabilities, 28*(4), 362–85.

Playschool (2006). *Big Ted and Friends.* Sydney: Harper Collins.

Poehlmann, J., Clements, M., Abbeduto, L., & Farsad, V. (2005). Family experiences associated with a child's diagnosis of Fragile X or Down syndrome: Evidence for disruption and resilience. *Mental Retardation, 43,* 255–67.

Pottenza, M. N., Holmes, J. P., Kanes, S. J., & McDougle, C. J. (1999). Olanzapine treatment of children, adolescents and adults with pervasive developmental disorders: An open labelled pilot study. *Journal of Clinical Psychopharmacology, 19,* 37–44.

Prendergast, M. (2000). A pragmatic approach to medication. InGillberg, C. & O'Brien, G. (eds). *Developmental Disability and Behaviour* (pp. 138–47). London: Mac Keith Press.

Prince, E., Frader, J., & Bosk, C. (1982). Hedging in physician-physician discourse. In Di Pietro, R. J. (ed.). *Linguistics and the Professions* (pp. 83–97). Norwood, NJ: Ablex.

Prizant, B.M., Meyer, E.C., & Lobato, D. J. (1997). Brothers and sisters of young children with communication disorders. Seminars in Speech and Language, 18, 263-281.

Prizant, B. M. & Wetherby, A. M (1990). Toward an integrated view of early language and communication development and socioemotional development. *Topics in Language Disorders, 10*(4), 1–16.

Prochaska, J. & DiClemente, C. (1986). Toward a comprehensive model of change. In Miller, W. & Heather, N. (eds). *Treating Addictive Behaviours: Processes of Change*. New York: Plenum Press.

Prochaska, J. O., Velicer, W. F., Rossi, J. S., Goldstein, M. G., Marcus, B. H., Rakowski, W., et al. (1994). Stages of change and decisional balance for 12 problem behaviors. *Health Psychology, 13*(1), 39–46.

Ptacek, J. T. & Eberhardt, T. L. (1996). Breaking bad news: A review of the literature. *Journal of the American Medical Association, 276*(6), 496–502.

Quine, L. & Pahl, J. (1985). Examining the causes of stress in families with severely mentally handicapped children. *British Journal of Social Work, 15*, 501–17.

Quine, L. & Pahl, J. (1991). Stress and coping in mothers caring for a child with severe learning difficulties: A test of Lazarus' transactional model of coping. *Journal of Community and Applied Social Psychology, 1*(1), 57–70.

Quinn, J. (2006). Illustrated interactions (unpublished information package). Sydney: NSW Department of Ageing Disability and Home Care.

Quinn, M., Carr, A., Carroll, L., & O'Sullivan, D. (2007). Parents Plus programme I: Evaluation of its effectiveness for preschool children with developmental disabilities and behavioural problems. *Journal of Applied Research in Intellectual Disabilities, 20*, 345–59.

Rapanaro, C., Bartu, A., & Lee, A. H. (2008). Perceived benefits and negative impact of challenges encountered in caring for young adults with intellectual disabilities in the transition to adulthood. *Journal of Applied Research in Intellectual Disabilities, 21*, 34–47.

Rapee, R., Lyneham, H., Schneiring, C., Wuthrich, V., Abbott, M., Hudson, J., & Wignall, A. (2005). *The Cool Kids Anxiety Program*. Sydney: Emotional Health Clinic, Macquarie University. Available from <http://www.psy.mq.edu.au/CEH/materials.html>.

Rapport, M. D., Quinn, S. O., DuPaul, G. J., Quinn, E. P., & Kelly, K. L. (1989). Attention deficit disorder with hyperactivity and methylphenidate: The effect of dose and mastery level on children's learning performance. *Journal of Abnormal Child Psychology, 17*, 669–89.

Ratcliffe, A. E. & Cress, C. J. (1998). Guidelines for enhancing reciprocal peer communication with adolescents who use augmentative/alternative communication. *Journal of Children's Communication Development, 20*(2), 25–35.

Ratcliffe, B., Grahame, V., & Wong, M. (2008). Pilot study of emotion-based social skills training (EBSST) for children with autism spectrum disorder and mild intellectual disability (unpublished raw data). Sydney: The Children's Hospital at Westmead.

Ratcliffe, B., Grahame, V., & Wong, M. (2010). *Emotion-Based Social Skills Training (EBSST) for Children with Autism Spectrum Disorder and Mild Intellectual Disability* (treatment manual and youth workbooks). Sydney: The Children's Hospital at Westmead.

Reber, S. (1995). *Dictionary of Psychology* (2nd edn). London: Penguin.

Reed, J. & Clements, J. (1989). Assessing the understanding of emotional states in a population of adolescents and young adults with mental handicaps. *Journal of Mental Deficiency Research, 33*, 229–33.

Reed, V. (2005). *An Introduction to Children with Language Disorders* (3rd edn). Boston: Pearson/Allyn & Bacon.

Reeves, S., Goldman, J., & Oandasan, I. (2007). Key factors in planning and implementing interprofessional education in health care steetings. *Journal of Allied Health, 36*(4), 231–5.

Reid, J., Patterson, G., & Snyder, J. (2002). Antisocial behaviour in children and adolescents: A developmental analysis and model for intervention. Washington, DC: American Psychological Association.

Reisman, J. E. & Hanschu, B. (1992). Sensory Integration Inventory-Revised for Individuals with Developmental Disabilities. Stillwater, MN: PDP Press.

Reiss, D. & Neiderhiser, J. (2000). The interplay of genetic influences and social processes in developmental theory: Specific mechanisms are coming into view. *Development and Psychopathology, 12*, 357–74.

Reiss, S., & Valenti-Hein, D. (1994). Development of a psychopathology rating scale for children with mental retardation. *Journal of Clinical and Clinical Psychology, 62*(1), 28–33.

Renwick, R., Brown, I., & Nagler, M. (Eds.) (1996). *Quality of Life in Health Promotion and Rehabilitation: Conceptualizations, Issues and Applications.* Thousand Oaks, CA: Sage.

Repetto, J. B. & Correa, V. I. (1996). Expanding views on transition. *Exceptional Children, 62*(2), 551–63.

Reynhout, G. & Carter, M. (2006). Social Stories for children with disabilities. *Journal of Autism and Developmental Disorders, 36*(4), 445–69.

Reynhout, G. & Carter, M. (2007). Social Story efficacy with a child with autism spectrum disorder and moderate intellectual disability. *Focus on Autism and Other Developmental Disabilities, 22*(3), 173–82.

Reynolds, S. & Lane, S. (2008). Diagnostic validity of sensory over-responsivity: A review of the literature and case reports. *Journal of Autism and Developmental Disorders, 38*(3), 516–29.

Reynolds, W. M. & Baker, J. A. (1988). Assessment of depression in persons with mental retardation. *American Journal on Mental Retardation, 93*, 93–103.

Ricci, L. A. & Hodapp, R. M. (2003). Fathers of children with Down's syndrome versus other types of intellectual disability: Perceptions, stress and involvement. *Journal of Intellectual Disability Research, 47*(4–5), 273–84.

Rhodes, P. (2000). A systemic approach to the assessment of challenging behaviour in group homes: Three case studies. Unpublished manuscript.

Rhodes, P. (2002). Mainstreaming intellectual disability into the history of family therapy. *Australian and New Zealand Journal of Family Therapy, 23*(4), 211–14.

Rhodes, P. (2003). Behavioural and family systems interventions in developmental disability: Towards a contemporary and integrative approach. *Journal of Intellectual and Developmental Disability, 28*(1), 51–64.

Rhodes, P. (2008). Amplifying deviations in family interactions: Guidelines for trainees in Post-Milan family therapy. *Australian and New Zealand Journal of Family Therapy, 29*(1), 34–9.

Riding, T., Swann, C., & Swann, B. (2005). *The Handbook of Forensic Learning Disabilities.* Oxford: Radcliffe Publishing.

Ring, H., Zia, A., Lindeman, S., & Himlok, K. (2007). Interactions between seizure frequency, psychopathology, and severity of intellectual disability in a population with epilepsy and learning disability. *Epilepsy and Behaviour, 11*(1), 92–7.

Roberts, C., Mazzucchelli, T., Studman, L., & Sanders, M. (2006). Behavioral family intervention for children with developmental disabilities and behavioral problems. *Journal of Clinical Child and Adolescent Psychology, 35*(2), 180–93.

Rodriguez, J. R., Geffken, G. R., & Morgan, S. B. (1993). Perceived competence and behavioral adjustment of siblings of children with autism. *Journal of Autism and Developmental Disorders, 23*, 665–74.

Roid, G. H. (2003). *Stanford-Binet Intelligence Scales* (5th edn). Itasca, IL: Riverside Publishing.

Rojahn, J. & Heisel, W. (1991). The aberrant behaviour checklist with children and adolescents with dual diagnosis. *Journal of Autism and Developmental Disorders, 21*(1), 17–28.

Rojahn, J. & Tassé, M. J. (1996). Psychopathology in mental retardation. In Jacobson, J. W. & Mulick, J. A. (eds). *Manual of Diagnosis and Professional Practice in Mental Retardation* (pp. 147–56). Washington, DC: American Psychological Association.

Romski, M. & Sevcik, R. A. (2003). Augmented input: Enhancing communication development. In Light, J. C., Beukelman, D. R., & Reichle, J. (eds). *Communicative Competence for Individuals Who Use AAC: From Research to Effective Practice* (pp. 147–62). Baltimore: Paul H. Brookes.

Rose, R., Howley, M., Fergusson, A., & Jament, J. (2009). Mental health and special education needs: Exploring a complex relationship. *British Journal of Special Education, 36*(1), 3–8.

Rosenstein, D.S. & Horowitz, H.A. (1996). Adolescent attachment and psychopathology. *Journal of Consulting and Clinical Psychology, 64,* 244–53.

Ross, P. & Cuskelly, M. (2006). Adjustment, sibling problems and coping strategies of brothers and sisters of children with autistic spectrum disorders. *Journal of Intellectual and Developmental Disability, 31,* 77–86.

Rossiter, L. & Sharpe, D. (2001). The siblings of individuals with mental retardation: A quantitative integration of the literature. *Journal of Child and Family Studies, 10,* 65–84.

Rowland, C. & Schweigert, P. D. (2003). Cognitive skills and AAC. In Light, J. C., Beukelman, D. R., & Reichle, J. (eds). *Communicative Competence for Individuals Who Use AAC: From Research to Effective Practice* (pp. 241–75). Baltimore: Paul H. Brookes.

Rowling, L. (2007). School mental health promotion: MindMatters as an example of mental health reform. *Health Promotion Journal of Australia, 18*(3), 229–36.

Royal College of Psychiatrists (2001). *The Diagnostic Criteria for the Psychiatric Disorders for Use with Adults with Learning Disabilities/Mental Retardation.* Occasional Paper 48 (pp. 1–128). London: Gaskell Press.

Runnion, V. M. & Wolfer, T. A. (2004). Relationship disruption in adults with cognitive disabilities. *Families in Society: The Journal of Contemporary Social Services, 85*(2), 205–13.

Rush, K. S., Bowman, L. G., Eidman, S. L., Toole, L. M. & Mortenson, B. P. (2004). Assessing psychopathology in individuals with developmental disabilities. *Behavior Modification, 28*(5), 621–37.

Russell, E. W. (1995). The accuracy of automated and clinical detection of brain damage and lateralization on neuropsychology. *Neuropsychology Review, 5,* 1–68.

Russo, D. (2004). Outside the square: Paediatric mental health speech pathologists. *ACQuiring Knowledge in Speech, Language and Hearing, 6*(2), 113–15.

Rutecki, P. A. & Gidal, B. E. (2002). Antileptic drug treatment in the developmentally disabled: Treatment considerations with newer antileptic drugs. *Epilepsy and Behaviour, 3*(6), S24–S31.

Rutter, M., LeCouteur, A., & Lord, C. (2003). Autism Diagnostic Interview – Revised (ADI-R). Los Angeles, CA Western Psychological Services.

Rutter, M., Maughan, B., Mortimore, P., Ouston, J., & Smith, A. (1980). *Fifteen Thousand Hours: Secondary Schools and their Effects on Children.* Cambridge, MA: Harvard University Press.

Rutter, M., Tizard, J., Yule, W., Graham, P., & Whitmore, K. (1976). Research report: Isle of Wight studies, 1964–1974. *Psychological Medicine, 6*(2), 313–32.

Saeed, S. A. (2008). Working with individuals with mental illness and developmental disabilities: Synthesizing the best information for the practicing clinician. *Psychiatry Quarterly, 79,* 153–5.

Salimen, A. L., Harra, T., & Lautamo, T. (2006). Conducting case study research in occupational therapy. *Australian Occupational Therapy Journal, 53*, 3–8.

Salmon, G. & Rapport, F. (2005). Multi-agency voices: A thematic analysis of multi-agency working practices with in the setting of a child and adolescent mental health service. *Journal of Interprofessional Care, 19*(5), 429–43.

Sameroff, A. J. (2000). Developmental systems and psychopathology. *Development and Psychopathology, 12*, 297–312.

Sanders, M. R. (1999). Triple P-Positive Parenting Program: Towards an empirically validated multilevel parenting and family support strategy for the prevention of behavior and emotional problems in children. *Clinical Child and Family Review, 2*(2), 71–90.

Sanders, M. R. & Markie-Dadds, C. L. (1996). Triple P: A multilevel family intervention program for children with disruptive disorders. In Cotton, P. & Jackson, H. (eds). *Early Intervention and Prevention in Mental Health* (pp. 59–87). Melbourne: Australian Psychological Society.

Sanders, M. R., Mazzucchelli, T. G., & Studman, L. J. (2003). *Practitioner's Manual for Standard Stepping Stones Triple P.* Milton, QLD: Triple P International Pty. Ltd.

Sanders, M. R., Mazzuccelli, T. G., & Studman, L. J. (2004). Stepping Stones Triple P: The theroretical basis and development of an evidence-based positive parenting program for families with a child who has a disability. *Journal of Intellectual and Developmental Disability, 4*(3), 265–83.

Sandman, C. A., Barron, J. L., & Coleman, H. (1990). An orally administered opiate blocker, naltrexone, attenuates self-injurious behaviour. *American Journal on Mental Retardation, 95*, 93–102.

Saunders, P. (2006). *The Costs of Disability and Incidence of Poverty.* Social Policy Research Centre Discussion Paper No 147. Retrieved 24 November 2009 from <http://www.sprc.unsw.edu.au/media/File/DP147.pdf>.

Sawyer, M. G., Arney, F. M., Baghurst, P. A., Clark, J. J., Graetz, B. W., Kosky, R. J., Nurcombe, B., Patton, G. C., Prior, M. R., Raphael, B., Rey, J., Whaites, L. C., & Zubrick, S. R. (2001). The mental health of young people in Australia: Key findings from the child and adolescent component of the National Survey of Mental Health and Well-being. *Australia and New Zealand Journal of Psychiatry, 35*(6), 806–14.

Scattone, D. (2007). Social skills interventions for children with autism. *Psychology in the Schools, 44*(7), 717–26.

Schaaf, R. C. & Miller, L. J. (2005). Occupational therapy using a sensory integrative approach for children with developmental disabilities. *Mental Retardation and Developmental Disabilities Research Reviews, 11*, 143–8.

Schaaf, R. C., Miller, L. J., Seawell, D., & O'Keefe, S. (2003). Children with disturbances in sensory processing: A pilot study examining the role of the parasympathetic nervous system. *American Journal of Occupational Therapy, 57*(4), 442–9.

Schaaf, R. C. & Nightlinger, K. M. (2007). Occupational therapy using a sensory integrative approach: A case study of effectiveness. *American Journal of Occupational Therapy, 61*, 239–46.

Schiffer, F., Teicher, M. H., & Papanicolaou, A. C. (1995). Evoked potential evidence for right brain activity during the recall of traumatic memories. *Journal of Neuropsychiatry and Clinical Neurosciences, 7*(2), 169–75.

Schore, A. N. (1994). *Affect Regulation and the Origin of Self: The Neurobiology of Emotional Development.* Hillsdale, NJ: Lawrence Erlbaum Associates.

Schore, A. N. (1996). The experience-dependent maturation of a regulatory system in the orbital prefrontal cortex and the origin of developmental psychopathology. *Development and Psychopathology, 8*, 59–87.

Schore, A. N. (2003). *Affect Regulation and the Repair of Self.* New York: W. W. Norton.

Schneider, J., Wedgewood, N., Llewellyn, G., & McConnell, D. (2006). Families challenged by and accommodating to the adolescent years. *Journal of Intellectual Disability Research, 50*(12), 926–36.

Schneider, M. L., Moore, C. F., Gajewski, L. L., Larson, J. A., Roberts, A. D., & Converse, A. K. (2008). Sensory processing disorder in a primate model: Evidence from a longitudinal study of prenatal alcohol and prenatal stress effects. *Child Development, 79*(1), 100–13.

School Therapy Services (2001). *Learning Through the Senses Resource Manual: The Impact of Sensory Processing in the Classroom.* Darwin: Department of Health and Community Services.

ScopeVic (n.d.). Communication aids. Retrieved 5 February 2009 from <http://www.scopevic.org.au/>.

Scott, S. (2008). Parenting programs. In Rutter, M., Bishop, D., Pine, D., Scott, S., Stevenson, J. S., Taylor, E. A. & Thapar, A. (eds). *Rutter's Child and Adolescent Psychiatry* (5th edn) (pp. 1046–61). Oxford: Blackwell.

Scott, S. & Dadds, M. R. (2009). Practitioner review: When parent training doesn't work: Theory-driven clinical strategies. *Journal of Child Psychology and Psychiatry, 50*(12), 1441–50.

Scottish Executive (2000). *The Same As You? A Review of Services for People with Learning Disabilities.* Edinburgh: Learning Disability Review, Scotland Government. Retrieved 30 January 2009 from <http://www.scotland.gov.uk/Resource/Doc/159140/0043285.pdf>.

Scottish Executive (2005). Delivering for health. Edinburgh: Scottish Executive. Retrieved 22 December 2009 from <http://www.scotland.gov.uk/Resource/Doc/76169/0018996.pdf>.

Seiler, L. (2008). *Cool Connections with Cognitive Behavioural Therapy: Encouraging Self-Esteem, Resilience and Well-Being in Children and Young People Using CBT Approaches.* London: Jessica Kingsley Publishers.

Seligman, M. & Darling, R. B. (2007). *Ordinary Families, Special Children: A Systems Approach to Childhood Disability* (3rd edn). New York: Guildford Press.

Seltzer, M. M., Greenberg, J. S., Krauss, M. W., Gordon, R. M., & Judge, K. (1997). Siblings of adults with mental retardation or mental illness: Effects on lifestyle and psychological well-being. *Family Relations*, *46*(4), 395–405.

Selvini-Palazzoli, M., Bosculu, L., Cecchin, G., & Prata, G. (1978). *Paradox and Counter-paradox*. New York: Jason Aronson.

Sensky, T. (1985). Family stigma and physical deformity. *General Hospital Psychiatry*, *7*, 385–6.

Servais, L. (2006). Sexual health care in persons with intellectual disabilities. *Mental Retardation and Developmental Disabilities Research Reviews*, *12*, 48–56.

Sevcik, R. A. (2006). Comprehension: An overlooked component in augmented language development. *Disability and Rehabilitation*, *28*(3), 159–67.

Scior, K. & Grierson, K. (2004). Service provision for young people with intellectual disabilities and additional mental health needs: Service-providers' perspectives. *Journal of Applied Research in Intellectual Disabilities*, *17*, 173–9.

Shaffer, D., Fisher, P., Lucas, C., Dulcan, M., & Schwab-Stone, M. (2000). NIMH Diagnostic Interview Schedule for Children, Version IV (NIMH DISC-IV): Description, differences from previous versions, and reliability of some common diagnoses. *Journal of the American Academy of Child and Adolescent Psychiatry*, *39*, 28–38.

Sharpe, D. & Rossiter, L. (2002). Siblings of children with a chronic illness: A meta-analysis. *Journal of Pediatric Psychology*, *27*, 699–710.

Sheehan, N. W. (1996). Management issues in service coordination: The experience of the resident services coordinator program. *Journal of Gerontological Social Work*, *26* (1–2), 71–86.

Shelton, T. L. & Stepanek, J. S. (1994). *Family-centered Care for Children Needing Specialized Health and Developmental Services* (3rd edn). Bethesda, MD: Association for the Care of Children's Health.

Shelton, T. L. & Stepanek, J. S. (1995). Excerpts from family-centred care for children needing apecialized health and developmental service. *Pediatric Nursing*, *21*(4), 362–4.

Sherwood, M. (2004). Working with BLADES: Adding meaning and interaction to language therapy. *ACQuiring Knowledge in Speech, Language and Hearing*, *6*(1), 10–13.

Shin, L. M., Orr, S. P., Carson, M. A., Rauch, S. L., Macklin, M. L., Lasko, N. B., Peters, P. M., Metzger, L. J., Lougherty, D. D., Cannistraro, P. A., Alpert, N. M., Fischman, A. J., & Pitman, R. K. (2004). Regional cerebral blood flow in the amygdala and medial prefrontal cortex during traumatic imagery in male and female Vietnam veterans with PTSD. *Archives of General Psychiatry*, *61*, 168–76.

Shine, S. A. (2009). *Friendships and Dating: Information about Relationships for Parents, Carers and Young People* (rev. edn) (booklet). Retrieved 12 November 2009 from <http://www.shinesa.org.au/?objectid=508918BE-C74E-1C07-C0B06A022A738ED8&topicCategory=&topicKeyword=Friendships+and+dating>.

Siever, L. J. & Davis, K. L. (1985). Overview: Toward a dysregulation hypothesis of depression. *American Journal of Psychiatry, 142,* 1017–31.

Sigafoos, J., Arthur, M., & O'Reilly, M. (2003). *Challenging Behaviour and Developmental Disability.* London: Whurr.

Simeonsson, R. J., Leonardi, M., Lollar, D., Bjorck-Akesson, E., Hollenweger, J., & Martinuzzi, A. (2003). Applying the international classification of functioning, disability and health (ICF) to measure childhood disability. *Disability and Rehabilitation, 25*(11–12), 602–10.

Simpson, A. (2007). The impact of team processes on psychiatric case management. *Journal of Advanced Nursing, 60*(4), 409–18.

Singh, N. N., Lancioni, G. E., Winton, A. S. W., Curtis, W. J., Wahler, R. G., Sabaawi, M., Singh, J., & McAleavey, K. (2006). Mindful staff increase learning and reduce aggression in adults with developmental disabilities. *Research in Developmental Disabilities, 27,* 545–58.

Siperstein, G. N. & Rickards, E. P (2004). *Promoting Social Success: A Curriculum for Children with Special Needs.* Baltimore: Paul H. Brookes.

Skotko, B. (2005). Mothers of children with Down syndrome reflect on their postnatal support. *Pediatrics, 115,* 64–80.

Slee, P. T., Lawson, M. J., Russell, A., Askell-Williams, H., Dix, K. L., Owens, L., Skrzypiec, & Spears, B. (2009). *KidsMatter–Primary Evaluation Final Report.* Adelaide: Centre for Analysis of Educational Futures, Flinders University. Retrieved 28 February 2010 from <http://www.kidsmatter.edu.au/wp/wp-content/uploads/2009/10/kidsmatter-exec-summary-report-web.pdf>.

Slevin, E., Truesdale-Kennedy, M., McConkey, R., Bar, O., & Taggart, L. (2008). Community learning disability teams: Developments, composition and good practice. A review of the literature. *Journal of Intellectual Disabilities, 12*(1), 59–79.

Sloper, P. (2004). Facilitators and barriers for co-ordinated multi-agency services. *Child: Care, Health and Development, 30*(6), 571–80.

Smidt, A., Balandin, S., Reed, V., & Sigafoos, J. (2007). A communication training programme for residential staff working with adults with challenging behaviour: Pilot data on intervention effects. *Journal of Applied Research in Intellectual Disabilities, 20*(1), 16–29.

Smiley, E., Cooper, S., Finlayson, J., Jackson, A., Allan, L., Mantry, D. et al. (2008). Genetics. In Rutter, M., Bishop, D., Pine, D., Scott, S., Stevenson, J. S., Taylor, E. A. & Thapar, A.. (eds). *Rutter's Child and Adolescent Psychiatry* (5th edn) (pp. 339–59). Oxford: Blackwell.

Smith, M. (2005). The dual challenges of aided communication and adolescence. *Augmentative and Alternative Communication, 21,* 67–79.

Smith, S. A., Press, B., Koenig, K. P., & Kinnealey, M. (2005). Effects of sensory integration intervention on self-stimulating and self-injurious behaviours. *American Journal of Occupational Therapy, 59,* 418–25.

Smith-Bird, E. & Turnbull, A. (2005). Linking behaviour support to family quality of life outcomes. *Journal of Positive Behaviour Interventions, 7*(3), 174–80.

Smyly, S. (2006). Who needs to change: Using systemic ideas when working with group homes. In Baum, S. & Lynggaard, H. *Intellectual Disabilities: A Systemic Approach* (pp. 142–63). London: Karnac Books.

Soper, G. & Thorley, C, R. (1996). Effectiveness of an occupational therapy program based on sensory integration theory for adults with severe learning disabilities. *British Journal of Occupational Therapy, 59*(10), 475–80.

Snow, P. (2008). Oral language competence in childhood and adolescence: The missing link in mental health promotion? Paper presented at Auckland: Joint New Zealand Speech Therapists Association and Speech Pathology Australia Conference, May. Retrieved on 24 June 2008 from <http://www.speechpathologyaustralia.org.au>.

Snowling, M. J., Bishop, D. V., Stothard, S. E., Chipchase, B., & Kaplan, C. (2006). Psychosocial outcomes at 15 years of children with a preschool history of speech-language impairment. *Journal of Child Psychology and Psychiatry, 47*(8), 759–65.

Solanto, M. V. & Wender, E. H. (1989). Does methylphenidate constrict cognitive functioning? *Journal of the American Academy of Child and Adolescent Psychiatry, 28*, 897–902.

Sonuga-Barke, E. J., Beckett, C., Kreppner, J., Castle, J., Colvert E., Stevens, S.,Hawkins, A., & Rutter, M. (2008). Is sub-nutrition necessary for a poor outcome following early institutional deprivation? *Developmental Medicine and Child Neurology, 50*(9), 664–71.

Soo, C. A. & Bailey, J. G. (2006). A review of functioning of attentional components in children with attention-deficit/hyperactivity disorder and learning disabilities. *Brain Impairment, 7*(2), 133–47.

Sorce, J. F. & Emde, R. N. (1982). The meaning of infant emotional expression: Regularities in caregiving responses in normal and Down's syndrome infants. *Journal of Child Psychology and Psychiatry, 23*, 145–58.

Sorgi, P., Ratey, J., Knoedler, D. W., Markert, R. J., & Reichman, M. (1991). Rating aggression in the clinical setting a retrospective adaptation of the Overt Aggression Scale: Preliminary results. *Journal of Neuropsychiatry, 3*, 552–6.

Sovner, R. & Hurley, A. (1986). Four factors affecting the diagnosis of psychiatric disorders in mentally retarded persons. *Psychiatric Aspects of Mental Retardation Reviews, 5*(9), 45–9.

Sparrow, S. S., Cicchetti, D. V., & Balla, D. A. (2005). *Vineland Adaptive Behavior Scale* (2nd edn). Circle Pines, MN: American Guidance Service.

Spence, S. H. (2003). Social skills training with children and young people: Theory, evidence and practice. *Child and Adolescent Mental Health, 8*(2), 84–96.

Spence, S. & Donovan, C. (1998). Interpersonal problems. In Graham, P. (ed.). *Cognitive Behaviour Therapy for Children and Families* (pp. 1–15). Cambridge: Cambridge University Press.

Sporn, J. & Sachs, G. (1997). The anticonvulsant lamotrigine in treatment-resistant manic-depressive illness. *Journal of Clinical Psychopharmacology, 17*, 185–9.

Spragg, P. A. (1988). Structured clinical interview. Unpublished instrument. Denver: University of Colorado Health Sciences.

Stagnitti, K., Raison, P., & Ryan, P. (1999). Sensory defensiveness syndrome: A paediatric perspective and case study. *Australian Occupational Therapy Journal, 46*(4), 175–87.

Stahl, S. M. (2008). *Stahl's Essential Psychopharmacology: Neuroscientific Basis and Practical Applications* (3rd edn). New York: Cambridge University Press.

Stainton, T. & Besser, H. (1998). The positive impact of children with an intellectual disability on a family. *Journal of Intellectual Disability, 23*(1), 57–70.

Stallard, P. (2002). *Think Good, Feel Good: A Cognitive Behaviour Therapy Workbook for Children and Young People*. New York: John Wiley.

Starling, J. (2003). Getting the message across: Safeguarding the mental health of adolescents with communication disorders. *ACQuiring Knowledge in Speech, Language and Hearing, 5*(1), 37–9.

Starling, J. & Dossetor, D. (2009). Pervasive developmental disorders and psychosis. *Current Psychiatry Reports, 11*(3), 190–6.

Steele, M. & Quinn, D. (2004). Recent advances in the treatment of ADHD and other comorbid disorders. *Canadian Child and Adolescent Psychiatric Review, 13*(2), 1–11.

Steitz, M. (2008). Access to services. Unpublished manuscript. Improved Service Access and Parenting for Families with Children and Adolescents with Intellectual Disability in NSW Project, Mental Health and Drug and Alcohol Office (MHDAO) of NSW and Hunter New England Area Health Service.

Sterkenburg, P. S., Janssen, C. G. C., & Schuengel, C. (2008). The effect of an attachment-based behaviour therapy for children with visual and severe intellectual disabilities. *Journal of Applied Research in Intellectual Disabilities, 21*, 126–35.

Sterling-Turner, H. E. & Jordan, S. S. (2007). Interventions addressing transition difficulties for individuals with autism. *Psychology in the Schools, 44*, 681–90.

Stevenson, A. (ed.) (2007). *Shorter Oxford English Dictionary* (6th edn). Oxford: Oxford University Press.

Stewart, D., Antle, B., Healy, H., Law, M., & Young, N. (2007). *Best Practice Guidelines for Transition to Adulthood for Youth with Disabilities in Ontario: An Evidence-Based Approach*. Retrieved 12 November 2007, from <http://www.canchild.ca/Default.aspx?tabid=1878>.

Stewart, D., Starvness, C., G., K., Antle, B., & Law, M. (2006). A critical appraisal of literature reviews about the transition to adulthood for youth with disabilities. *Physical and Occupational Therapy in Pediatrics, 26*(4), 5–24.

Stifter, C. A., Spinrad, T. L., & Braungart-Rieker, J. M. (1999). Toward a developmental model of child compliance: The role of emotion regulation in infancy. *Child Development, 70*, 21–32.

Stigler, K. A., Posey, D. J., & McDougle, C. J. (2004). Case report: Aripiprazole for maladaptive behaviour in pervasive developmental disorder. *Journal of Child Adolescent Psychopharmacology, 14*, 455–63.

Stokes, D., Matthews, R., & Shafik-Eid, R. (2006). Developing an allied health code set: The indicator for intervention. *Health Information Management Journal, 35*(2), 46–8.

Stonefelt, L. & Stein, F. (1998). Sensory integrative techniques applied to children with learning disabilities: An outcome study. *Occupational Therapy International, 5*, 252–72.

Stoneman, Z. (1997). Mental retardation and family adaption. In McLean, Jr, W. E. (ed.). *Ellis' Handbook of Mental Deficiency: Psychological Theory and Research* (3rd ed.) (pp. 405–37). Mahwah, NJ: Lawrence Erlbaum Associates.

Stoner, J. B., Angell, M. E., House, J. J., & Bock, S. J. (2007). Transitions: Perspectives from parents of young children with Autism Spectrum Disorder (ASD). *Journal of Developmental and Physical Disabilities, 19*(1), 23–39.

Strohm, K. (2002). *Siblings: Brothers and Sisters of Children with Special Needs.* Kent Town, SA: Wakefield Press.

Sturm, J. M. & Clendon, S. A. (2004). Augmentative and alternative communication, language, and literacy: Fostering the relationship. *Topics in Language Disorders, 24*(1), 76–91.

Sugai, G., Horner, R. H., Dunlap, G., Hieneman, M., Lewis, T.J., Nelson, C.M., Scott, T., Liaupsin, C., Sailor, W., Turnbull, A. P., Turnbull, H. R., Wickham, D., Wilcox, B., & Ruef, M. B. (2000). Applying positive behavioural support and functional behavioural assessments in schools. *Journal of Positive Behavioural Interventions, 2*, 131–43.

Summers, S. J. & Jones, J. (2004). Cross-cultural working in community learning disabilities services: Clinical issues, dilemmas and tensions. *Journal of Intellectual Disability Research, 48*(7), 687–94.

Svensson, T. H. (1987). Peripheral, autonomic regulation of locus coeruleus noradrenergic neurons in brain: Putative implications for psychiatry and psychopharmacology. *Psychopharmacology, 92*(1), 1–7.

Swan, L. & Alderman, N. (2004). Measuring the relationship between overt aggression and expectations: A methodology for determining clinical outcomes. *Brain Injury, 18*, 143–60.

Swanson, H. L. (2001). Research on interventions for adolescents with learning disabilities: A meta-analysis of outcomes related to higher order processing. *Elementary School Journal, 101*(3), 331–45.

Swanson, J. L. & Fouad, N. A. (1999). Applying theories of person–environment fit to the transition from school to work. *Career Development Quarterly, 47*, 337–47.

Szymanski, E. M. (1994). Transition: Life-span and life-space considerations for empowerment. *Exceptional Children, 60*(5), 402–11.

Talay-Ongan, A. & Wood, K. (2000). Unusual sensory sensitivities in autism: A possible crossroads. *International Journal of Disability, Development and Education, 47*(2), 201–12.

Tanguay, P., Robertson, J., & Derrick, A. (1998). A dimensional classification of autism spectrum disorder by social communication domains. *Journal of American Academy of Child and Adolescent Psychiatry, 37*, 271–7.

Taunt, H. M. & Hastings, R. P. (2002). Positive impact of children with developmental disabilities on their families: A preliminary study. *Education and Training in Mental Retardation and Developmental Disabilities, 37*, 410–20.

Taylor, J. L., Lindsay, W. R., & Willner, P. (2008). Client group applications. CBT for people with intellectual disabilities: Emerging evidence, cognitive ability and IQ effects. *Behavioural and Cognitive Psychotherapy, 36*, 723–33.

Teeters Myers, C. (2006). Exploring occupational therapy and transitions for young children with special needs. *Physical and Occupational Therapy in Pediatrics, 26*(3), 73–88.

Tew, B. & Lawrence, K. M. (1975). Some sources of stress found in mothers of spina bifida children. *British Journal of Preventative Social Medicine, 29*, 27–30.

Thapar, A. & Rutter, M. (2008). Genetics. In Rutter, M., Bishop, D., Pine, D., Scott, S., Stevenson, J. S., Taylor, E. A. & Thapar, A. (eds). *Rutter's Child and Adolescent Psychiatry* (5th edn) (pp. 339–58). Oxford: Blackwell.

Thorin, E., Yovanoff, P., & Irvin, L. (1996). Dilemmas faced by families during their young adults' transition to adulthood. *Mental Retardation, 34*, 117–20.

Tiet, Q. Q., Bird, H. R., Hoven, C. W., Moore, R., Wu, P., Wicks, J.,Jensen, P., Goodman, S., & Cohen, P. (2001). Relationship between specific adverse life events and psychiatric disorders. *Journal of Abnormal Child Psychology, 29*(2), 153–64.

Todd, S. & Jones, S. (2005). Looking at the future and seeing the past: The challenge of the middle years of parenting a child with intellectual disabilities. *Journal of Intellectual Disability Research, 49*(6), 389–404.

Todd, S. & Shearn, J. (1996). Struggles with time: The careers of parents with adult sons and daughters with learning disabilities. *Disability and Society, 1*(3), 341–66.

Tomanik, S., Harris, G. E., & Hawkins, J. (2004). The relationship between behaviours exhibited by children with autism and maternal stress. *Journal of Intellectual and Developmental Disability, 29*, 16–26.

Tonge, B., & Einfeld, S. (2000). The trajectory of psychiatric disorders in young people with intellectual disabilities. *Australian and New Zealand Journal of Psychiatry, 34*(1), 80–4.

Torr, J., Iacono, T., Graham, M., & Galea, J. (2008). Checklists for general practitioner diagnosis of depression in adults with intellectual disability. *Journal of Intellectual Disability Research, 52*(11), 930–41.

Torr, J., Lennox, N., Cooper, S., Rey-Conde, T., Ware, R., Galea, J., & Taylor, M. (2008). Psychiatric care of adults with intellectual disabilities: Changing perceptions over a decade. *Australian and New Zealand Journal of Psychiatry, 42*(10), 890–7.

Trimble, M. R. (1990). Anticonvulsants in children and adolescents. *Journal of Child Adolescent Psychopharmacology, 1*, 107–24.

Triple P International (n.d.). *Triple P–Positive Parenting Program®*. Retrieved 25 February 2010 from <http://www1.triplep.net/>.

Trott, M. A. (2002). *Oh Behave! Sensory Processing and Behavioural Strategies: A Practical Guide for Clinicians, Teachers, and Parents*. San Antonio: Psychological Corporation.

Trute, B. & Hiebert-Murphy, D. (2002). Family adjustment to childhood developmental disability: A measure of parental appraisal of family impacts. *Journal of Pediatric Psychology, 27*(3), 271–80.

Tsakanikos, E., Bouras, N., Costello, H., & Holt, G. (2007). Multiple exposure to life events and clinical psychopathology in adults with intellectual disability. *Social Psychiatry and Psychiatric Epidemiology, 42*(1), 24–8.

Tsiantis, J., Diareme, S., Dimitrakaki, C., Kolaitis, G., Flios, A., Christogiorgos, S., Weber, G., Salvador-Carulla, L., Hillery, J., & Costello, H. (2004). Care staff awareness training in mental health needs of adults with learning disabilities. *Journal of Learning Disabilities, 8*(3), 221–34.

Tsiouris, J., Cohen, I., Flory, M., Freedland, R., Brown, W., & Pettinger, J. (2008). Association of psychiatric diagnoses to medical illness, etiological diagnoses and degree of ID. *Journal of Intellectual Disability Research, 52*(8–9), 730.

Tsiouris, J. A., Cohen, I. L., Patti, P. J., & Korosh, W. M. (2003). Treatment of previously undiagnosed psychiatric disorders in persons with developmental disabilities decreased or eliminated self-injurious behavior. *Journal of Clinical Psychiatry, 64*(9), 1081–90.

Tsiouris, J. A., Mann, R., Patti, P. J., & Sturmey, P. (2003). Challenging behaviours should not be considered as depressive equivalents in individuals with intellectual disability. *Journal of Intellectual Disability Research, 47*(1), 14–21.

Tur-Kaspa, H. (2002). The socioemotional adjustment of adolescents with LD in the kibbutz during high school transition periods. *Journal of Learning Disabilities, 35*(1), 87–96.

Tyrer, P., Oliver-Africano, P. C., Bouras, N., Cooray, S., Ahmed, Z., Hare, M., Murphy, D., Meade, M., Reece, B., Kramo, K., Bhaumik, S., Harley, D., Karatela, S., Regan, R., Thomas, D., Rao, B., North, B., Eliahoo, J., Soni, A., & Crawford, M (2008). Risperidone, haloperidol and placebo in the treatment of aggressive challenging behaviour in intellectual disability: Randomised controlled trial. *Lancet, 371*(9606): 57–63.

University of Cambridge (2002). *Mind Reading: The Interactive Guide to Emotions* (CD-ROM). London: Jessica Kingsley Publishers.

VandenBerg, N. (2001). The use of a weighted vest to increase on task behavior in children with attention difficulties. *American Journal of Occupational Therapy, 55*, 621–28.

van Mourik, M. & Roberts, B. (2003). Language for learning: A checklist for language difficulties at the secondary level. *Acquiring Knowledge in Speech, Language and Hearing, 5*(1), 33–6.

Vernon, A. (1989). *Thinking, Feeling, Behaving: An Emotional Education Curriculum for Adolescents. Grades 7–12*. Champaign, IL: Research Publishing.

Vernon, A. (2002). *What Works When with Children and Adolescents: A Handbook of Individual Counselling Techniques*. Champaign, IL: Research Publishing.

Wagner, A. P. (2004). *Up and Down the Worry Hill: A Children's Book about Obsessive-Compulsive Disorder and its Treatment*. Mobile, AL: Lighthouse Press Inc.

Walker, L. S., Van Slyke, D. A., & Newbrough, J. R. (1992). Family resources and stress: A comparison of families of children with cystic fibrosis, diabetes and mental retardation. *Journal of Pediatric Psychology, 17*(3), 327–43.

Wallander, J. L., Dekker, M. C., & Koot, H. M. (2006). Risk factors for psychopathology in children with intellectual disability: A prospective longitudinal population-based study. *Journal of Intellectual Disability Research, 50*(4), 259–68.

Wallander, J. L. & Noojin, A. B. (1995). Mother's report of stressful experiences related to having a child with a physical disability. *Children's Health Care, 24*(4), 245–56.

Wechsler, D. (2002). *Wechsler Preschool and Primary Scale of Intelligence (WPPSI–III)* (3rd edn). San Antonio, TX: Psychological Corporation.

Wechsler, D. (2003). *Wechsler Intelligence Scale for Children (4th ed.) (WISC-IV)*. San Antonio, TX: Psychological Corporation.

Westby, C. (2010). Multiliteracies: The changing world of communication. *Topics in Language Disorders, 30*(1), 64–71.

Whalen, C. (1989). Does stimulant medication improve the peer status of hyperactive children? *Journal of Consulting and Clinical Psychology, 57*, 545–9.

Whalen, C. K. & Henker, B. (1992). The social profile of attention-deficit hyperactivity disorder. *Child and Adolescent Psychiatry Clinics of North America, 1*, 395–410.

Whalen, C. K., Henker, B., & Granger, D. A. (1990). Social judgment processes in hyperactive boys: Effects of methylphenidate and comparisons with normal peers. *Journal of Abnormal Child Psychology, 18*, 297–316.

While, A., Forbes, A., Ulman, R., Lewis, S., Mathes, L., & Griffiths, P. (2004). Good practices that address continuity during transition from child to adult care: Synthesis of the evidence. *Child: Care, Health & Development, 30*(5), 439–52.

Whitaker-Azmita, P. M. (2001). Serotonin and brain development: Role in human developmental diseases. *Brain Research Bulletin, 56*(5), 479–85.

White, D. L (2001). The effect of a sensory-based communication program on the challenging behaviours and engagement levels of individuals with intellectual disabilities and severe communication impairments. Unpublished Masters thesis. Sydney: Macquarie University.

White, D. L. (2011). Communication assessment for individuals with intellectual disability and criminal justice system involvement: A protocol for speech pathologists. Revised unpublished document. Epping, NSW: Ageing, Disability & Home Care, Department of Human Services, NSW.

White, D., Dossetor, D., & Whatson, L. (2007). Unpublished raw data. Developmental Psychiatry Clinic, 2006–07.

White, D., Dossetor, D., Whatson, L., & Farah, J. (2009). A framework for professional practice: A partnership in the development of an educational program for professionals in child mental health and intellectual disability. Paper presented: Hobart: 44th ASSID Conference, November.

White, M. (1989). The externalizing of the problem and reauthoring of lives and relationships. *Dulwich Centre Newsletter,* Summer, 3–21.

White, M. & Epston, D. (1990). *Narrative Means to Therapeutic Ends.* New York: Norton.

Whitehouse, A. J. O., Watt, H. J., Line, E. A., & Bishop, D. V. M. (2009). Adult psychosocial outcomes of children with specific language impairment, pragmatic language impairment and autism. *International Journal of Communication Disorders, 44*(4), 511–28.

Whitehouse, R. M., Tudway, J. A., Look, R., & Kroese, B. S. (2006). Adapting individual psychotherapy for adults with intellectual disabilities: A comparative review of the cognitive-behavioural and psychodynamic literature. *Journal of Applied Research in Intellectual Disabilities, 19*(1), 55–65.

Whitehurst, T. (2008). Impact of mental health training for frontline staff working with children with severe intellectual disabilities. *Journal of Policy and Practice in Intellectual Disabilities, 5*(1), 6–11.

Wiese, M.Y., Stancliffe, R.J., & Hemsley, B. (2005). *Positive Behaviour Support Programs for Families.* Sydney: Centre for Developmental Disability Studies.

Wiggins, J. S. (1981). Clinical and statistical prediction: Where are we and where do we go from here? *Clinical Psychology Review, 1,* 3–18.

Wikler, L., Haack, J., & Intagliata, J. (1984). Bearing the burden alone? Helping divorced mothers of children with developmental disabilities. *Family Therapy Collections, 11,* 44–62.

Wilbarger, P. (1984). Planning a 'sensory diet': Application of sensory processing theory during the first year of life. *Zero to Three, 5*(1), 7–12.

Wilbarger, P. (1995). The sensory diet: Activity programs based on sensory processing theory. *Sensory Integration Special Interest Section Newsletter, 18*(2), 1–4.

Wilbarger, P. & Wilbarger, J. (1991). *Sensory Defensiveness in Children Aged 2–12: An Intervention Guide for Parents and Other Caretakers*. Panorama City, CA: Avanti Educational Programs.

Wilbarger, J. & Wilbarger, P. (2002). Wilbarger approach to treating sensory defensiveness and clinical application of the sensory diet. In Bundy, A. C., Murray, E. A., & Lane, S. (eds). *Sensory Integration: Theory and practice* (2nd edn). Philadelphia: F. A. Davis.

Wilbarger, P. & Wilbarger, J. (2007, April). Sensory defensiveness: A comprehensive treatment approach. Presented at a workshop organised by Sensory Tools Australia, Sydney.

Wilkinson, K. M. & Hennig, S. (2007). The state of research and practice in augmentative and alternative communication for children with developmental/intellectual disabilities. *Mental Retardation and Developmental Disabilities Research Reviews, 13*, 58–69.

Williams, M. S. & Shellenberger, S. (1994). The Alert Program™ for self-regulation. *American Occupational Therapy Association Sensory Integration Special Interest Section Newsletter, 17*, 1–3.

Williams, M. S. & Shellenberger, S. (1996). *'How Does Your Engine Run?'. A Leader's Guide to the Alert Program™ For Self-regulation*. Albuquerque, NM: TherapyWorks.

Williamson, G. & Anzalone, M. (2001). *Sensory Integration and Self Regulation in Infants and Toddlers*. Washington, DC: Zero to Three: National Center for Infants, Toddlers and Families.

Willis, T. J. & LaVigna, G. W. (1996). Behavioural assessment: An overview. *Positive Practices, 1*(2), 1, 8-15.

Willis, T. J., LaVigna, G. W., & Donnellan, A. M. (1993). *Behavior Assessment Guide*. Los Angeles: Institute for Applied Behavior Analysis.

Wilson, K. (2009. A parent's perspective. Paper presented at the High Functioning Autism and Asperger's Syndrome Seminars for Parents and Carers, Newcastle, September. The Children's Hospital at Westmead.

Wilson, M. A. & Tonegawa, S. (1997). Synaptic plasticity, place cells and spatial memory: Study with second generation knockouts. *Trends in Neurosciences, 20*, 102–6.

Wing, L. (1982). Schedule of handicaps, behaviors and skills. Unpublished manual. London: Institute of Psychiatry.

Wing, L. & Gould, J. (1978). Systematic recording of behaviors and skills of retarded and psychotic children. *Journal of Autism and Childhood Schizophrenia, 8*(1), 79–97.

Wing, L. & Gould, J. (1979). Severe impairments of social interaction and associated abnormalities in children: Epidemiology and classification. *Journal of Autism and Developmental Disorders, 9*(1), 11–29.

Winnicott, D. (1960). The theory of the parent-infant relationship. *Journal of Psycho-Analysis, 41*, 585–94.

Winnicott, D. (1996). *Thinking about Children*. London: Karnac Books.

Wong, M., Lopes A., & Heriot, S. (2004). Emotion-Based Social Skills Training (EBSST). Unpublished treatment manual. Sydney: The Children's Hospital at Westmead.

Wong, M. & Heriot, S. (2009,) Emotion-Based Social Skills Training (EBSST) for children with high functioning autism and asperger's syndrome: A randomized-controlled trial. Paper presented at Sydney: Asia Pacific Autism Conference, August.

Wong, S. Y., Wong, T. K. S., Martinson, I., Lai, A. C., Chen, W. J., & He, Y .S. (2004). Needs of Chinese parents of children with developmental disability. *Journal of Learning Disabilities, 8*(2), 141–58.

Wonnacott, S. (1997). Presynaptic nicotinic ACh receptors. *Trends in Neurosciences, 20*, 92–8.

Woolfson, L. & Grant, E. (2006) Authoritative parenting and parental stress of pre-school and older children with developmental disabilities. *Child: Care, Health and Development, 32*(2), 177–84.

Woolley, H., Stein, A., Forrest, G. C., & Baum, J. D. (1989). Imparting the diagnosis of life threatening illness in children. *British Medical Journal, 298*, 1623–6.

World Health Organization (WHO) (1948). *Preamble to the Constitution of the World Health Organization as Adopted by the International Health Conference, New York, 19–22 June 1946; signed on 22 July 1946 by the representatives of 61 States* (Official Records of the World Health Organization, no 2, p. 100) and entered into force on 7 April 1948.

World Health Organization (WHO, 2002). *Towards a Common Language for Functioning, Disability and Health: ICF: The International Classification of Functioning, Disability and Health.* Retrieved 22 December 2009 from <http://www.who.int/classifications/icf/training/icfbeginnersguide.pdf>.

World Health Organization (WHO) (2004). *Prevention of Mental Disorders: Effective Interventions and Policy Options: Summary Report: A Report of the World Health Organization, Department of Mental Health and Substance Abuse in collaboration with the Prevention Research Centre of the Universities of Nijmegen and Maastricht* (pp. 42–3). Retrieved 2 December 2009 from <http://www.who.int/mental_health/evidence/en/prevention_of_mental_disorders_sr.pdf>.

World Health Organization (WHO) (2007). *International Statistical Classification Of Diseases And Related Health Problems* (10th rev. edn). Geneva: World Health Organization.

Worrall-Davies, A., Kiernan, K., Anderton, N., & Cottrell, D. (2004). Working with young people with complex needs: Practitioners views. *Child and Adolescent Mental Health, 9*(4), 180–6.

Xyrichis, A. & Lowton, K. (2008). What fosters or prevents interprofessional teamworking in primary and community care? A literature review. *International Journal of Nursing Studies, 45*, 140–53.

Yin, R. (2003). *Applications of Case Study Research* (2nd edn). Thousand Oaks, CA: Sage.

Yuan, S. (2003). Seeing with new eyes: Metaphors of family experience. *Mental Retardation, 41*(3), 207–11.

Zametkin, A. J. & Rapoport, J. L. (1987). Noradrenergic hypothesis of attention deficit disorder with hyperactivity: A critical review. In Meltzer, H. Y. (ed.). *Psychopharmacology: The Third Generation of Progress* (pp. 837–42). New York: Raven Press.

Zametkin, A., Rapoport, J. L., Murphy, D. L., Linnoila, M., & Ismond, D. (1985). Treatment of hyperactive children with monoamine oxidase inhibitors: Clinical efficacy. *Archives of General Psychiatry, 42*(10), 962–6.

Zimmerman, A. & Popynick, M. (2003). Program evaluation of a behaviour therapy group for parents of children with developmental disabilities ages four to seven. *Journal on Developmental Disabilities, 10*, 151–8.

Zimmerman, F. & Christakis, D. (2007). Associations between content types of early media exposure and subsequent attentional problems. *Pediatrics, 120*(5), 986–92.

Zubrick, S. R., Ward, K. A., Silburn, S. R., Lawrence, D., Williams, A. A., Blair, E., Robertson, D., & Sanders, M. R. (2005). Prevention of child behavior problems through universal implementation of a group behavioral family intervention. *Prevention Science, 6*(4), 287–304.

Index

Note: A high percentage of the following entries could be cross-referenced to the subjects of book's title, 'children' and/or 'adolescents with intellectual and developmental disabilities'. Therefore the reader should assume such cross-referencing, except where otherwise clearly shown.